Organization *of* School Health Programs

SECOND EDITION

Organization *of* School Health Programs

KERRY REDICAN

Virginia Polytechnic Institute and State University

LARRY OLSEN

Penn State Univesity

CHARLES BAFFI

Virginia Polytechnic Institute and State University

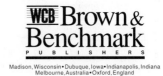

WCB Brown & Benchmark
PUBLISHERS

Madison, Wisconsin • Dubuque, Iowa • Indianapolis, Indiana
Melbourne, Australia • Oxford, England

Book Team

Editor *Chris Rogers*
Developmental Editor *Susan J. McCormick*
Production Editor *Scott Sullivan*
Designer *Eric Engelby*
Art Editor *Rachel Imsland*
Photo Editor *Robin Storm*

Visuals/Design Developmental Consultant *Marilyn A. Phelps*

WCB Brown & Benchmark

A Division of Wm. C. Brown Communications, Inc.

Vice President and General Manager *Thomas E. Doran*
Executive Managing Editor *Ed Bartell*
Executive Editor *Edgar J. Laube*
Director of Marketing *Kathy Law Laube*
National Sales Manager *Eric Ziegler*
Marketing Manager *Pamela Cooper*
Advertising Manager *Jodi Rymer*
Managing Editor, Production *Colleen A. Yonda*
Manager of Visuals and Design *Faye M. Schilling*

Design Manager *Jac Tilton*
Art Manager *Janice Roerig*
Production Editorial Manager *Vickie Putman Caughron*
Publishing Services Manager *Karen J. Slaght*
Permissions/Records Manager *Connie Allendorf*

Wm. C. Brown Communications, Inc.

Chairman Emeritus *Wm. C. Brown*
Chairman and Chief Executive Officer *Mark C. Falb*
President and Chief Operating Officer *G. Franklin Lewis*
Corporate Vice President, Operations *Beverly Kolz*
Corporate Vice President, President of WCB Manufacturing *Roger Meyer*

Cover photo © Steven Burr Williams/The Image Bank

Copyedited by Linda L. Gomoll

Contents

v

Preface

The second edition of *Organization of School Health Programs* represents years of collaborative efforts between the authors. In this second edition some material was deleted (first aid procedures) and some new material was added. For example, a whole new chapter was devoted to drugs, AIDS and adolescent pregnancy. Other chapters contain relevant and timely material incorporated into them.

The student is the focal point of this text. Further, all activities on the part of school personnel that are designed to protect, promote, or improve the health of the students are presented in a manner that will operationalize content and process in order to increase the chances of meeting the many needs and interests of students.

The second edition of this text is still organized into the following four sections: Foundations, Environment, Services, and Instruction. The Foundations section explains the basics necessary for the development of sound school health programs. Topics such as the growth and development characteristics of students, the needs and interests of students, and legal aspects of school health programs are discussed. The Environment section explains the prerequisites for a sound physical plant, maintenance, and emotional climate.

The Health Services chapters should help prospective school personnel or public health personnel currently working in a school setting to understand their roles with regard to the health appraisal, screening, and referral of students. We have included several chapters that focus on such topics as counseling and interpretation, child abuse, communicable disease control, and some of the special medical problems found in the classroom including drugs, AIDS, and adolescent pregnancy.

The chapters comprising the Health Instruction section provide a good foundation for the presentation of necessary content and activities that will help in developing sound school health curricula. These chapters succinctly present concepts in a pragmatic and easy-to-implement manner.

Finally, we feel that the school health program and the public health program have a great many contributions to make to help school-age students attempt to maximize their educational experiences. We believe that a healthy student has a better opportunity to utilize fully all of his or her educational experiences. Therefore, whenever applicable we've approached the school health program as an extension of the public health program. Both programs working in harmony should significantly contribute to the health and well-being of our nation's most precious resource—our school-age youth.

ACKNOWLEDGMENTS

A number of people have helped us in completing this text. Specifically, we would like to thank Ms. Susie McCormick, developmental editor at Brown & Benchmark for her expert help. We would also like to thank Mr. Chris Rogers for his help and encouragement. We would like to thank Dr. Ronald Bos, Division Director of Health, Physical Education and Recreation at Virginia Tech, and Dr. James Buffer, Dean of the College of Education at Virginia Tech, for their support in the preparation of this text. Also, we would like to recognize and thank Dr. Rick Loya, Cal State–Long Beach; Dr. Dennis Smith, University of Houston; and Dr. Rhonda Rodamer, James Madison University, who reviewed the text. Finally, we would like to thank our families: Barbara, Kelly, and Kyle Redican; Mary Anne, Nicholas, and Andrew Baffi; and Larry and Laura Olsen for their patience, support, understanding, and encouragement through the process of writing this text.

K. J. R.
L. K. O.
C. R. B.

Organization of School Health Programs

Introduction

1

Generally speaking, the health of the school-age child is a community concern. That is to say, the responsibility for providing the student with an environment that nurtures positive health and well-being is jointly shared by all members, groups, organizations, and institutions of the community in which the student resides. Specifically, the community agents carrying most of the responsibility for the student's health status are the student; the family; the community organizations and institutions concerned with the health and well-being of all residents of the community; and the school, including district supervisors, administrators, principals, and teachers. Collectively, these individuals and community groups play an important role in providing an atmosphere in which students are able and are encouraged to participate in a variety of life experiences that help protect, promote, or improve their health.

It is most unfortunate, however, that for a number of reasons, many of which are beyond the community control, the environment within a community is not always conducive to support for good health. The result is that much of the burden of responsibility for providing for the student's health rests with the school. The mechanism utilized by schools in meeting this charge varies in the degree that it functions and is effective. This mechanism is called the school health program, and the requirements for a sound school health program are the subject of this text.

This text provides the information necessary to develop and organize a sound school health program. It is the hope of the authors that the student and professional will be able to utilize this information in the development, organization, and evaluation of existing or newly emerging school health programs.

The school health program should be viewed as one of the basic responsibilities of the school, at both the local school level and the district level. One should consider that between 25 and 85 percent of the students in a school, depending upon the socioeconomic level of the community, enter schools with a variety of health defects. These defects may be manifested in a variety of areas, including hearing, vision, or emotional problems.

The school health program could be viewed as an extension of the public health program, designed to reach a specific population group. The public health program deals with a wide variety of groups, whereas the school health program concentrates almost exclusively on students.

Prevention of health problems is not the sole concern of the school health program. Rather, the school health program should have a comprehensive framework wherein the overall purpose or ultimate objective is to protect, promote, and improve the health status of students. Personnel involved in the school health program should be trained to do one or more of the following:

1. Incorporate the major foundation areas into the school health program.
2. Assist in all activities designed to provide a healthful school environment.
3. Identify potential health problems of students.
4. Conduct or assist in health appraisal of students.
5. Counsel students and parents concerning health-related problems.
6. Utilize a sound health referral system, including participation in follow-up.
7. Assist in all activities designed to control communicable diseases in the school setting.
8. Assist in all activities designed to improve the health status of handicapped students.
9. Provide emergency care when needed for both students and school personnel.
10. Implement comprehensive health education at all grade levels.

One must keep in mind that the school health program must be functional; it should be student-oriented. It must also be flexible enough to incorporate the growth and development characteristics of students, their needs and interests, and any legal aspects imposed by the local county or state. This program is a comprehensive one that is made up of many different areas.

A schematic of the school health program as developed by Johns is presented in Figure 1.1. The focal point of the school health program is the school-age student. Important influences in his or her life are family, peers, and community. These influences in some cases can be so powerful that they can literally render the school health program ineffective.

Also important to note is the relationship that exists between the school and community health councils. These councils immediately influence the school-age student. Their functions and purposes will be discussed in Chapter 4. Another important element is the "Foundations" category, which includes the important elements upon which the school health program is essentially built.

The last three sections of the model represent the three main areas of the school health program: healthful school environment, health services, and health instruction. It is these three areas and the many points included in these three areas that comprise the operational component of the school health program.

Before any component in Figure 1.1 can become truly operational, it takes planning time and concerted effort on the part of a variety of individuals. These individuals are often referred to as the school health team; the team includes parents; students; teachers; curriculum specialists; administrators; medical

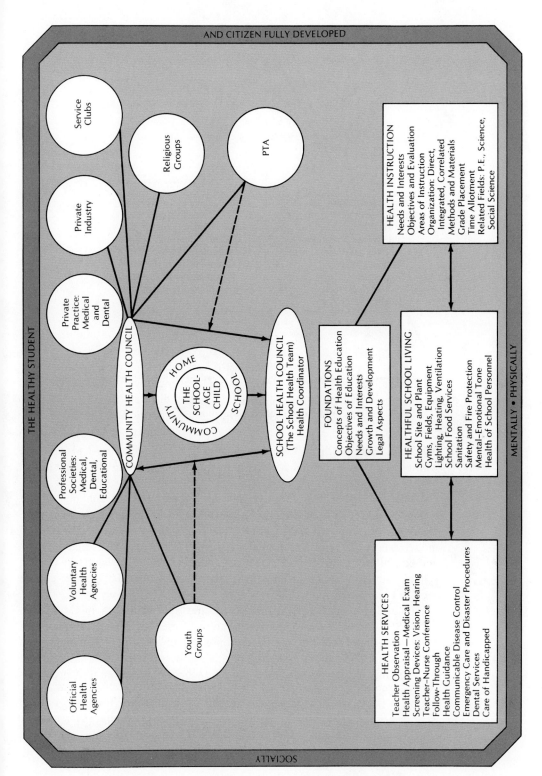

FIGURE 1.1

A concept of a school health program.
Developed by Edward B. Johns, Ed.D., Professor Emeritus, School of Public Health, University of California, Los Angeles.

Politics of terminology

3

FIGURE 1.2

A school health model
for the 1990s.
*Reprinted with permission
from* Journal of School
Health. *Access: Keystones
for School Health
Promotion. Vol. 60, No. 8,
September 1990, p. 299.
Copyright 1990. American
School Health Association,
Kent, OH 44240.*

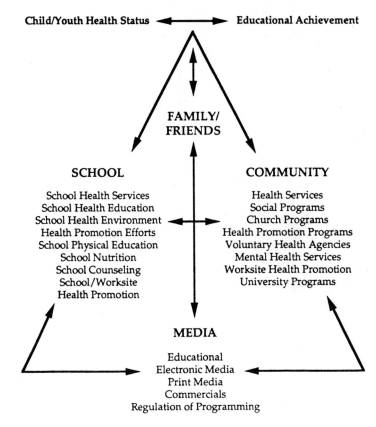

personnel; and auxiliary school personnel, including janitors and cafeteria workers. All these people have responsibilities in helping to maintain the school health program.

The school health program model developed by Johns contains all the necessary ingredients of a comprehensive school health program. Recently, Nader (1990) proposed a 1990 school health model which builds upon Johns' model. Nader's school health model suggests that "the child's health status and educational achievements are placed at the apex of a triangle of family, school, and community systems" (Stone, 1990, p. 299). This model can be seen in Figure 1.2.

In addition to Nader's model, another school health model called ACCESS, which focuses on administration, community, curricula, environment, and school services, has been proposed. From Figure 1.3 it can be seen that the ACCESS model provides for a broad-based organizational structure for planning, implementing, and evaluating school health promotion programs (Stone, 1990). An important element of the ACCESS model is its emphasis on health promotion programs. According to Stone (1990), the health promotion component of the model reflects the promotion of healthy behavior, a major tenet of public health. According to Kolbe (1986), the distinction

Organization of School Health Programs

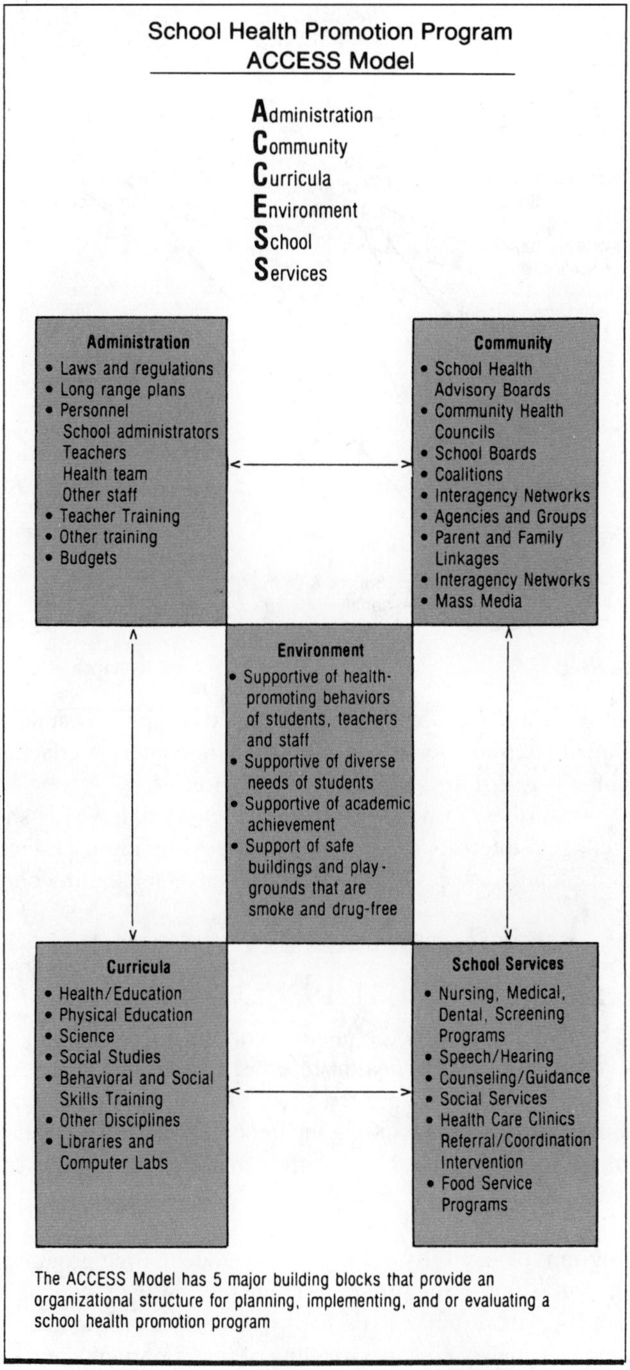

School Health Promotion Program
ACCESS Model

Administration
Community
Curricula
Environment
School
Services

Administration
- Laws and regulations
- Long range plans
- Personnel
  School administrators
  Teachers
  Health team
  Other staff
- Teacher Training
- Other training
- Budgets

Community
- School Health
  Advisory Boards
- Community Health
  Councils
- School Boards
- Coalitions
- Interagency Networks
- Agencies and Groups
- Parent and Family
  Linkages
- Interagency Networks
- Mass Media

Environment
- Supportive of health-
  promoting behaviors
  of students, teachers
  and staff
- Supportive of diverse
  needs of students
- Supportive of academic
  achievement
- Support of safe
  buildings and play-
  grounds that are
  smoke and drug-free

Curricula
- Health/Education
- Physical Education
- Science
- Social Studies
- Behavioral and Social
  Skills Training
- Other Disciplines
- Libraries and
  Computer Labs

School Services
- Nursing, Medical,
  Dental, Screening
  Programs
- Speech/Hearing
- Counseling/Guidance
- Social Services
- Health Care Clinics
  Referral/Coordination
  Intervention
- Food Service
  Programs

The ACCESS Model has 5 major building blocks that provide an
organizational structure for planning, implementing, and or evaluating a
school health promotion program

FIGURE 1.3

School health promotion
ACCESS model.
*Reprinted with permission
from* Journal of School
Health. *Access: Keystones
for School Health
Promotion. Vol. 60, No. 8,
September 1990, p. 300.
Copyright 1990. American
School Health Association,
Kent, OH 44240.*

FIGURE 1.4

School health program
components and
outcomes.
*Kolbe, L. "Education and
Promotion," Gochman,
D.S. (ed.), Health
Behavior: Emerging
Research Perspectives,
Figure 2, p. 387, New York:
Plenum Press, 1988.*

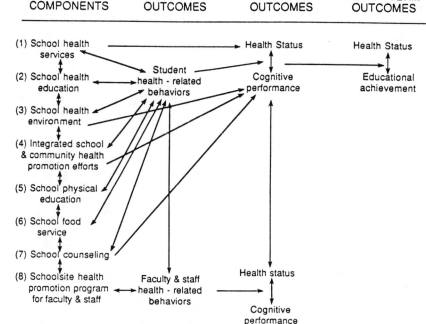

between health promotion and health education is best depicted by examining immediate, short-term, and long-term outcomes. A conceptual framework for Kolbe's assertion can be found in Figure 1.4.

Regardless of which model is preferred all have the student and his or her needs and interests as their central focus. In addition, these models have the elements of services, instruction, and environment in common.

SCHOOL HEALTH TEAM RESPONSIBILITIES

Parents have perhaps the most important role in helping students maintain a level of high-quality health. In order for parents to be effective members of the school health team, they should be willing to learn as much as possible about good health, including the importance of early diagnosis and subsequent follow-up of identified health problems. Essentially, this requires the parents' understanding of the function and importance of health screening in the schools. Parents can be a valuable resource in all phases of the school health program. If they fully understand the focus of the program, they will be more likely to support the program in whatever ways they can.

The school nurse is perhaps the member of the health team who has the most well-balanced understanding of the importance of the health status of the student as well as the medical knowledge to make sound referrals. The nurse is also able to relate the specifics of the problems found in the schools to parents and to other medical personnel.

Some of the major responsibilities of the school nurse as a member of the school health team include:

1. Constructing and/or maintaining health records of all students.
2. Periodically reviewing records to make sure they are accurate and up-to-date.
3. Dispensing medication to students in accordance with health policies.
4. Providing in-service training on health observation of students to all school personnel.
5. Conducting ongoing follow-up on students referred to health professionals for a potential medical problem.
6. Participating actively in the development of school health policies.
7. Providing or arranging for health counseling for students.
8. Reporting suspected cases of child abuse and/or neglect.
9. Acting as medical resource person for health education teachers.
10. Identifying students with special medical problems and educating school personnel in how to deal with the student.
11. Identifying and using community resources for school health services.

The responsibilities of the school administrator are important to the functioning of a comprehensive school health program. The school administrator should:

1. Demonstrate a thorough understanding of the key components to a healthful school environment, sound school health services program, and comprehensive health education.
2. Support all activities related to the school program.
3. Coordinate all phases of the school health program (if the school does not have a health coordinator).
4. Be a liaison between community health and social agencies and the school.
5. Allocate resources, including funds, so that the optimal operation of the school health program will be ensured.
6. Act as a functional member of the school health team, including participation on the school health council.
7. Establish a mechanism for an ongoing evaluation of the total school health program.

Perhaps the most important member of the school health team is the teacher. Since the teacher spends so much time with the student, the teacher can be the best source for identifying health problems or defects. Responsibilities of the teacher in the school health program are incorporated throughout the text. Each area is treated with the responsibilities of the teacher in mind.

Mayshark and Shaw identify some key responsibilities of the teacher in the school health program. Some of these responsibilities include the following:

1. Motivate and assist students in establishing good health habits.
2. Encourage students to evaluate their own health behavior and to take responsibility for its improvement.
3. Integrate life's experiences into health instruction.
4. Plan a thorough and progressive direct health instruction program.
5. Identify those students who suffer from remediable health problems and refer to proper source for correction; follow up reported cases to ensure correction and proper adjustment of student.
6. Identify obstructions to the healthful school environment and seek to improve unhealthful situations.
7. Counsel individual students with respect to health problems or concerns [1975, pp. 117–118].

Other members of the school health team, who have their own responsibilities include medical personnel such as the speech pathologist and the audiologist, as well as community members. The community members include representatives from the public health department, voluntary health agencies, physicians, and social service personnel. These community members should also be involved in both the school and community health councils.

If specific job duties or responsibilities of some of the members of the school health team are not spelled out by the school or district, then certainly one of the main responsibilities of the community or school health councils could be to detail the responsibilities of these auxiliary and yet important members of the school health team.

TERMINOLOGY

In organizing a school health program, it is important that all members of the school health team have an understanding of school health and community health terminology. Some of the more common terms and definitions as developed by the Joint Committee on Health Education Terminology include the following:[1]

---

1. Reprinted by permission from Ameriance Alliance for Health Education. *Journal of Health Education,* March/April, 1991, vol. 22, no. 2.

A. Contextual Definitions

Health education takes place within the broad context of health. Certain health terms are defined to clarify how health education functions. These are:

Health

There are many definitions written for the word "HEALTH". Three examples are provided.

"A state of complete physical, mental, and social well-being, and not merely the absence of disease and infirmity." (6)

"A quality of life involving dynamic interaction and independence among the individual's physical well-being, his (sic) mental and emotional reactions, and the social complex in which he (sic) exists." (7)

"An integrated method of functioning which is oriented toward maximizing the potential of which the individual is capable. It requires that the individual maintain a continuum of balance and purposeful direction with the environment where he (sic) is functioning." (8)

Health Promotion and Disease Prevention

Health promotion and disease prevention is the aggregate of all purposeful activities designed to improve personal and public health through a combination of strategies, including the competent implementation of behavioral change strategies, health education, health protection measures, risk factor detection, health enhancement and health maintenance.

Healthy Lifestyle

A healthy lifestyle is a set of health-enhancing behaviors, shaped by internally consistent values, attitudes, beliefs and external social and cultural forces.

Official Health Agency

An official health agency is a publicly supported governmental organization mandated by law and/or regulation for the protection and improvement of the health of the public.

Voluntary Health Organization

A voluntary health organization is a non-profit association supported by contributions dedicated to conducting research and providing education and/or services related to particular health problems or concerns.

(Note: Private voluntary organization—PVO is the term used outside the U.S.A. to denote a voluntary health organization; in some countries and in connection with the United Nations, the term non-governmental organization—NGO—is used.)

Private Health Agency

A private health agency is a profit or non-profit organization devoted to providing primary, secondary, and/or tertiary health services which may include health education.

B. Primary Health Education Definitions

Certain health education terms are generic and are defined here, as follows:

Health Education Field

The health education field is that multidisciplinary practice, which is concerned with designing, implementing, and evaluating educational programs that enable individuals, families, groups, organizations, and communities to play active roles in achieving, protecting, and sustaining health.

Health Education Process

The health education process is that continuum of learning which enables people, as individuals and as members of social structures, to voluntarily make decisions, modify behaviors, and change social conditions in ways which are health enhancing.

Health Education Program

A health education program is a planned combination of activities developed with the involvement of specific populations and based on a needs assessment, sound principles of education, and periodic evaluation using a clear set of goals and objectives.

Health Educator

A health educator is a practitioner who is professionally prepared in the field of health education, who demonstrates competence in both theory and practice, and who accepts responsibility to advance the aims of the health education profession.

Examples of settings for health educators and the application of health education include, but are not limited to, the following:

- Schools
- Communities
- Post-secondary educational institutions
- Medical care institutions
- Voluntary health organizations
- Worksites (business and industry)
- Rehabilitation centers
- Professional associations
- Governmental agencies
- Public health agencies
- Environmental agencies
- Mental health agencies

Certified Health Education Specialist (CHES)

A Certified Health Education Specialist (CHES) is an individual who is credentialed as a result of demonstrating competency based on criteria established by the National Commission for Health Education Credentialing, Inc. (NCHEC).

Health Education Coordinator

A health education coordinator is a professional health educator who is responsible for the management and coordination of all health education policies, activities, and resources within a particular setting or circumstance.

Health Education Administrator

A health education administrator is a professional health educator who has the authority and responsibility for the management and coordination of all health education policies, activities, and resources within a particular setting or circumstance.

Health Information

Health information is the content of communications based on data derived from systematic and scientific methods as they relate to health issues, policies, programs, services, and other aspects of individual and public health, which can be used for informing various populations and in planning health education activities.

Health Literacy

Health literacy is the capacity of an individual to obtain, interpret, and understand basic health information and services and the competence to use such information and services in ways which are health enhancing.

Health Advising**

Health advising is a process of informing and assisting individuals or groups in making decisions and solving problems related to health.

C. Definitions Related to Community Settings

The terms that relate more specifically to community or public health education are defined here, as follows:

Community Health Education

Community health education is the application of a variety of methods that result in the education and mobilization of community members in actions for resolving health issues and problems which affect the community. These methods include, but are not limited to, group process, mass media, communication, community organization, organization development, strategic planning, skills training, legislation, policy making, and advocacy.

Community Health Educator

A community health educator is a practitioner who is professionally prepared in the field of community/public health education who demonstrates competence in the planning, implementation, and evaluation of a broad range of health promoting or health enhancing programs for community groups.

D. Definitions Related to Educational Settings

The terms that relate more specifically to school health education are defined here, as follows:

** The Committee believes that Health Counseling is a term that should be defined by the health counseling profession.

Comprehensive School Health Program

A comprehensive school health program is an organized set of policies, procedures, and activities designed to protect and promote the health and well-being of students and staff which has traditionally included health services, healthful school environment, and health education. It should also include, but not be limited to, guidance and counseling, physical education, food service, social work, psychological services, and employee health promotion.

School Health Education

School health education is one component of the comprehensive school health program which includes the development, delivery, and evaluation of a planned instructional program and other activities for students preschool through grade 12, for parents and for school staff, and is designed to positively influence the health knowledge, attitudes, and skills of individuals.

School Health Services

School health services are that part of the school health program provided by physicians, nurses, dentists, health educators, other allied health personnel, social workers, teachers and others to appraise, protect and promote the health of students and school personnel. These services are designed to insure access to and the appropriate use of primary health care services, prevent and control communicable disease, provide emergency care for injury or sudden illness, promote and provide optimum sanitary conditions in a safe school facility and environment, and provide concurrent learning opportunities which are conducive to the maintenance and promotion of individual and community health.

School Health Educator

A school health educator is a practitioner who is professionally prepared in the field of school health education, meets state teaching requirements, and demonstrates competence in the development, delivery, and evaluation of curricula for students and adults in the school setting that enhance health knowledge, attitudes, and problem-solving skills.

Comprehensive School Health Instruction

Comprehensive school health instruction refers to the development, delivery and evaluation of a planned curriculum, preschool through 12, with goals, objectives, content sequence, and specific classroom lessons which includes, but is not limited to the following major content areas:

- Community health
- Consumer health
- Environmental health
- Family life
- Mental and emotional health
- Injury prevention and safety
- Nutrition
- Personal health
- Prevention and control of disease
- Substance use and abuse

Post-Secondary Health Education Program

A post-secondary health education program is a planned set of health education policies, procedures, activities, and services that are directed to students, faculty and/or staff of colleges, universities, and other higher education institutions. This includes, but is not limited to:

- general health courses for students
- employee and student health promotion activities
- health services
- professional preparation of health educators and other professionals
- self-help groups
- student life

1. Mabel Rugen. (1972). *A fifty year history of the public health section of the American Public Health Association, 1922–1972.* American Public Health Association, Inc. Washington, DC, p. 9.
2. Jesse Feiring Williams (Chair). (1934, Dec. 10). Report of the Health Education Section of the American Physical Education Association. Definitions of terms in health education, *Journal of Health and Physical Education,* 5(16–17), 50–51.
3. Bernice Moss (Chair). (1950). Joint Committee on Health Education Terminology. *Journal of Health and Physical Education,* 21(41).
4. Robert Yoho (Chair). (1962, Nov.). Joint Committee on Health Education Terminology. Health education

terminology, *Journal of Health, Physical Education, Recreation,* 33(27–28).
5. Edward B. Johns (Chair). (1973, Nov/Dec). Joint Committee on Health Education Terminology. Report of the Joint Committee on Health Education Terminology, *Health Education,* 4(6), p. 25.
6. World Health Organization. (1946). *Constitution of the World Health Organization.* Geneva, World Health Organization.

7. *Health education: A conceptual approach to curriculum design, school health education study.* Washington, DC: 3M Education Press, p. 10.
8. Halbert Dunn. (1967). *High level wellness.* Virginia: R. W. Beatty, 4–5.

Source: 1990 Joint Committee on Health Education Terminology, "Report of the 1990 Joint Committee on Health Education Terminology," from *Health Education,* Vol. 22, No. 2, 1991.

It is important to note that these terms are used throughout this text, and familiarity with them will enhance understanding of the organization of the various components of the school health program.

As a final introductory point, it is important that the student or practitioner recognize that the school health program is a viable part of the total school program. Through the coordination of health services, the provision of a healthful school environment, and the development of sound, comprehensive health instruction, students can best profit from the total school experience.

The following sections and chapters will focus directly on the health of the school environment, school health services, and health instruction. It is hoped that after reading these chapters the student and/or practitioner will develop a well-founded theoretical as well as a practical operational basis for the development and implementation of a sound school health program.

REFERENCES

Joint Committee on Health Education Terminology. Report of the 1990 Joint Committee on Health Education Terminology. *Journal of Health Education* 22:3 (May–June 1991), pp. 173–184.

Kolbe, L., "Education and Promotion." In Gochman, D. S., *Health Behavior: Emerging Research Perspectives.* New York: Plenum Press, 1988.

Mayshark, C., and D. Shaw. *Administration of School Health Programs.* St. Louis, Mo.: C. V. Mosby, 1975.

Stone, E. "ACCESS: Keystones for School Health Promotion." *Journal of School Health* 60:7 (September 1990), p. 299.

PART I

Foundations

The School-Age Child

2

N o two people are the same. People differ with respect to the color of their eyes, hair, and skin, as well as in their body build, physical and mental abilities, energy, behavior, and interests. No one is perfect, and despite these obvious differences, most people are healthy. The trick is to be able to identify those differences, those imperfections, that cause people to deviate too far from what is generally expected.

The purpose of this chapter is to enable teachers to better understand the social, psychological, and physical growth and development needs of students.

CHARACTERISTICS OF THE HEALTHY STUDENT

Erik H. Erikson, a psychologist interested in how healthy personalities develop, has proposed that the human develops in eight stages. These are summarized in Table 2.1. To become a well-adjusted adult, a child must progress through each of the stages in a manner that expands, enlarges, and enriches his or her personality (Sorochan and Bender, 1979, p. 52).

Children enter school somewhere between the locomotor–genital stage and the latency stage. Depending upon exactly when they enter school, children who are developing in a healthful manner will be curious, alert, and active. They will also come to school with a constellation of socially approved behaviors, and they will acquire more behaviors and refine those with which they arrived. These behaviors are acquired via the process of socialization. The healthy child shows signs that he has "acquired the knowledge, skills and dispositions, and learns to play the social roles necessary for effective participation in society" (Needle, 1973, p. 6).

Healthy students, by the time they enter school, will have developed a basic trust for others. This characteristic develops out of the child's having experienced love and affection and having had his basic needs satisfied in early infancy (Stage 1). Healthy primary-grade students will express a sense of self-worth and of autonomy. They also will have developed an effective and useful imagination. The primary-grade teacher can help students develop a sense of responsibility, a sense of duty, and a sense of industry by assigning them tasks, showing them how to keep busy, and requiring them to complete their assigned tasks. Healthy students will continue to improve their social skills and the ways in which they deal with conflict and tension (Sorochan and Bender, 1975, pp. 55–56).

TABLE 2.1

Erikson's Stages of the Development of Man

Age	Stage	Characterization of Stage	Value Strengths of Man
0–1	Oral-sensory	Basic trust vs. shame	Hope and drive
2–3	Muscular-anal	Autonomy vs. shame, doubt	Willpower and self-control
4–5	Locomotor-genital	Initiative vs. guilt	Purpose and direction
6–12	Latency	Industry vs. inferiority	Competence and method
13–19	Puberty and adolescence	Identity vs. role confusion	Fidelity and devotion
20–30	Young adulthood	Intimacy vs. isolation	Love and affiliation
30–64	Adulthood	Generativity vs. stagnation	Care and production
65+	Maturity	Ego integrity vs. despair	Wisdom and renunciation

From *Teaching Elementary Health Science* 2d ed. by Walter Sorochan and Stephen J. Bender (Reading, MA: Addison-Wesley, 1979), p. 51; adapted from *Childhood and Society,* 2d ed. (New York: W. W. Norton, 1963), revised by Erik H. Erikson. Reprinted by permission of W. W. Norton & Co., Inc.

As students reach junior high school, they will begin to experiment with different social roles in an attempt to attain a sense of identity. Adolescence is a period of rapid physical, sexual, and intellectual change. As their sense of identity grows stronger, the adolescents will view themselves as distinct individuals (Conger, 1979, p. 10). For most adolescents, however, there is a feeling of inconsistency as they play roles that change from situation to situation. Their interests are expanding during this period, and they become increasingly capable of organizing their own activities. Also, daydreaming is common, as are rapid changes in mood and emotions.

Senior high students are idealistic and insecure. The peer group becomes a dominant force in their lives, and they seek the approval of this group by conforming to its expectations and demands. Students in this group are becoming more and more independent from their parents as they seek to solidify and stabilize their identity.

Students who for one reason or another have not adequately resolved the developmental conflicts identified by Erikson often will:

1. Be jealous.
2. Be shy and withdrawn.
3. Be inhibited.

4. Be distrusting of others.
5. Be unable to establish meaningful relationships.
6. Avoid displays of love, affection, and intimacy.

These students will also generally find learning more difficult and are more likely to experience failure and think of themselves as failures than are healthy students.

The ability to make sound moral judgments, to be able to distinguish good from bad, is another characteristic of the healthy student. A leading authority in the development of moral judgments in children is Kohlberg. He advocates a cognitive developmental framework within which moral development occurs in three levels: preconventional, conventional, and postconventional (Craig, 1976, p. 108). The maturation of the student's reasoning ability appears to play an important role in his or her movement from one level to the next.

The first level, preconventional, is characterized by an awareness on the part of the student of reward and punishment. At this level the individual acts to avoid punishment. The student's major concern at this level is with outcomes, not intention (Craig, 1976, p. 108). The second level, conventional, on the other hand, recognizes the importance of intention. At this level the focus is on getting the approval of others by performing good behaviors. There is also recognition of societal rules and authority. The third and highest level, postconventional, is characterized by behavior that conforms to societal standards and displays an awareness and respect for personal values. This level is further "motivated by conscience and is built around the desire to conform to avoid self-condemnation." Here "moral principles, rather than rigid cultural do's and don'ts, determine values and the aim is justice and respect for others" (Craig, 1976, p. 110). In each of these levels, Kohlberg identifies two stages; the result is a model with three levels and six stages. This model of moral development is summarized in Table 2.2.

PHYSICAL, SOCIAL, AND COGNITIVE DEVELOPMENT

Children develop physically, socially, and mentally at their own rates. When it is said that a child is developing normally, it merely means that he or she is progressing along some dimension (physical, social, or cognitive) within an acceptable range of possibilities from a standard point of reference, or an average. Not all children measure up to this average; they vary with regard to behavior, intelligence and intellectual interests, body build, and physical abilities. Some of these variations are obvious to all of us, and some will be obvious only to the trained eye. In part, it is the teacher's responsibility to identify those children who deviate too far from the established norm. These children should be referred to the school nurse. Being able to discern between acceptable and nonacceptable growth and development requires that a teacher be observant and receive training in needs and characteristics of students.

TABLE 2.2

Kohlberg's Six Stages of Moral Development

Preconventional Level

Stage 1:

Punishment and obedience orientation. The physical consequences of an action determine whether it is good or bad. Avoiding punishment and bowing to superior power are valued positively.

Stage 2:

Instrumental relativist orientation. Right action consists of behavior that satisfies one's own needs. Human relations are viewed in marketplace terms. Reciprocity occurs, but is seen in a pragmatic way, i.e., "you scratch my back and I'll scratch yours."

Conventional Level

Stage 3:

Interpersonal concordance (good boy—nice girl) orientation. Good behaviors are those that please or are approved by others. There is much emphasis on conformity and being "nice."

Stage 4:

Orientation toward authority ("law and order"). Focus is on authority or rules. It is right to do one's duty, show respect for authority, and maintain the social order.

Postconventional Level

Stage 5:

Social-contract orientation. This stage has a utilitarian, legalistic tone. Correct behavior is defined in terms of standards agreed upon by society. Awareness of the relativism of personal values and the need for consensus is important.

Stage 6:

Universal ethical principle orientation. Morality is defined as a decision of conscience. Ethical principles are self-chosen, based on abstract concepts (e.g., the Golden Rule) rather than concrete rules (e.g., the Ten Commandments).

Source: Liebert/Wicks-Nelson/Kail, *Developmental Psychology,* 4e, © 1986, p. 336. Reprinted by permission of Prentice Hall, Englewood Cliffs, New Jersey.

Physical Growth and Development

Growth in height and weight is a dynamic process that reflects progress toward optimal physical maturity. The period of childhood usually referred to as middle childhood ranges from approximately 5 to 12 years of age and is a period of slow growth. During this period, growth is cyclic and not predictable.

A method for recording the growth in height and weight of school-age children has been with us since the 1870s, when H. P. Bowditch developed the first growth charts for average height and weight for American children. This chart and these averages were based on data he collected while studying Boston school children. Research in the growth patterns of U.S. school children continued during the ensuing years; however, much was still unknown about the variations in physical growth as well as about the growth patterns of infants and early preschoolers (Hamill and Moore, 1981, p. 1). By 1921, charts for these latter groups were developed, and since then, the development of growth charts has proliferated (Baldwin–Wood, Wetzel, Stuart–Meredith, NEA–AMA, and Reed–Stuart, to name a few) (Hamill and Moore, 1981, pp. 1–4). While measuring growth in increments, today these charts are also used to help provide reference data for attained status at given age; further, they remain an important screening tool used in child health supervision.

It is quite apparent that throughout the life course, differences in body type exist. A popular way to describe these differences is in morphological terms. Three terms commonly used are (1) ectomorph, referring to the person who is thin, with small muscles and long arms and legs; (2) mesomorph, meaning the muscular, solidly built person; and (3) endomorph, describing the fleshy or stocky person (Jenne and Greene, 1976, p. 211). Although it is unlikely that teachers will be trained to, or will have the time to somatotype their students, this technique, developed by Sheldon in 1940, has some descriptive utility (Hamill and Moore, 1981, pp. 1–4). Somatotyping has shown us that the healthy or normal student cannot be characterized by a singular label. Normal variations in body build do exist, and the teacher and health professional concerned with the physical growth and development of students should take this fact into consideration when screening children for growth and development defects.

The discussion of physical growth to this point has focused on external growth. This should not lead one to conclude that, during this middle childhood period, external growth is the only type of physical growth occurring, for growth and development of the internal organs and systems are also taking place. Table 2.3 depicts the growth and development of organs at different ages. In general, growth and development of all the body systems occurs during the period of middle childhood.

Important variables that influence physical growth and development are nutritional status, family socioeconomic status, and illness.

Nutritional Status

Generally, students who eat daily meals that are nutritionally sound and well balanced are likely to be growing and developing in a healthful manner. Children who are malnourished and have diets low in calories and proteins are likely to experience some deficiency in growth and development. Usually this deficiency in growth can be reversed by placing the child on a diet high in proteins and calories. The severity of the deficiency and the length of time it takes to reverse the situation depend upon how long the child has been malnourished (Jenne and Greene, 1976, p. 213).

TABLE 2.3

Average Weights of Organs at Different Ages (g)

	Newborn	1 yr	6 yr	Puberty	Adult
Brain	350	910	1,200	1,300	1,350
Heart	24	45	95	150	300
Thymus	12	20	24	30	0–15
Kidneys (both)	25	70	120	170	300
Liver	150	300	550	1,500	1,600
Lungs (both)	60	130	260	410	1,200
Pancreas	3	9	20	40	90
Spleen	10	30	55	95	155
Stomach	8	30	50	80	135

Reprinted with permission from George H. Lowrey, *Growth and Development of Children,* 7th ed., p. 232. Copyright © 1978 by Year Book Medical Publishers, Chicago.

Family Socioeconomic Status

Almost always, low socioeconomic status is accompanied by low status in other factors in a person's life. For example, people who are at or below the poverty level, as established by the U.S. government, are usually less well educated than are those persons whose incomes place them above the poverty level. Just as socioeconomic status relates to all other aspects of a person's life, it also is associated with poor health and deficiencies in the growth and development of children. Children born into poor families, when compared to children born to middle- and upper-class families, generally have lower intelligence test scores as measured by standardized intelligence tests and are slower to grow and develop.

Illness

There is an inverse relationship between the severity of an illness and the growth and development of a child. The more severe the illness, the less growth and development occur.

Social Growth and Development

Effective growth and development as a social being requires that the child successfully move from one developmental stage to the next. The ultimate end is passage into adulthood. Play is the vehicle that children most often use to pass through the various stages of social development. Play serves many important purposes in this regard, as it affords children the opportunity to test reality and to learn to distinguish between fantasy and reality. Play provides children with an opportunity to practice various mental and physical skills; to learn to cooperate; to try on various social roles, such as sex roles; to develop

Organization of School Health Programs

TABLE 2.4

Social Stage and Play

Social-Developmental Stage	Type of Play
Toddler (1.5–3 years of age)	Solitary play and parallel play
Early preschool (approximately 3–4 years of age)	Parallel play continues; associative play begins
Late preschool (approximately 4.5–5 years of age)	Cooperative play begins and continues throughout life

Adapted from Catherine T. Best and Lauren Julius Harris, ''Childhood,'' *Psychology 84/85* (Guilford, CT: Dushkin Publishing Group, Inc., 1984).

a sense of self-identity; to exercise their imagination; and to learn to compromise and adjust in order to get along with others. They learn that not everyone has the same thoughts, feelings, and beliefs about different topics and, perhaps most important, they enhance their friendship-making skills.

Children at the toddler stage will be found to engage in play that best utilizes their imaginative skills. The play session is characterized predominantly by solitary play. When another child is around, the toddler will often play next to but not with this other child. Around the age of three, the child begins to mimic the play of others around him, although he continues to play essentially ''alone.'' This type of play generally continues until the child is about four and a half years old. At this time play begins to reflect cooperative activities. Rules will be established, and children will begin to practice various roles. This type of play becomes more refined as the child gets older. By the time puberty is reached, the child has acquired the skills necessary for the establishment and maintenance of friendships throughout a lifetime (Best and Harris, 1984, pp. 163–166). The social developmental stage and the type of play occurring are summarized in Table 2.4.

Cognitive Development

Mental traits are acquired in a progressive manner. As children develop, their thoughts and behaviors become increasingly influenced by their understanding of language. The more sophisticated their language skills become, the more they are able to follow instructions and display behavior appropriate to the situation.

Between 6 and 8 years of age, the child has a short attention span and thus finds it very difficult to accomplish long, time-consuming tasks. His or her memory, however, is becoming stronger and more accurate. By the time the student is 9 years of age, he or she is able to spend longer periods of time on specific tasks. The ability to work cooperatively with others is improved, and time can now be organized reliably toward more constructive ends. These capacities continue to increase as the child approaches adolescence. During this period, the child applies more logical approaches to solving relatively complex problems. Reading speed and comprehension are increasing. At 15 years of age, the child's logical skills are developed to the point that he or she is able to make formal logical deductions and is also better able to organize his or her life in a meaningful and constructive manner.

Piaget offers another way of viewing mental development. He suggests that mental growth and development occur via the processes of accommodation and assimilation. Accommodation is a process whereby the child adjusts its perception of the world to accommodate new information that it receives about the world. Assimilation occurs when the child interprets this new information in light of his or her understanding of the world based on past learning. Piaget refers to the processing of information as schemata. Schemata change as we grow and, according to Piaget, this change occurs in four periods: sensorimotor, preoperational, concrete operations, and formal operations.

During the sensorimotor period (birth to 2 years), the infant begins to construct reality through at first the unplanned and then later the deliberate use of its senses and bodily movements. As this period ends, the preoperational period (2 to 7 years of age) begins. This period is characterized by the child's use of speech and the developing awareness that objects can be represented by words. The child is also beginning to deal with complex problems during this period (Craig, 1979, p. 34).

From about 7 to 11 years of age, the child is developing his ability to think in an orderly and logical fashion. This is the concrete operations period. During this period the child is able to organize his world better than he could during the preoperational period. Finally, during the formal operations period (11 to adulthood), the ability to think abstractly and to understand logical contradictions becomes refined (Craig, 1979, p. 34).

INFLUENCES

A number of variables impact on a child's development. Some, however, have a profound impact; they are (1) family, (2) school, (3) peers.

Family

From birth the child's family interacts with him or her in such a way that he or she begins to draw conclusions about others based on these familial interactions. The family sets the stage for childhood development of a sense of basic trust in others, a sense of autonomy, and a sense of purpose and initiative. The child also learns the basic social skills necessary to establish lasting, meaningful relationships. It is through the family that the child attaches meaning and value to relationships by observing other family members. From these relationships with other family members, the child develops concepts of and attitudes toward people.

Organization of School Health Programs

Familial influences on the physical well-being of children are equally profound. The child's basic beliefs about and attitudes toward health are conceived through early interactions with parents, siblings, and other members of the family. The family will also be directly responsible for the child's health behaviors as well—it is the parents who take the child to the dentist; they also decide if and when the child should see a physician. The child observes the personal health habits of parents and other family members and, through repeated exposure to their habits, the child will begin eventually to assume these behaviors, regardless of whether or not they are good habits.

Does the child see the family eating well-balanced meals with limited snacking in between? Do they exercise or exhibit other positive health behaviors? Whether or not a child is exposed to a home atmosphere that is conducive to the development of healthful habits will be a determining factor in whether or not, as an adult, he or she displays appropriate health behaviors.

School

The school has the responsibility for providing the student with the most appropriate conditions for learning and growing and developing. In order for the school to meet this responsibility, it must provide the student with a total health program. This means that the school must do everything necessary to maintain and improve the health of its students. It must teach the student to become a partner in establishing his or her own fate. They must learn to accept some of the responsibility for their own health status. The school's health program must be well rounded. It is composed of three interdependent areas: services, environment, and instruction.

School health services are dedicated to maintaining the students' well-being and moving them in the direction of optimal health. The school must provide the student with well-trained personnel and well-designed, relevant services.

The environment is concerned with (1) the school's emotional climate, (2) the physical plant, and (3) maintenance. Each of these aspects of the environment is essential for the maintenance of an optimal health status. Everyone in the school system has some degree of responsibility for ensuring a healthful school environment.

It is the purpose of the instruction aspect of the school health program to provide students with worthwhile learning experiences that will enhance their attitudes and behaviors toward health. It should also favorably influence health knowledge. The teacher is in an ideal position to promote optimal health through imparting knowledge, developing motivational techniques, providing meaningful learning activities, and displaying positive personal health habits.

Peers

As children approach adolescence, they become more dependent on their peers and less dependent on their parents. With this growing dependence on peers, adolescents use the peer group to help establish an identity. This further solidifies the dependent bond forming between the individual and the peer group. The adolescent's conforming to the group's wishes often takes the form of inappropriate health behaviors. Smoking cigarettes, drinking alcoholic beverages, and using drugs are all examples of the behaviors that students may begin to display as a result of peer-group interrelationships.

SUMMARY

People grow and develop physically, emotionally, and socially at different rates. Psychologists, most notably Erikson, Kohlberg, and Piaget, have attempted to explain psychoemotional growth and development. Each of these scholars has developed a hierarchical approach to this phenomenon. In order for a child to become a psychologically healthy adult, according to Erikson, he must pass successfully through several developmental stages. The individual must resolve the conflicts that exist at each stage before he can move to the next stage of development.

For Kohlberg, the intellectual growth and development of the child contribute to his or her development of moral judgments. For Piaget, mental growth and development occur as a result of the processes of accommodation and assimilation.

A student's physical and social growth and development also occur in stages. These stages are relatively clearly defined. If teachers are to be effective in helping the total student, they must understand these growth stages. Teachers must also be aware of the numerous variables that affect physical and social growth, such as nutritional status, family socioeconomic status, illness, and peers.

REVIEW QUESTIONS

1. How do Erikson and Piaget explain psychoemotional growth and development?
2. What is the relationship between the development of moral judgments in children and their developing healthy personalities?
3. What is normal development? What is the responsibility of the teacher and the school with regard to the physical, social, and cognitive development of students?
4. What impact do nutritional status, family socioeconomic status, and illness have on the physical growth and development of students?
5. What role do accommodation and assimilation play in cognitive development?

REFERENCES

Best, C. T., and L. J. Harris. "Childhood." Annual Edition: *Psychology 84/85*. Guilford, Conn.: The Duskin Publishing Group, Inc., 1984.

Conger, J. *Adolescence*. New York: Harper & Row, 1979.

Craig, G. J. *Human Development*. Englewood Cliffs, N.J.: Prentice-Hall, 1979.

Dinkmeyer, D., and R. Dreikurs. *Encouraging Children to Learn: The Encouragement Process.* Englewood Cliffs, N.J.: Prentice-Hall, 1963.

Erikson, G. H. *Childhood and Society.* New York: W. W. Norton, 1963.

Glover, J. A., and R. H. Bruning. *Educational Psychology: Principles and Applications,* 3d ed. Glenview, Ill.: Scott, Foresman/Little, Brown Higher Education, 1990.

Gordon, D. J. *Human Development.* New York: Harper & Row, 1962.

Hafen, B. Q., et al., eds. *Adolescent Health: For Educators and Health Personnel.* Salt Lake City: Brighton Publishing Company, 1978.

Hamill, P. V. V., and W. M. Moore. ''Contemporary Growth Charts: Needs, Construction, and Application.'' Ross Growth and Development Program, Ross Laboratories, Columbus, Ohio, June 1981.

Jenne, F. H., and W. H. Greene. *School Health and Health Education,* 7th ed. St. Louis, Mo.: C. V. Mosby, 1976.

Keniston, K., and Carnegie Council on Children. *All Our Children: The American Family under Pressure.* New York: Carnegie Corporation of N.Y., 1977.

Liebert, Robert M., R. W. Poulos, and G. S. Marmor. *Developmental Psychology,* 2d ed. Englewood Cliffs, N.J.: Prentice-Hall, 1977.

Martinson, F. M. *Infant and Child Sexuality: Sociological Perspective.* St. Peter, Minn.: The Book Mark, Gustavus Adolphus College, 1973.

Needle, R. H. *The Relationship between Sexual Behavior and Ways of Handling Contraception among College Students.* Unpublished doctoral dissertation, University of Maryland, 1973.

Roche, A. F., and J. H. Himes. ''Incremental Growth Charts.'' *American Journal of Clinical Nutrition* **33**:9 (September 1980), pp. 2041–2052.

Schickedanz, J. A., K. Hansen, and P. D. Forsyth. *Understanding Children.* Mountain View, Ca.: Mayfield Publishing Company, 1990.

Schultz, D. *Growth Psychology: Models of the Healthy Personality.* New York: Van Nostrand Reinhold, 1977.

Sorochan, W. D., and S. J. Bender. *Teaching Elementary Health Science,* 2d ed. Reading, Mass.: Addison-Wesley, 1979.

Stone, D. B., L. B. O'Reilley, and J. D. Brown. *Elementary School Health Education: Ecological Perspectives.* Dubuque, Ia.: Wm. C. Brown Publishers, 1976.

Willgoose, C. E. *Health Teaching in Secondary Schools,* 3d ed. Philadelphia: Saunders, 1982.

Bases for Development of a School Health Program

3

I t is the purpose of this chapter to provide the reader with some insight concerning the bases of a school health program. We hope that, after reading this chapter, you will be able to answer such questions as:

1. What is the philosophical basis of the school health program?
2. How is the total school health program organized?
3. What are the objectives of the school health program?
4. Who is responsible for the school health program?
5. What is the relationship between needs and interests?
6. How does one determine students' needs and interests?

PHILOSOPHY

No school is an island. All schools exist in and are integral parts of communities. Issues and points of concern in one often appear symptomatically in the other. For example, drunk driving and acts of violence in the community affect the schools; student drug use in the schools affects the well-being of the community. John Hanlon, in *Principles of Public Health Administration,* states that the school health program and its education component are merely parts of the larger total community health program (Hanlon, 1984, p. 424). Because of the essential role each plays in the functioning of the other, there should be a great deal of collaboration between the schools and all other community parts. In fact, over thirty years ago, a general recommendation of the Los Angeles Area School Health Education Evaluative Study (Johns, ed., 1959) was that community agencies and schools should jointly conduct health education research to improve the health of humankind. Thus, not only must schools provide students with quality instruction; there should also be total support for and commitment to the school health program from school administrators, teachers, the school nurse, the school housekeeping staff, food service personnel, parents, local health and medical agencies and personnel, and other community members. It also means that parents ''must encourage the practice of health habits learned in school, and they should also follow up on needed and recommended health services for children'' (Mayshark, Shaw, and Best, 1977, p. 134).

The philosophy of the school health program should be developed as a joint effort of school and community members and should reflect and complement the beliefs and values of the community in general and the community's total health program in particular. ''The success and effectiveness of the [school health] program depends in large measure upon the common understanding on the part of each group and each individual involved as to

(1) the precise scope of its sphere of action, (2) its role in the total community health picture, and (3) the need for consistent cooperation in its implementation'' (Hanlon, 1984, p. 424).

The school health program that makes the greatest possible contribution to the long-term health and welfare of its students is one that has formulated and applies health policies consistent with the philosophy of the community's health program. It will likely be found that from state to state the philosophical underpinnings of the school health program in each of the schools in each state may vary. It is more probable, however, that in general there will be agreement with regard to basic philosophical beliefs. Smolensky and Bonvechio have identified some generalized basic philosophic statements:

1. "Health is a means to an end and is not an end in itself."
2. "Health is a dynamic and not a static condition."
3. "Health is a many-sided subject matter field which draws upon many interdisciplinary fields for its content and approach. It includes the physical, mental, emotional, social and moral aspects of the human organism."
4. "The intermediate and long range goals of health instruction should be the intelligent self-direction of one's own health behavior and that of his or her community."
5. "The health of the school-age population is the responsibility of all community members" (Smolensky and Bonvechio, 1966, pp. 6–7).
6. Health determines one's ability to function efficiently as a community member.
7. The effects of a good school health program extend beyond the school to the home and the community and into adult life.
8. The school health program should collaborate with local public health programs to ensure continuity of services.
9. The most important influence on the student's total well-being and growth and development is his or her relationship with his or her parent(s).
10. The school health program should reinforce the parents' responsibility for their child.
11. The purpose of the school health program is to enable the child to achieve maximum potential for learning, growth, and development.

ORGANIZATION OF THE TOTAL SCHOOL HEALTH PROGRAM

The purpose of the total school health program is to assist in the improvement, maintenance, and understanding of the health of both the students and the entire school staff. To carry out these functions, the total school health program is commonly divided into three related areas: services, environment, and instruction. The scope of the school health service program is to promote, protect, and appraise the health status of students. It is accomplished through (1) teacher observation, (2) health screenings and appraisals, (3) counseling with those involved in the health screenings and appraisals, (4) prevention and control of disease, (5) suggestions and recommendations to the student's family regarding needed health services, and (6) emergency care for students who have become ill or been injured. The healthful school environment involves (1) the organization of a healthful school day, (2) provision of a well-designed and adequately sized physical plant, and (3) maintenance of the physical plant. Health instruction is the "process of providing a sequence of planned and spontaneously originated learning opportunities comprising the organized aspects of health education in the school or community" (Green, 1972–73, p. 36). Each of these areas contributes to the total welfare of the student, and they are so interrelated that for the program to be good, consideration must be equally distributed among all three areas.

Goals and Objectives

The overall goal of the total school health program is to promote, maintain, and contribute to the understanding of the student's health. It accomplishes this by supporting each of its three areas—services, environment, and instruction—with equal fervor, as well as by engaging all community health personnel to pool their efforts with those of the school's so that the end result is an integrated school and community health program directed at helping the student achieve optimal health status.

The objectives of the three component parts of the school health program are interrelated. The objectives of the school health services aspect of the program are (1) to promote, maintain, and contribute to the understanding of the health of the student; (2) to appraise the health status of the student through screening tests and health examinations; (3) to adjust school programs to meet the needs of special groups; (4) to provide emergency services for students who have been injured or who have become ill at school; (5) to counsel and advise students, parents, and teachers regarding health or behavioral problems; and (6) to coordinate its efforts with those of all community health groups interested in the health of the student.

The purposes of maintaining a healthful school environment are: (1) to promote, maintain, and contribute to the understanding of the health of the student; (2) to provide an environment that is healthful and safe and one that contributes to student learning; and (3) to organize the school day in a healthful manner.

Finally, the objectives of health instruction are (1) to promote, maintain, and contribute to the understanding of the health of the student; (2) to promote the development of sound health knowledge, practices, and attitudes; (3) to provide instruction that is well planned; (4) to provide instruction that meets the growth and development needs and interests of the students.

Responsibility for the School Health Program

Although the major responsibility for the health of children belongs to the family, the prime responsibility for the school health program belongs to the school administrator. Sharing in this responsibility are teacher, nurses, physicians, dentists, counselors and psychologists, social workers, the health coordinator, food-service personnel, custodians, parents, community health agencies, local public health officials, and the student. Collectively this group is often referred to as the school health team.

Some of the responsibilities of the team members are detailed here.

Administrators

The administrator is important to the school health program from several standpoints. First, the administrator is the representative of the school board, and as such, is responsible for distributing the funds allocated by the school board to the various areas of the school in an equitable manner. It is also this person's responsibility to petition the school board for additional funding.

Second, the administrator has the responsibility for ensuring that only qualified, highly trained personnel will be hired. Third, the administrator must see to it that teachers are provided with an atmosphere that is conducive to teaching and that the equipment, materials, and facilities necessary for sound health instruction are available. Fourth, the administrator must work with the school board in providing students with all necessary medical services. Fifth, it is the administrator's responsibility to foster healthy relationships between all team members and the school board. Finally, the administrator is assigned the task of providing the students and school personnel with a healthful and safe school environment.

Teachers

Teachers play a key role in the success or failure of the school health program. The teacher guides the child's learning and is responsible for motivating the student to develop appropriate health habits. Other responsibilities of the teacher include: (1) to understand the growth and development characteristics and needs of the students; (2) to continually observe the students to determine their health status; (3) to serve as a model of good health habits for the students; (4) to develop a meaningful instruction program—one that blends students' needs and interests; (5) to confer with school medical personnel when the status of a child's health is in question; (6) to conduct screening tests for vision, hearing, height, and weight; (7) to practice satisfactory disease-control measures.

Nurses

To be effective, the nurse must establish a working relationship with the rest of the school health team. Basic responsibilities for the school nurse may include:

1. Participating in obtaining a health history.
2. Performing physical appraisals.
3. Evaluating developmental status.
4. Advising and counseling children, parents, and others.
5. Helping in the management of technologic, economic, and social influences affecting child health.

6. Participating in appropriate routine immunization programs.
7. Assessing and managing certain minor illnesses and accidents of children.
8. Planning to meet the health needs of children in cooperation with physicians and other members of the health team. [American Nurses' Association, 1973, pp. 594–597].

Physicians

The relationship of the physician to the school health program and the school health team is one that Rash and Pigg (1979, p. 42) have labeled as cooperative. Generally, the physician serves as a technical consultant to teachers in planning health education curricula. The physician works cooperatively with and as an advisor to the school nurse, administrator, and other team members.

Dentists

Usually, most of the dental care in schools is provided by the dental hygienist. The dentist, on the other hand, functions in much the same capacity in the school as does the physician—an advisory one. Mayshark points out that the dentist in the school health program should have the following responsibilities:

1. Organize and conduct dental examinations of the students.
2. Supervise and conduct preventive and restorative dental work.
3. Supervise or carry out oral prophylaxis.
4. Assist the superintendent, principal, and faculty members responsible for health instruction in the selection and preparation of curriculum material in dental education. [Mayshark, Shaw, and Best, 1977, p. 314].

Counselors, Psychologists, and Social Workers

The primary responsibilities of counselors, psychologists, and social workers are to identify and counsel students who are experiencing mental or emotional problems. They also serve in an advisory capacity to the school staff, particularly with regard to problems that these persons may have with students. Counselors and psychologists have the responsibility of consulting with parents of children who are experiencing problems in school that are directly related to school activities or problems that are symptomatic of difficulties at home. Social workers are primarily responsible for and interested in the relationships that exist between the students, the school, and the community.

Health Coordinator

The health coordinator plays an important part in the school health program. It is his or her primary responsibility to coordinate the efforts of and act as a liaison between the school, the family, and the community with respect to achieving optimal health for the student. The health coordinator is also responsible for arranging in-service instruction for the staff, coordinating health fairs, and planning the health program with the administrator. Additional responsibilities for the health coordinator are included in Table 3.1.

TABLE 3.1

Responsibilities, or Opportunities, of the Coordinator

1. Planning ways to create a closer working relationship between teachers and the health service and custodial personnel.

2. Encouraging all teachers to inform others of their plans for health teaching and to find out what is being taught by other teachers.

3. Participating in and encouraging curriculum planning for health education and helping develop long-range plans for health instruction, a course of study to ensure that important points not be neglected and that there not be needless repetition between related techniques (e.g., biology and health) or from year to year (e.g., repetition in high school of what is taught in the lower grades).

4. Promoting the use of community resources and facilities in the health instruction program and aiding in such use by making appropriate contacts and assisting in scheduling speakers, planning field trips, and keeping teachers informed of developments in the community.

5. Providing essential instructional materials, screening new publications and new materials, and making appropriate ones available to members of the school health team.

6. Fostering interpersonal relationships to promote a closer working relationship of all members of the school health team.

Reprinted by permission from Keogh Rash and Morgan Pigg, *The Health Education Curriculum* (New York: John Wiley & Sons, 1979), p. 44.

Food Service Personnel

The main responsibility of food service personnel is to ensure that the student is getting nutritious meals that contribute to the total nutritional status of the student. These people can also supplement the health instruction program.

Custodians

The custodian is responsible for the physical aspects of the school building. Some specific responsibilities of the custodian include: (1) to maintain an environment that is safe; (2) to maintain an environment that is sanitary; (3) to ensure the safe and efficient operation of the heating, ventilating, and water systems; (4) to provide for the safe storage of all materials used in maintaining the school.

Parents

The parents have the main responsibility for the health of their child. Parents are responsible for the emotional and mental well-being of their child. They are also responsible for reinforcing the health practices taught in the school, as well as for following up on health services recommended for the child. Generally speaking, the parents are responsible for cooperating with all the school health team members in their striving for the provision of a school health program that will promote, protect, and maintain the health of the child.

Organization of School Health Programs

Community Health Agencies

The responsibilities of community health agencies include: (1) to conduct community health needs assessments; (2) to provide services to meet existing, identified needs; (3) to support and conduct research, in conjunction with the school, that is designed to improve the health and safety of the school-age student; (4) to educate; (5) to support and promote public health programs; (6) to promote health legislation.

Public Health Officials

One of the most basic responsibilities of public health officials is to establish local public health policy. It is their responsibility and prerogative to determine the direction a public health program is to take. Another important responsibility of these persons is the direct safeguarding of the health of the community.

Students

Students share in the responsibility for their health. In many ways, through their actions, they contribute to the maintenance of a school environment that is:

1. Conducive to proper growth and development.
2. Healthful.
3. Emotionally and intellectually stimulating.
4. Safe.

Legal Aspects

Teachers and schools have a moral and sometimes legal responsibility for the safety and well-being of their students. ''The legal responsibility that teachers and schools have for their students is called *tort liability*. In this form of liability, the teacher or the school is legally accountable for any wrongful acts (torts) that result in injuries to students, their property, or their reputations'' (Mroz, 1978, p. 175).

Torts include acts of (1) malfeasance—performing an illegal act, (2) misfeasance—performing the correct act incorrectly, and (3) nonfeasance—not performing a legal responsibility. Teachers who are remiss in their duty of supervising their students are placing themselves in a position from which they can be charged with nonfeasance. For example, if an aquatics instructor leaves students unsupervised in the swimming pool and one of the students is injured, the instructor can be charged with nonfeasance.

Before someone can win a judgment against either a teacher or a school for a school-related injury, that person must demonstrate that the teacher or the school failed to act in a reasonably prudent manner. Failure to act in such a manner is called *negligence*.

The first step the court takes in deciding whether the teacher or school was negligent is to establish exactly what ''acting in a reasonably prudent manner'' means. Once it has done so, it then seeks to determine whether or not the individual or school could have foreseen the consequences of the acts. If so, guilt is determined.

The liability laws regarding the relationship between the student and the teacher or school vary from state to state.

Needs and Interests

It has been said countless times that health instruction, in order to be effective, should be relevant to students' lives. One way to ensure relevancy is to assess the needs and interests of the students, as expressed by the students, prior to curriculum development. It is generally held to be true by many health professionals that the health needs and the health interests of students are interdependent. These professionals also note that there are, however, important differences between needs and interests that should be considered when deciding what to teach about health.

Needs are inherent, whereas interests are the by-products of learning. This distinction is an important one to note when deciding what to teach the students regarding their health. For example, according to Humphrey et al. (1975, p. 55) it is possible that ''a student might express interest in a certain practice that is not compatible with his or her needs at a certain age level.'' The nine-year-old may be interested in driving an automobile, but this practice might result in injury (Humphrey et al., 1975, p. 55). The successful health teacher is one who is able to determine what health topics the students are interested in learning about, as well as what they need to know about their health. The teacher then strives to establish a balance between these two. The prudent health teacher also realizes that if the students do not express an interest in a topic, it does not mean that the topic should be avoided. It should be noted that there is a relationship between having been exposed to a topic area and expressing an interest in that area. Gaines reports that when students are lacking in knowledge about a subject, they also tend to indicate a lack of interest about the subject (Gaines, 1983, p. 12).

A good guide to use in determining the balance of needs and interests is the age level of the students. At the elementary school level, interests should play a lesser role than needs. As the students grow older, interests become a more substantial part of the curriculum. By at least senior high school, and very definitely at the college level, interests should be the basis for much of what is being taught in the health curriculum. However, student needs cannot be totally discounted. At this level, it will often be found that the students' health needs and health interests coincide.

There are several ways in which the health needs and the health interests of students have been assessed in the past. Needs have been determined through teacher observation of student behavior, through teacher-student interviews and discussions, and through understanding and analysis of growth and development characteristics of students. Also, a careful study of school

Organization of School Health Programs

records will give observant health teachers a good sense for the health needs of their students. Tests designed to measure subject knowledge might also be useful tools for teachers in their attempt to determine the health needs of their students.

Interests often will serve as a motivational springboard for student learning. Student interest in a topic very often contributes to the student's enjoyment of the topic, as well as development of a sense of the meaningfulness of what he or she is doing. Interests might be assessed as follows:

1. Observation. An observant teacher will pick up on things that are of interest to his students by being alert to their behaviors and listening to what they have to say. Further, the questions students ask will often give the same insight (Humphrey et al., 1975, p. 71).

2. Questionnaires and checklists. This method of information gathering has been used since the early part of this century. Its results have varied (Humphrey et al., 1975, p. 72).

3. Expository writing. Allowing students to write about areas of health that they would find interesting to pursue further can be a valuable method (Humphrey et al., 1975, p. 72).

SUMMARY

Although the health of the student is the responsibility of the family, responsibility for the school health program is jointly shared by the school and community alike. Community participation in the school health program comes mainly via the school health team. The ideal health program is an integrated school–community program in which each supports and reinforces the activities of the other, in an attempt to attain the desired goal of promoting, maintaining, and contributing to the understanding of the health of the student. This goal is achieved by school and community support for the three areas of the school health program—services, instruction, and environment.

REVIEW QUESTIONS

1. What is the relationship between the school health program and the larger total community health program?
2. How important to the successful achievement of the goals and objectives of the school health program is its philosophical base?
3. What is the purpose of the school health program and how does the organization of the school health program enhance or inhibit its meeting its purpose?
4. Compare the various responsibilities of the school health team members for the school health program.
5. Why are the needs and interests of the students important to the success of health instruction?

REFERENCES

American Nurses' Association and the American School Health Association. "Recommendations on Educational Preparation and Definition of the Expanded Role and Functions of the School Nurse Practitioner." *Journal of School Health* 43 (November 1973), 594–597.

Anspaugh, D. J., and G. O. Ezell. *Teaching Today's Health,* 3d ed., NY: Merrill Pub. Co., 1990.

Creswell, W., and I. Newman. *School Health Practice.* St. Louis, Mo.: C. V. Mosby Co., 1989.

Gaines, J. M. "On the Health Interests of College Students." In Hudson, E., *Assessing the Health Interests of College Students.* Unpublished masters project, Virginia Polytechnic Institute and State University, 1983.

Green, L. W. "New Definitions: Report of the 1972–73 Joint Committee on Health Organizations," *Health Education Monographs,* no. 33, 1973, pp. 33–37.

Hanlon, J. J. *Principles of Public Health Administration,* 8th ed. St. Louis: C. V. Mosby Co., 1984.

Humphrey, J. H., W. R. Johnson, and D. R. Nowarch. *Health Teaching in Elementary Schools.* Springfield, Ill.: Charles C Thomas, 1975.

Johns, E. B., ed. *The School Health Education Evaluative Study.* Los Angeles: Los Angeles County Tuberculosis and Health Association, 1959.

Mayshark, C., D. D. Shaw, and W. B. Best. *Administration of School Health Programs.* St. Louis: C. V. Mosby, 1977.

Mroz, J. H. *Safety in Everyday Living.* Dubuque, Iowa: Wm. C. Brown Publishers, 1978.

Rash, K., and M. Pigg. *The Health Education Curriculum.* New York: John Wiley & Sons, 1979.

Smolensky, J., and L. R. Bonvechio. *Principles of School Health.* Boston: D. C. Heath and Company, 1966.

Washington State Medical Association. *School Health Policy,* Olympia, Washington, 1965.

School and Community Health Councils

4

Promoting the health of the school-age child is no easy task. It cannot effectively be accomplished through the singular efforts of an individual, a school, or an agency. Often these groups find themselves duplicating services and competing with each other while working toward a similar goal. What is needed to serve the public health effectively is sympathetic cooperation between the many individuals, schools, agencies, and organizations in the community. One way to direct the efforts of these groups and to effect a cooperative relationship between them is by establishing school and community health councils.

The purpose of this chapter is to introduce the reader to the notion of health councils and to answer the following questions: What are their purposes? What are their responsibilities? Who makes up these councils? In what activities are they involved? What effects do these councils have on school–community relationships?

PURPOSE OF THE SCHOOL HEALTH COUNCIL (SHC)

There are many community agencies and school personnel interested in the health and well-being of students. Often these groups will be found working independently rather than together. A bonding agent is needed to bring them together so that their efforts are coordinated. One such agent is the school health council. Kilander writes that the primary purpose and goal of the school health council "is simply to mobilize all the health resources of the school and the community to meet the health needs" (Kilander, 1962, p. 401).

The utility of these councils has been identified by a number of community and school groups and, with the urging of PTAs, state Departments of Health and Education, official and voluntary health agencies, school health coordinators, teachers, school administrators, nurses, and custodians, many school districts have organized school health councils.

The school health council may also have a representative elected to the community health council and thus will serve in a linking capacity between the school and community health programs.

It is important to realize that this council functions only in an advisory capacity. It does not have official sanction within the school system and is not designed to supplant the specific duties of the school administration in the health program. Further, whether or not each school in a particular school district has a council depends on the size of the district.

RESPONSIBILITIES OF THE SCHOOL HEALTH COUNCIL

Essentially, the school health council advises the district or the school about the school health program. More specifically, it:

1. Identifies the health needs of students.
2. Makes recommendations regarding school health policies and the school health program.
3. Evaluates the school health program.
4. Makes recommendations for and aids in the implementation of school health policies.
5. Coordinates the efforts of community members interested in the health and well-being of students with those of the school's staff.
6. Seeks parental support and participation in school health activities.
7. Stresses the primacy of family responsibility for the health of the students.
8. Supports existing school health programs and the development of health programs when none exist.
9. Helps school personnel in working out solutions to existing health problems.
10. Keeps the community informed with regard to school health programs.

MEMBERSHIP OF THE SCHOOL HEALTH COUNCIL

The school health council will vary in size and complexity, depending upon the size of the school and its needs. It is good practice, however, to make sure that the council is thoroughly representative of the school staff. Following is a list of suggested members:

- School principal.
- Health teacher (or coordinator).
- Physical education teacher.
- Guidance counselor.
- Food service personnel—dietician.
- Chief custodian.
- Teachers.
- Nurse (school physicians or dentists, when available, should be on the council).
- Parents.
- Students (high school).

Council meetings should be held once each month during the academic year. If necessary, emergency meetings should be called. Some of the afore-mentioned council members might not be able to attend regularly scheduled meetings; in such cases, those persons should serve the council as consultants, and replacements should be sought. Ideally, the council should be chaired by the health teacher or coordinator.

ACTIVITIES OF THE SCHOOL HEALTH COUNCIL

In general, the activities of the school health council pertain to at least one of the following areas: (1) healthful school environment, (2) health services, (3) health instruction, and (4) general activities.

1. Healthful School Environment
   a. "Conduct a survey of the school's physical environment (i.e., lighting, ventilation, maintenance of the plant, adequacy of the school's water supply, and so on)."
   b. "Conduct a survey of the school's emotional climate."
   c. "Develop communicable disease policies."
   d. "Conduct an examination of the safeness of the school."
   e. "Examine playground and gymnasium safety policies."
   f. "Examine the adequacy and safeness of all playground, gym-nasium, and athletic apparatus."
2. Health Services
   a. "Improvement of classroom screening activities."
   b. "Improvement of physical examinations for students."
   c. "Improvement of preschool screening and examination activities."
   d. "Improvement of the dental health program."
   e. "Improvement of the ways in which emergency injuries or ill-nesses are handled."
   f. "Improvement of the school's nutritional program."
   g. "Improvement of the nurses' health room facilities."
   h. "Improvement of health examination follow-up procedures."
   i. "Improvement of health recordkeeping."
   j. "Improvement of counseling facilities and procedures."
   k. "Improvement of referral policy."
   l. "Expansion of services offered to students with special problems."
   m. "Evaluation of the school's communicable disease prevention and control practices."
   n. "Establishment of teacher–parent–nurse conferences regarding the health care of the student."

An activity of the school health council is the examination of playground safety policies.

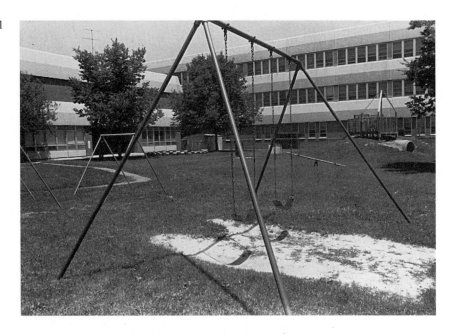

3. Health Instruction
   a. "Improve the coordination of all health education activities."
   b. "Develop a comprehensive health education curriculum for grades K–12."
   c. "Improve health instruction."
   d. "Support teacher in-service training."
   e. "Develop a library for health instructional materials and arrange for adult health education classes."
   f. "Evaluate health education texts, pamphlets, and instructional audiovisual material."
4. General Activities
   a. "Improve coordination of the school health program."
   b. "Improve coordination of the activities of the school and various community agencies."
   c. "Improve parent participation in and cooperation with the activities of the school health program" (Kilander, 1962, pp. 405–407).

In the same manner that the community health council becomes the health voice of the community in health matters, the school health council becomes the health voice of the school. It can become an excellent forum for receiving input from parents, interested groups, and other citizens on matters affecting the health of the school-age individual or the school staff.

Often the school health council becomes a means for conducting some phases of the community health program. Those activities that have a direct bearing on the health of the school-age child, such as sickle cell screening, lead screening, immunization programs, and many others, could be coordinated by the school and community health councils.

PURPOSE OF THE COMMUNITY HEALTH COUNCIL (CHC)

If the school health program is to attain optimal success, cooperative planning between the school and community is necessary. It should be obvious that as the school and community health programs work more closely together, benefit will accrue to each in a greater fashion than if each worked in isolation.

It is only logical to assume that the purpose of the community health council is to coordinate the various health-related activities of community agencies. In like manner, it provides a viable link between the school health program and community health program. This linkage helps assure that the school health program will be responsive to community health needs.

In addition to this general purpose, the CHC has the following purposes:

1. To provide indirect services to the community.
2. To coordinate the efforts of member agencies.
3. To organize various agencies into a cohesive action-taking force.
4. To promote, protect and maintain the public health.
5. To eliminate needless duplication of services.
6. To aid in formulating public opinion regarding public health needs, programs and legislation.
7. To serve as a sounding board for community health complaints [National Committee of Health Council Executives, p. 1].

Some of the services that the council provides are:

1. Helps in the control of communicable diseases.
2. Lobbies locally for the provision of medical, dental, mental health, and family planning clinics.
3. Coordinates the efforts of individuals and groups interested in the health of students.

MEMBERSHIP OF THE COMMUNITY HEALTH COUNCIL

The community health council should be composed of a representative sample of the various groups existing in and working for the health of the community. Although it is likely that the exact composition will vary between communities, its members might include representatives from:

- Voluntary health agencies.
- Occupational and industrial health groups.
- Local health departments.
- State extension services.

- Agricultural groups.
- Social welfare department.
- Local medical and allied health personnel and societies.
- Church and youth groups.
- Parents.
- Service clubs and other civic-minded organizations.
- School administrators.
- Members of the school's health council.
- District-wide school health personnel.
- Teachers.
- Police and fire departments.
- School health council representatives.
- Business and industry representatives.
- General citizenry.

The community health council should be as representative of the community as possible, and it should be organized as simply as possible. An effective way to organize the council is to have one head group coordinating the activities of many subgroups operating at the neighborhood level.

OBJECTIVES OF THE COMMUNITY HEALTH COUNCIL

Smolensky suggests that the community health council has the following objectives:

1. Bringing together medical, allied professional, and other interested groups for discussion and interchange of opinions.
2. Serving as a clearing house for health and medical care problems and programs, facilitating joint planning where it is needed to speed up approved projects and to reduce duplication of efforts.
3. Encouraging, stimulating, fostering, and actively supporting the establishment of health and medical care programs designed to improve the health of the people in the community.
4. Gathering and analyzing information on medical care and health needs already obtained from surveys and initiating additional studies or surveys.
5. Devising means for reaching all the people, with particular attention to the extension of projects into rural areas and people living outside of cities and towns. [Smolensky, 1977, pp. 67–68]

Some other objectives are:

6. To encourage lay participation.
7. To find solutions to common problems through citizen study, planning, and action.
8. To promote an efficient and economical way of spending health and welfare dollars.

9. To help agencies coordinate their services to fill gaps and prevent duplication.
10. To stimulate public understanding and support in meeting community needs.

HEALTH ANALYSIS

Before the community health council can responsibly take action, it must have some understanding of the community's health needs and the resources it has at its disposal to meet these needs. This analysis can be done by:

1. Observation.
2. Studying the vital and communicable disease statistics of the community.
3. Examining the health budget.
4. Comparing the existing health program with those in other communities.
5. Comparing health services, activities, and facilities of the community with those of similar communities. [Smolensky, 1977, p. 67]

IMPROVEMENT OF SCHOOL–COMMUNITY RELATIONSHIPS

When people and groups are united in their efforts to reach a common goal, often the following are likely to result:

1. An elimination of needless duplication of services.
2. An increase in the sensitivity that each group and individual has regarding the needs of the other.
3. A sense of communality.
4. A feeling of cohesiveness.
5. An economy of effort, resulting in an increased likelihood of success.
6. More effective services.
7. An improved emotional climate for both the school and the community.
8. Greater support for the school by the community and vice versa.

SUMMARY

The promotion, protection, and maintenance of the health and well-being of the student require the orchestrated efforts of many school and community individuals and groups. To ensure that the efforts of these individuals and groups enhance the quality and effectiveness of the health services provided to both the student and the community at large, health councils are developed. These councils have the specific purposes of:

1. Coordinating the efforts of the school and the community to effectively serve the public.
2. Eliminating unnecessary duplication of services.

3. Ensuring a more efficient and effective manner of spending health and welfare funds.
4. Promoting citizen support for and participation in health programs.
5. Advising the school and the community with regard to their health activities.

REVIEW QUESTIONS

1. Differentiate between the purposes of the school and community health councils.
2. Who makes up the membership of the school and community health councils?
3. In what activities are the school and community health councils involved?

REFERENCES

Cox, F. M., J. L. Erlich, J. Rothman, and J. E. Tropman. *Strategies of Community Organization: A Book of Readings,* 3d ed. Itasca, Ill.: F. E. Peacock, 1979.

Green, L., and Anderson, C. L. *Community Health,* 5th ed. St. Louis: Mosby, 1986.

Greene, W. H., and B. G. Simons-Morton. *Introduction to Health Education.* New York: Macmillan, 1984.

Hiscock, I. V. *Community Health Organization,* 4th ed. New York: Commonwealth Fund, 1950.

Kilander, H. F. *School Health Education: A Study of Content, Methods and Materials.* New York: Macmillan, 1962.

Milio, N. *The Care of Health in Communities.* New York: Macmillan, 1975.

Murrell, S. A. *Community Psychology and Social Systems: A Conceptual Framework and Intervention Guide.* New York: Behavioral Publications, 1973.

National Commission on Community Health Services. *Health Is a Community Affair.* Cambridge, Mass.: Harvard Univ. Press, 1966.

National Committee of Health Council Executives. ''Principles Essential for Effective Organization and Functioning of a CHC.'' Chicago: Association of Health Council Executives, 1978.

Smolensky, J. *Principles of Community Health,* 4th ed. Philadelphia: W. B. Saunders, 1977.

PART II

Environment

Planning of the Physical Plant

5

T he planning of a school's physical plant is a complex process that requires the efforts of many people. The physical plant should be designed so that it enhances the student's quality of life. The responsibility for providing such an atmosphere is shared by all community and school members. Failure to provide such an environment results in less than optimal growth and development for the student.

PLANNING FOR A HEALTHFUL SCHOOL ENVIRONMENT

A school that is well planned and well maintained fosters an environment that enables teaching and learning to be enjoyable and nonstressful experiences. Such an environment is supportive of the students' health and their quality of life. It also promotes safety and reduces the likelihood of accidental injury.

A healthful environment is one that supports the holistic nature of students by providing them with health services, food services, gymnasiums and play areas for physical activity, and satisfactory classroom instruction. This environment sets the stage for health education and the development of sound health habits.

The planning of a healthful environment requires a great deal of premeditation on the part of the school planners. It is a well-organized, deliberate effort of a committee of individuals representing the school, the community, state and local governments, the board of education, medical and business persons, religious leaders, politicians, teachers, parents, and anyone else who has an interest in the school. In other words, the planning for a healthful school environment is a well-orchestrated community effort. Having all segments of the community involved in this process provides the school with a broad base of support that is likely to be useful in future planning efforts.

A formal committee, representative of most community and school groups, should be formed. This committee's responsibilities might be: (1) to assist in the selection of the architect who will design the school; (2) to review budgetary items, particularly cost-cutting proposals (Jenne and Greene, 1976, p. 187); (3) to serve in an advisory capacity to the architect, builder, and local board of education; (4) to inspect the building during and after construction, keeping on the alert for obvious safety violations and structural defects (Jenne and Greene, 1976, p. 188).

Although it is today's children who are using the school, the planning of a healthful school environment should keep in mind tomorrow's children as well.

A school site should be large enough to accommodate present and projected student population adequately.

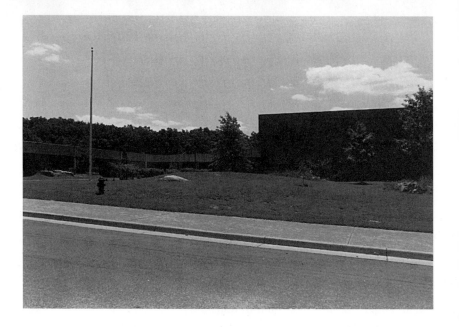

LOCATION

The location of a school directly affects the safety, well-being, and educational experience of the student. If a school site is selected in a haphazard manner, the educational experience for both the teacher and the student is likely to be less than optimal. Those involved in the selection process should think carefully about the following:

1. What are the present and projected student populations?
2. Is the site accessible by public transportation?
3. Are an acceptable water supply and sewage system available locally? If not, can the area support a deep well and a septic tank?
4. Is the site located near a major thoroughfare, railroad, or airport?
5. Was the site ever a landfill?
6. Will air pollution be a problem?
7. How much of the natural ground cover, such as trees and shrubs, can be preserved?
8. Will the school be near landfills, a dump, refineries, industrial or manufacturing plants? Locating a school near structures such as these will affect the safety and well-being of the students.
9. Is the site quiet? Does the noise level exceed 70 decibels? (NEA, 1966, p. 148; HEW, 1961, pp. 1–2; Jenne and Greene, 1976, pp. 189–90).

Organization of School Health Programs

SIZE OF SITE AND GROUNDS

A school site should be large enough to accommodate the present and projected student populations comfortably. Students tend to consider schools that are spacious, or that give the appearance of being so, to be pleasant. The site should not make them feel crowded or cramped. There is no one nationally accepted school site size, but generally, the size of the site and ground depends on whether the school is located in a large city, a suburban area, or a rural area. The specific site size is usually determined jointly by the local board of education and the state departments of education and health.

It is usually easier to obtain a spacious site in a rural or suburban area than it is to obtain one in a large city. This, however, will vary among cities and states. For elementary schools, it is recommended that there be a minimum of 10 acres, 20 acres for a junior high school, and 30 acres for a senior high school. Furthermore, one acre should be added for every additional 100 students (Jenne and Greene, 1976, p. 190). Thus, for a high school comprised of 500 students, there should be at least 35 acres.

SAFETY CONSIDERATIONS

In the United States, accidents are the fourth leading cause of death for persons of all ages, killing over 100,000 people a year and resulting in more than 10 million disabling injuries. In addition, when insurance costs, medical and hospital costs, lost days at work, lost wages, and property damage are considered, the bill amounts to over $40 billion annually. "For people between the ages of 15 and 24, accidents account for more deaths than all other causes combined" (Olsen (ed.), 1983, p. 544). Thus, the responsibility for providing students with a maximally safe site is an important one.

Although maintaining the safety of a school is usually not the responsibility of one person, it is advisable to have one person in the school to whom all hazards and accidents must be reported. It is also recommended that, in junior and senior high, the school administrator establish a student safety committee. The responsibility of this committee is to keep on the alert for hazards and safety violations, as well as for situations that have the potential of becoming dangerous to the well-being of the students. These hazards should be reported to the school safety officer.

Safety considerations can be divided into two general sections: the internal environment and the external environment. Internally, all stairways, corridors, lavatories, classrooms, gymnasiums, shower rooms, pools, cafeterias, auditoriums, and shops are potential hazards to the student. Each of these areas, as well as the remainder of the building, should be constructed in compliance with the fire safety code as established by the office of the state fire marshal. These areas should also be free of obstruction, should be well

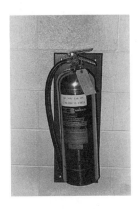

The location of fire extinguishers throughout the school is an important safety consideration.

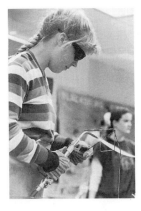

Shop teachers should establish procedures designed to prevent accidents.

lighted and ventilated, and should have clearly marked entrances and exits. The exit doors should all open outward and be equipped with a cross-bar release. Shop teachers, physical education teachers, and athletic coaches should inspect their facilities to eliminate hazards and establish procedures designed to prevent accidents.

Externally, the amount of traffic is an important consideration. The site should be away from railroads, airports, water hazards (such as washes and drainage and irrigation ditches), and heavily traveled roads. Students should not have to cross major thoroughfares to get to the school. If the traffic adjacent to a school is hectic, adult traffic directors should either be provided to the school by the local police department, or teachers should be assigned traffic-directing tasks on a rotating basis. The responsibility of these traffic directors is to ensure the safety of the student, to direct traffic, and to report traffic violations to the police department. Traffic lights might also be made available.

For those children who walk or ride bicycles to school, the distances should not be such that their lives and well-being are endangered. It is recommended that elementary school children not be expected to walk more than half a mile from home to school; beyond this distance, it has been found that traffic accidents increase. Although children of this age group are usually physically able to walk this distance and farther, they do tend to lose concentration and pay less attention to bypassing traffic than they should. The walking distance for junior high students should not exceed one mile, and the walking distance for senior high students should not exceed two miles. At distances greater than these, junior and senior high students spend too much of their time traveling to and from school.

Special consideration should also be given to the safe construction of playgrounds and athletic fields.

BUILDING

With regard to school buildings, the National Committee on School Health Policies of the National Education Association and the American Medical Association suggests that the building "should provide an environment that encourages good teaching, permits healthful practices, and protects health." It further suggests that the "facilities should be adapted to the ages of the children and the program of instruction" (National Committee on School Health Policies, 1966, p. 23).

New buildings should be designed by, and the remodeling of older buildings should be supervised by, an architect who specializes in or who has experience in the design and remodeling of school buildings. As mentioned in the introduction to this chapter, the architect should be assisted by a school building planning committee in designing a useful, safe, and aesthetically pleasing building. This committee serves in an advisory capacity and is comprised of representatives of the school and the community. Members might

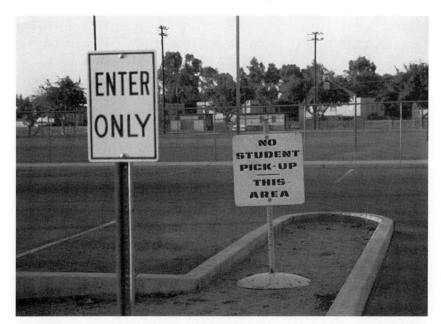

There should be specially designated areas for picking up and dropping off students.

include school board members; the superintendent of schools or a representative; school staff members; community leaders; medical personnel; members of industry and business; state and local construction officials; safety, sanitation, lighting, heating, and ventilation experts. The committee, in addition to its advisory function, should oversee the construction of the building, making sure that it complies with state and local requirements and fire safety codes.

The building should be constructed and decorated such that its classrooms, offices, and other areas are of different sizes, shapes, and colors, as this tends to reduce the occupants' feelings of monotony.

The building should be designed and built so that much of the natural beauty and landscape of the terrain is preserved. If needed, landscaping should be handled by professional landscapers to make the site aesthetically pleasing to the students and to protect the students and the building from flying debris, dust, pollution, and winds. Also, the building should be placed on the site in such a way as to take advantage of natural light and ventilation.

The school should be constructed with the future in mind. Projected student populations should be taken into consideration when planning the school. There should be adequate room for expansion. Other considerations of the planning committee during the development stage are water supply, sewage disposal; solid waste disposal and the plumbing system; food service facilities, lighting, heating and ventilation, acoustics, and other safety factors (U.S. Department of HEW, 1961, p. 2).

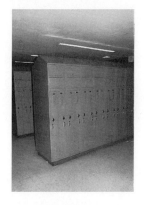

Students lockers should be plentiful.

Landscaping should
receive special
consideration.

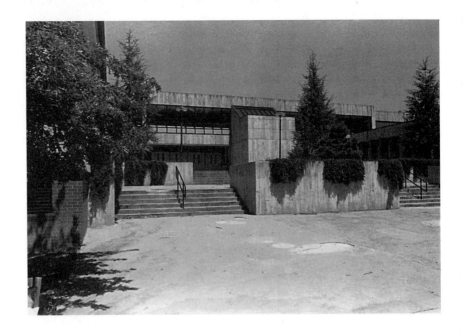

SIDEWALKS AND DRIVES

Sidewalks should be wide enough to accommodate several passersby at any given moment. These sidewalks should not only lead up to the front entrance of the school but should provide access to the school on the least traveled side, that is, the side away from the main street.

"Walks should be a safe distance from the wall of the building in areas where there is danger of heavy snow slides" or where there is water runoff from the roof. "Walks leading from outside doorways should be nearly as level with the floor within the doorway as possible" (U.S. Department of HEW, 1961, p. 63).

"Driveways should be planned so that trucks and other vehicles will not cross the play areas or in other ways create a safety hazard to the students. Driveways should not cut across the school grounds leading from one street to another." The driveway should lead to delivery areas only (Shapiro, 1965, pp. 46–47).

SPECIAL GROUP REQUIREMENTS

The physical plant must be designed to meet the needs of handicapped students. Any structural barriers to their effective participation in school should be eliminated. Ramps should lead up to the entrances, the doors of which should be wide enough to accommodate a wheelchair. These doors should be electronically controlled by the individual. Bathrooms should be accessible to these persons, and toilet compartments should have handrails.

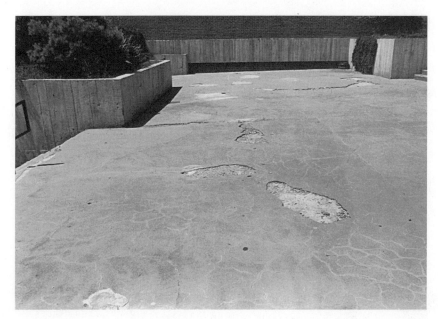

Sidewalks should be maintained so as to ensure the safety of passersby.

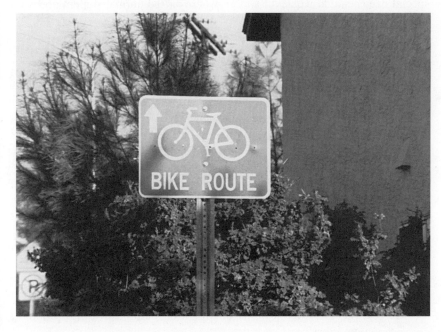

Bicycle routes should be clearly marked.

Wheelchair lifts are a special group consideration.

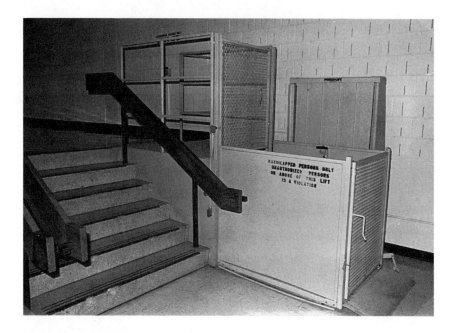

Outside the building, it is recommended that there be "loading platforms with readily accessible driveways . . . so that school buses, [vans,] private cars, and taxicabs can load and unload students in or with their wheelchairs" (Clark, 1975, pp. 143–144).

Basically, the school plant should be designed so that the student with special needs can do whatever and go wherever the normal student does and goes.

SUMMARY

The concern for and awareness of the relationship among a healthful school environment, learning, and student well-being are not new. The planning for a school plant such that it provides students with an environment that supports their mental, physical, and emotional needs requires much forethought by the architect and planning committee. They should give some thought to the following: Where will the school be located? How large is the school site? How much of the natural beauty on the site can be preserved? Are the grounds and physical plant safe? Is the building supportive of intellectual and physical growth and development? Will the building be large enough to accommodate future projected student populations? Will the building and its grounds meet the needs of special students?

REVIEW QUESTIONS

1. What is meant by the statement, "A healthful environment is one that supports the holistic nature of the student"?
2. What are the responsibilities of school building planning committees?

3. How does the physical location of a school affect the safety, well-being, and educational experience of students?
4. What is the recommended acreage for an elementary, junior high, and senior high school, each of which has 750 students?
5. How do the internal and external school environments affect the health, safety, and well-being of students?

REFERENCES

American Association for Health, Physical Education and Recreation. *School Safety Policies with Emphasis on Physical Education, Athletics and Recreation.* Washington, D.C.: National Educational Association, 1968.

American Automobile Association. *Teacher's Guide for the Safest Route to School Project.* Falls Church, Va.: AAA, 1979.

American Medical Association. *Healthy Youth 2000.* Chicago, Ill.: AMA, Dept. of Adolescent Health, 1990.

Clark, N. C. "Safety Education as Preventive Medicine." *The Journal of the Arkansas Medical Society* (August 1975), 143–144.

Florio, A. E., W. F. Alles, and G. T. Stafford. *Safety Education,* 4th ed. New York: McGraw-Hill, 1979.

Institute for Traffic Engineers. *A Program for School Crossing Protection.* Washington, D.C.: Institute for Traffic Engineers, 1971.

Jenne, F. H., and W. H. Greene. *Turner's School Health and Health Education.* St. Louis: C. V. Mosby, 1976.

Kigin, D. J. *Teacher Liability in School-Shop Accidents.* Ann Arbor, Mich.: Prakken Publications, 1973.

Los Angeles City School Districts. *Handbook of Safety Rules and Regulations from the Administrative Guide.* Los Angeles: L.A. City Board of Education, 1959.

Mroz, J. H. *Safety in Everyday Living.* Dubuque, Iowa: Wm. C. Brown Publishers, 1978.

National Committee on School Health Policies of the NEA and the AMA. *Suggested School Health Policies.* Chicago: Joint Committee on Health Problems in Education of the NEA and the AMA, 1966.

National Education Association. *Who Is Liable for Pupil Injuries?* Washington, D.C.: NEA, 1963.

Olsen, L. K. (ed.). *Health Today.* New York: Macmillan, 1983.

Punke, H. A. "Safety and Early Childhood Education." *Journal of School Health* (March 1971): 146–153.

Shapiro, F. S. "Your Liability for Student Accidents." *NEA Journal* (March 1965): 46–47.

U.S. Department of HEW. *Environmental Engineering for the School: A Manual of Recommended Practice.* Washington, D.C.: U.S. Dept. of HEW, 1961.

Willgoose, C. *Health Education in the Elementary School.* Philadelphia: W. B. Saunders, 1974.

Maintenance

6

School plant maintenance focuses primarily upon (1) providing the student with a healthful school environment and (2) supporting an optimum health status. Plant maintenance is the specific charge of the custodial staff. Additionally, the teachers, the school nurse, and the administrator have a responsibility to see to it that these goals are achieved. The result of the joint efforts of these individuals should be a school plant that is well maintained and that is conducive to the growth and development of the student.

ILLUMINATION

The productive conduct of the daily activities of a school is largely dependent upon a properly lighted school plant. A school plant that is properly lighted makes valuable contributions to student health, well-being, learning, and the successful performance of any visual tasks. It also greatly aids in the conservation of the eyesight of all its users; and it plays a significant part in the development, maintenance, and improvement of both worker and student esprit, satisfaction, and cooperation.

Illumination is a highly technical matter; thus, it is always advisable to consult either an experienced illumination engineer or an architect when trying to determine whether a school plant has sufficient lighting. There are, however, certain general features regarding illumination with which school administrators, teachers, planners, and maintenance personnel should be familiar. Conceptually, these features are related to the reflectance, the quantity, and the quality or brightness of light. Each of these lighting features has some direct influence on the performance of visual tasks, as well as contributing to the development of feelings of enjoyment, warmth, and comfort in the school environment.

The reflect factor is the amount of light that deflects from a surface. This factor can be determined by dividing the quantity of light by its brightness. Light quantity and brightness are expressed in specific units of measurement called footcandles and foot-lamberts, respectively. A footcandle is a unit of illuminance and is an expression of the amount of light on one square foot of surface, all parts of which are exactly one foot away from a standard candle (Joint Committee on Health Problems in Education, 1969, p. 164). Some of this light will be absorbed by the surface; the rest will be reflected. The amount of light that is reflected from this one-square-foot surface area is expressed in foot-lamberts.

Generally speaking, the source of light in schools is natural, artificial, or both. The sun, or the reflection of its rays from surfaces external to the classroom, such as automobiles, glass, and pavement, serves as the main source of

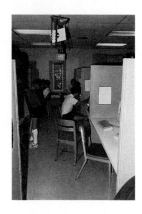

Lighting should be sufficient to allow adequate task performance.

natural light. Buildings should be designed in such a way to best utilize this inexpensive, efficient light source. However, if natural light is used, care must be taken to control glare. Proper placement of student desks and the use of window shades will aid greatly.

Another type of light source is artificial. Rooms that are intended to be used solely during daylight hours might require some minimal amount of artificial light. Rooms that are intended to be used both day and evening, or during the evening alone, will require much more artificial illumination. The most common source of artificial light in U.S. schools is fluorescent. Although the initial cost of installing fluorescent fixtures is high, over time these fixtures repay the high initial expenditure. Fluorescent fixtures should prove to be a very controllable, efficient, inexpensive, and desirable form of artificial lighting. The lights should not be directly visible; rather, they should be covered. Care must be taken so that glare from artificial light is avoided.

It should be remembered that the primary criterion to be used in judging the adequacy of a lighting source, regardless of whether it is natural or artificial, is whether or not it provides sufficient illumination for the performance of the task at hand. The effectiveness of any lighting system can be reduced by the amount of glare in the room. *Webster's New Collegiate Dictionary,* 7th edition, defines *glare* as a ''harsh uncomfortably bright light'' that results not only in some discomfort for the room's occupants but also in some difficulty in their seeing well. Glare in a classroom occurs very commonly when light from a bright source, such as the sun or a lighting fixture, reflects off a shiny surface, such as desk tops, glossy paper, chalkboard, windows, walls, highly waxed and polished floors, and so on.

One way to cut down on the amount of glare in a classroom is by the use of light colors on walls, ceilings, and window casings. Surfaces painted with dark colors tend to absorb more light than do surfaces painted with light colors. Light-colored surfaces not only reflect most of the light falling upon them, but they also contribute a pleasant feeling to a classroom. Paint manufacturers are generally willing to supply information regarding the glare-reduction and reflectance qualities of their paints.

The question then becomes, ''What can a teacher do?'' The National Education Association and the American Medical Association, in their joint publication *Healthful School Environment,* suggest the following:

Regarding pupils, the teacher can

1. Permit pupils to arrange or change seats whenever this will provide better conditions for seeing.
2. Arrange for pupils with eye difficulties to sit in places considered best from the standpoint of their specific defects.
3. Arrange seats and desks so that no pupil will face a window or work in his or her own shadow.
4. Try to alternate periods of close eye work with activities that are visually less demanding. [Joint Committee on Health Problems in Education, 1969, p. 170]

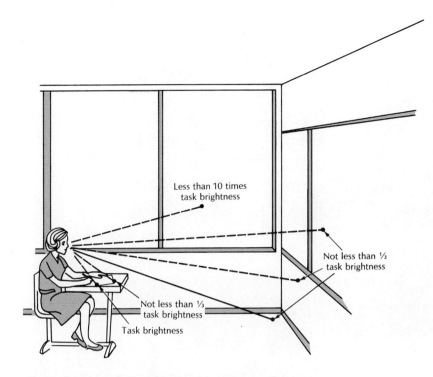

FIGURE 6.1
Surface brightness.
Source: American Institute of Architects, Illuminating Engineering Society, National Council on Schoolhouse Construction. American Standard Guide for School Lighting. *New York: Illuminating Engineering Society, 1962, p. 11.*

Less than 10 times task brightness

Not less than ⅓ task brightness

Not less than ⅓ task brightness

Task brightness

Regarding materials and equipment, the teacher can

1. Insist that the minimum type-size of textbooks be 10-point type. Young children should have books with larger type.
2. Make sure that all duplicated materials are of good quality.
3. Eliminate books, charts, and maps that have become so soiled that the contrast between print and paper is poor.
4. Use only matte-finished papers of high reflectance and a good degree of opacity for both workpaper and printed material.
5. Encourage the use of nonglossy inks.
6. Write on chalkboard in large clear letters, in the line of pupils' vision.
7. Keep chalkboard clean; white chalk of good quality is preferable.
8. Stand or sit in positions with direct pupils' view away from windows.
9. Avoid hanging posters and charts between windows.
10. Make sure that electric lights are turned on whenever the illumination falls below standard in any part of the room. (Some schools are equipped with photoelectric cells that do this automatically.)
11. Report failed lamps and see that they are replaced immediately. See that lighting equipment is cleaned periodically and thoroughly. [Joint Committee on Health Problems in Education, 1969, p. 171]

If these suggested procedures are followed, a pleasant, comfortable, supportive environment very likely will result.

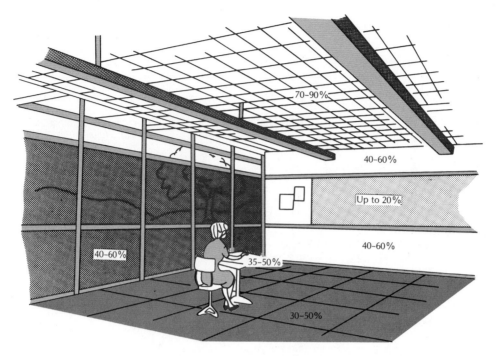

70-90%

40-60%

Up to 20%

40-60%

40-60%

35-50%

30-50%

FIGURE 6.2

Recommended reflectances for surfaces and furnishings in the classroom.

Source: American Institute of Architects, Illuminating Engineering Society, National Council on Schoolhouse Construction. American Standard Guide for School Lighting. *New York: Illuminating Engineering Society, 1962, p. 12.*

VENTILATION, HEATING, AND AIR CONDITIONING

Thermal control is often overlooked as a factor that contributes to a healthful classroom environment. Ventilation, heating, and air conditioning are important because they very directly affect the comfort and the general sense of well-being of the users of the school. Persons who are not physically comfortable generally will not learn as well as those who are comfortable.

In schools an often ignored phenomenon is that of human heat loss. Humans continuously give off heat and, for those interested in school ventilation, the control of this heat loss is important. The main consideration in this instance is the removal of this heat from the ambient air so that the air in the classrooms, buildings, and all of the other structures within the school plant remains comfortable.

Another function of ventilation is the removal of odors, especially those that are foul and present a nuisance to the building's occupants. This is generally accomplished by ensuring that the proper amount of air required to remove both heat and odors is available. The task requires an efficient and properly functioning ventilation system, as well as knowledge of certain facts, such as the cubic feet of air per person that are required for comfort and the level of odors found in the classrooms, labs, offices, and so on at any given moment. (See Tables 6.1 and 6.2.)

TABLE 6.1

Minimum Amounts of Air to Be Circulated per Minute Through
Schoolrooms, by Type

Type of Schoolroom	Cubic Feet of Fresh Air per Minute per Square Foot of Floor Area
Classrooms: study, reading, relaxation rooms, and libraries	0.5
Gymnasiums, locker rooms, and toilet rooms	2.0
Laboratories (no exhaust system on hoods)	2.0
Laboratories (exhaust system on hoods)	1.0
Lunchrooms	1.5
Kitchens	equal to the amount of air exhausted by mechanical exhaust systems in hoods over cooking equipment

Source: American School and University. *American School and University* 36:37; February 1964.

Ideally, classroom temperature will be between 68° and 73° F, the closer to 68° F the better. Gymnasiums and other rooms in which the level of activity is high can stand a temperature of approximately 65° F. The comfort of the room's occupants with regard to temperature will depend on their sex and age, the season of the year, and other factors. In general, it will be found that the cooler the room, the more active the occupants will be, with warm rooms resulting in diminished levels of activity. Students who are warm are more likely to daydream, become listless, and find it difficult to pay attention. To avoid this situation, teachers should open windows or regulate the thermostat when they find the air movement in the room stagnating. Children of grade-school age don't need as much environmental heat as do teachers; lowering the temperature may force teachers to wear sweaters or jackets, but it should result in a more active classroom.

Another factor that contributes to classroom comfort is the degree of dampness or moisture in the air. Usually referred to as humidity, the more air moisture, or the higher the humidity, the more the thermostat should be lowered. It is recommended that the relative humidity be kept at least at 45 percent. This is especially recommended if the heating system is the kind that recirculates the ambient air. If the classroom humidity reads below 45 percent, the air tends to be dry and the environment becomes uncomfortable.

TABLE 6.2

Minimum Outdoor Air Requirements to Remove Objectionable
Body Odors Under Laboratory Conditions

Type of Occupants	Air Space per Person in Cubic Feet	Outdoor Air Supply per Person per Minute in Cubic Feet
Sedentary adults of average socioeconomic status	100	25
	200	16
	300	12
	500	7
Laborers	200	23
Grade school children of lower socioeconomic status	200	38
Grade school children of average socioeconomic status	100	29
	200	21
	300	17
	500	11
Children attending private grade school	100	22

Source: American Society of Heating, Refrigerating and Air Conditioning Engineers. *ASHRAE Guide and Data Book: Fundamentals and Equipment for 1965 and 1966.* New York: The Society, 1965, p. 102.

An excellent way to control environmental humidity and air apportionment is through the use of air conditioners. Although air conditioners are not a necessity, may be expensive to maintain, and may not be found in all schools, they are a very good means for ensuring a comfortable, cheery, and productive environment. In schools where air conditioners are not available, teachers should open doors and windows to allow for proper air circulation, and if fans are available, they should be used in conjunction with the opening of doors and windows.

ACOUSTICS

Hearing that is unencumbered by poor acoustics, an inordinate amount of noise, or both is important to satisfactory performance in school. Noise is any disagreeable or unwanted sound. It is created by teachers, students, staff, and machinery (such as photocopiers), as well as by outside elements. External noise is produced by heavily traveled streets, factories, automobiles and trucks, airplanes, playgrounds, trains, and so on. Optimally, the external noise level should not be in excess of 70 decibels; thus, in choosing a site for a school, the external noise level is a prime consideration. Table 6.3 lists

TABLE 6.3

Acceptable Noise Levels in School Areas

Type of Room	Acceptable Noise Levels in Decibels
Classrooms	35 to 40
Cafeterias	50 to 55
School sites (outdoor noise levels)	Less than 70
Health rooms	Less than 45
Hearing test rooms	Less than 40
Music rooms	Less than 40

Source: Public Health Service: Division of Environmental Engineering and Food Protection, General Engineering Branch and the Office of Education Division of State and Local School Systems, School Administration Branch. *Environmental Engineering for the School: A Manual of Recommended Practice* (PHS Pub. No. 856). Washington, D.C.: U.S. Department of Health, Education, and Welfare, 1961.

acceptable noise levels (i.e., the highest level of noise that will not disturb the occupants in a school building).

Usually sound is measured in terms of its intensity and pitch. There are three units commonly used in sound measurement:

1. Decibel (db)—According to *Webster's New World Dictionary,* a decibel is "a unit for measuring the volume of a sound. It is equal to the logarithm of the ratio of the intensity of the sound to the intensity of an arbitrarily chosen standard sound." For each increase in intensity of 10 db, the actual sound pressure increases ten times. For example, sound that is measured at 60 db is 10 times greater than sound measured at 50 db and 100 times greater than sound measured at 40 db.

2. Hertz (Hz)—*Webster's* calls a hertz "the international unit of frequency, equal to one cycle per second."

3. Pitch—According to *Webster's,* pitch is "that quality of a tone or sound determined by the frequency of vibration of the sound waves reaching the ear; the greater the frequency the higher the pitch."

Ordinary conversation varies from about 40 to 60 db or 500 to 5000 Hz at a distance of about three feet.

If at all possible, classrooms should be constructed on the least noisy side of the site. Also, meticulous enforcement of rules with regard to hallway and classroom conduct will aid in reducing noise. So too will the use of noise-filtering material in the construction of the school building(s), such as acoustical ceiling tile and carpeting.

SEWAGE DISPOSAL

All school buildings require a system that effectively, efficiently, and sanitarily carries off human excrement. Human excrement serves as an important link in the transmission of disease; therefore, any system used should be closed.

The best way to dispose of sewage is via the public or municipal sewer system. When this is not possible, an alternative disposal vehicle, such as a chemical holding tank or a septic or Imhoff tank, is necessary.

Chemical holding tanks can be rented from commercial firms. These businesses have the necessary equipment to properly and sanitarily remove wastes. The removal of these wastes is done at least weekly (Cornacchia et al., 1984, p. 48).

Septic or Imhoff tanks, on the other hand, function a bit differently, as they retain sewage for varying periods of time to permit the settlement of solids. The solids will accumulate and will anaerobically decompose. Professional supervision is required for the proper maintenance of these tanks and for the sanitary removal of the solid wastes.

The precipitate of these tanks presents itself in the form of sludge. This material must be removed properly and in accord with public health requirements. Often commercial firms are employed specifically for this task. The disposal of this matter by these firms must also follow any federal, state, or local regulations. Failure to do so could result in the creation of an environment conducive to the proliferation of organisms that cause disease.

When septic tanks are used, soil percolation tests are necessary. These tests measure the rate at which the liquid seeps through the soil. Ideally, septic tanks will be constructed at a distance of 10 to 20 feet below ground surface. When wells provide the primary source of water, the septic tanks must be constructed below the well-water level.

REFUSE OR SOLID WASTE DISPOSAL

Schools must properly dispose of refuse. Generally, "refuse or solid waste includes all garbage, rubbish and other wastes exclusive of sewage" (Joint Committee on Health Problems in Education, 1969, p. 217).

An end result of proper refuse disposal is a clean school site. A site that is free of fire hazards and is not a haven for rodents and insects requires a sufficient number of storage bins or dumpsters with tight lids. Trash receptacles must be present both inside and outside the school. The number of receptacles necessary depends on the amount of daily refuse and the frequency of collection of this refuse. Each classroom, office, and laboratory should be provided with trash baskets. These baskets should be emptied at least once a day. Cafeterias and lavatories should also be provided with lidded baskets, which might need to be emptied more than once daily.

At all times refuse should be contained in the most cost-efficient and least noxious manner. This, in part, mandates that all receptacles be kept clean. One way this might be accomplished is by manually cleaning them or by using a commercially produced water and steam sprayer. It is advisable that the cleaning be done in an area that has good floor drainage and that is removed from the other school facilities.

ENVIRONMENTAL POLLUTANTS

Environmental pollutants have become a major source of concern in the United States over the past twenty years. The threat to our well-being presented by these pollutants stretches beyond our urban areas to the remotest regions of our country. Just as the family shares in the responsibility for protecting its members from environmental pollutants, schools share in the responsibility for protecting students, staff and faculty from environmental pollutants. While in some instances this may be a tall order, in the cases of some pollutants, such as lead and radon, it may be easier than many professionals realize. For example, to protect students from the possible negative effects of electromagnetic fields generated by computer screens, teachers should make sure that students are sitting at least two feet away from their terminals. In addition, teachers should be aware that some permanent felt-tip markers, rubber cement and glues, and paints that are often used in putting together student projects may be hazardous to their health. Teachers should know which supplies may be toxic and ban their use in the classroom. Parents should be warned of the potential threat some of the supplies they purchase for their children may pose (*U.S. News and World Report,* March 4, 1991).

Two pollutants that many schools may be confronted with today and from which students should be protected are radon and lead. School officials should take every precaution necessary to ensure students, parents, faculty, and staff that the school has taken steps to protect their well-being. Every attempt must be made by school officials to rid the school of these and other environmental contaminants, regardless of the costs.

Radon

Radon is an odorless and invisible radioactive gas that cannot be detected by human senses. It can be found in school buildings where it enters through structural defects from the earth's crust (Probart, 1989). This indoor radon represents a significant source of exposure to ionizing radiation in the environment. In fact according to the EPA, it represents an exposure source that is " . . . greater than all other sources combined, including background radiation, medical and dental X rays, and radioactivity escaping into the environment from the production of nuclear energy and weapons" (Probart, 1989).

Individual health consequences due to exposure to radon are cumulative. The major effect to students, faculty, and staff of exposure to high levels of radon in the school is an increased likelihood of lung damage and cancer.

Young children are especially "at increased risk for radon-induced lung damage because they have smaller lung capacity and higher breathing rates, increasing the amount of radioactive particles inhaled. In addition, immature lungs may be less efficient in removing foreign particles, increasing potential for radiation damage . . ." (Probart, 1989).

EPA-approved radon detectors are available at a minimal financial cost. Schools should purchase these kits and periodically monitor the facility for radon leaks. Probart offers the following five recommendations to schools to help them address their responsibility in this area.

1. A radon testing program should become a priority for schools . . . if funding is not available to purchase testing devices for all classrooms, the program should be implemented gradually, testing a portion of rooms each year, starting with the rooms estimated to be at highest risk.
2. Community volunteer groups and PTAs should be involved in education efforts and perhaps the purchase of the testing devices, if appropriate.
3. Radon information should be incorporated into the school curriculum as an environmental health topic.
4. Inservice education programs should be developed for school personnel. Personnel should understand the nature of the potential threat, the importance of accurate testing protocol. For instance, the best results are obtained if doors and windows remain closed as much as possible during the testing period.
5. Because radon control continually evolves as new information becomes available, school administrators should maintain contact with appropriate officials, usually the state radiation control officers, to obtain latest information on testing and mitigation." [Probart, 1989]

Lead

Lead poisoning is not just an issue for our nation's urban poor. Countless millions of older schools have lead-based paint and lead-tainted water. Lead poisoning is far more widespread than realized. According to a *U.S. News and World Report* article (March 4, 1991), "Even levels of lead in the blood once widely believed to be too low to matter can reduce a child's intelligence, memory, concentration and coordination without producing obvious signs of poisoning." The Center for Disease Control has lowered the threshold for lead poisoning from 25 micrograms of lead per 0.1 liter of blood to 10 micrograms. It is estimated that this change will result in approximately 17 percent of all U.S. children under the age of six considered lead poisoned.

It is important that school officials have the water taps and all painted surfaces tested for lead by local private experts or by experts from the health department. It is further recommended that parents of the highest risk group, preschool children, have their children tested for lead as early as age 1 by their pediatricians or local health department. School officials may want to

TABLE 6.4

Minimum Supply of Water to Be Provided for Public Schools	
Use	Quantity of Gallons per Pupil per Day
Basic minimum quantity	2
Building equipped with flushometer or flush fixtures but having no showers or kitchen	20
Building fully equipped, including showers and kitchen facilities	25

Source: Public Health Service: Division of Environmental Engineering and Food Protection, General Engineering Branch and the Office of Education Division of State and Local School Systems, School Administration Branch. *Environmental Engineering for the School: A Manual of Recommended Practice* (PHS Pub. No. 856). Washington, D.C.: U.S. Department of HEW, 1961.

consider developing a policy that requires all six- and seven-year-olds to be tested for lead before they are allowed in school.

WATER SUPPLY

Water is consumed daily in large amounts by humans. It is the responsibility of the school district to provide a safe water system. Ideally, the water supply should be obtained from town or municipal sources. When this is not possible, wells should be drilled.

The amount of water provided, regardless of whether the source is a well or a municipal system, should be in sufficient quantities to meet the daily demand (see Table 6.4).

Water systems must be checked and analyzed for coliform bacteria and other contaminants at least once a month. Depending upon the area served, the water supply may require more frequent analysis. The coliform bacterial group is found in the intestinal tracts of animals and humans; its presence in the water supply is an indication that the supply has been infected by sewage. State or local health authorities should be consulted for technical information and advice regarding the bacteriological quality of water. Analysis should also be conducted to monitor the levels of the chemicals found in water (Public Health Service, 1961).

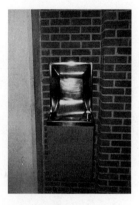

Drinking fountains placed in wall recesses help minimize safety hazards.

DRINKING FOUNTAINS

Sanitary drinking fountains should be strategically placed throughout a school building. These fountains should be easily accessible to persons in wheelchairs and should be placed in such a way as to minimize safety hazards. It is better if drinking fountains are placed in wall recesses rather than projecting into hallways. The fountains should be of the "jet" type as opposed to "bub-

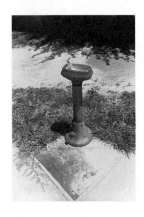

Outside water fountains should be away from play areas.

blers.'' Further, the drinking fountains should be designed for easy cleaning; this cleaning should occur several times daily.

There should be a sufficient number of fountains throughout the facility to meet the daily demands. There should be at least one fountain per floor and at least one fountain for every one hundred students. Although chilled water is desirable, it is not essential. The water should stream from the outlet jet under enough pressure that the student can drink the water without having to place his or her mouth too close to the jet.

LAVATORY FACILITIES

Like drinking fountains, lavatory facilities should be conveniently located throughout the school and should allow easy access by persons who are handicapped or who move about in a wheelchair. Lavatories should contain wash basins with hot and cold running water, soap dispensers, and towel dispensers. Commodes should be constructed to ensure privacy. Minimum requirements for lavatories and commodes, or water closets are shown in Tables 6.5 and 6.6. For preschool and kindergarten students, toilet and hand-washing facilities may be provided in the classroom. Urinals should be provided for boys in both elementary and secondary schools and should be cleaned daily.

SHOWER FACILITIES

In schools where swimming pools and gymnasiums exist, facilities for showering with warm water and soap should be provided. Ideally, these showers will be adjacent to pools and gyms. There should be an area outside the shower and removed from the locker area specifically set aside for drying. This will tend to decrease the amount of water on the locker room floors, thus reducing the hazards associated with wet floors.

There should be enough shower heads available to accommodate almost all of those who might be using the facility at any given time. The showers should have nonslip ceramic tile floors. These tiles are easy to clean and disinfect. The shower facility should be cleaned every day. Shower walls should be lined with moisture-resistant materials. The same ceramic tiles used for the shower floors might also be used for the walls. Ceilings should be insulated against condensation, and adequate drainage should be provided by having a slope to the floors.

Clean towels should be available to all students. On physical education or swim days, students might be required to bring their own towels, or the school may provide the students with clean towels. This would require the school to have laundry facilities on the school grounds or to contract with commercial laundry services to clean the towels. Students should be advised against leaving wet towels and bathing suits or soiled gym clothes in their lockers in order to prevent unpleasant odor.

Organization of School Health Programs

TABLE 6.5

Minimum Lavatory Facilities for Schools

Type of Schools	Fixture-to-Pupil Ratio
Elementary schools	1:30 pupils, up to 300 pupils
Secondary schools	1:40 pupils, for all above 300

Source: Public Health Service: Division of Environmental Engineering and Food Protection, General Engineering Branch and the Office of Education Division of State and Local School Systems, School Administration Branch. *Environmental Engineering for the School: A Manual of Recommended Practice* (PHS Pub. No. 856). Washington, D.C.: U.S. Department of HEW, 1961.

TABLE 6.6

Minimum Number of Water Closets for Schools

Type of Schools	Minimum Ratio Water Closets to Pupils	
	Boys	Girls
Elementary schools	1:40	1:35
Secondary schools	1:75	1:45

Source: Public Health Service: Division of Environmental Engineering and Food Protection, General Engineering Branch and the Office of Education Division of State and Local School Systems, School Administration Branch. *Environmental Engineering for the School: A Manual of Recommended Practice* (PHS Pub. No. 856). Washington, D.C.: U.S. Department of HEW, 1961.

LOCKER ROOMS

In addition to providing students with lockers for storing their books, coats, and lunches, junior and senior high schools might want to provide them with gym lockers as well. If possible, gym lockers should be full length; however, to economize on space, box lockers or basket-type lockers might be provided.

All locker rooms should be well lighted, well ventilated, clean, warm in the winter, and cool in the warmer months. Trash bins and toilet facilities should also be available. Benches in front of the lockers should be provided, and there should be enough of them to seat the largest class comfortably.

Gymnasiums should have plenty of floor space. They should also be constructed with enjoyment, comfort, and safety in mind.

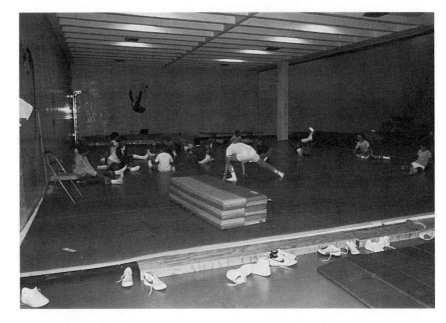

GYMNASIUMS

Gymnasiums should be large enough to provide adequate space for the largest physical education class, certain athletic events, and select recreational activities. The gymnasium should be constructed with enjoyment, comfort, and safety in mind. Floor space should be plentiful. There should be enough space between various apparatuses, such as basketball baskets, horse vaults, trampolines, ropes, and so on, and the surrounding walls to ensure students' safety. Also, the facility should be designed to meet the physical education needs of the handicapped or anyone else who might need remedial or special activities.

Doorways should be well lighted and marked and should allow persons in wheelchairs or on crutches easy and safe exit and entrance. The facility must always be kept clean and free of debris.

CUSTODIAL CARE

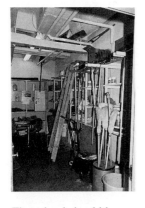

The school should be kept clean and sanitary by a well-equipped and dedicated custodial staff.

The prime responsibility of the school's custodial crew is to maintain the school facility, both inside and outside, in an attractive and sanitary manner. To contribute positively to the health and well-being of the students, schools must be kept free of dirt, filth, bacteria, and vermin. Also, a clean physical environment contributes to student esprit and cheerfulness. Positive mental and emotional well-being will thus be enhanced.

It helps, in keeping a school clean and sanitary, to have a dedicated custodial staff. The custodial staff should be given every opportunity to keep abreast of modern maintenance techniques and machinery. Workshops and demonstrations by commercial producers of housekeeping equipment and supplies should be periodically made available to all members of the custodial staff.

Organization of School Health Programs

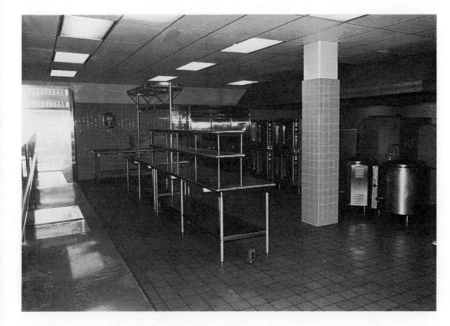

Kitchen equipment should be made of material that is easily cleaned and durable.

Custodial staff responsibilities may be categorized as follows:

1. Maintaining a clean and sanitary environment.
2. Maintaining a safe environment.
3. Vector control.
4. Environmental comfort and well-being.

FOOD SANITATION AND CAFETERIAS

Involvement of the federal government in school food services dates back to 1935, to PL 74–320 (the Agricultural Adjustment Act). Throughout the ensuing years, various laws have been passed (such as PL 79–396, the National School Lunch Act and PL 89–642, the Child Nutrition Act) in an attempt to safeguard the health of our children and assist them in developing appropriate attitudes toward nutrition.

The U.S. Department of Agriculture, the governmental agency primarily responsible for overseeing federally mandated and supported nutrition programs, has established as a priority of school food services the provision of meals that are balanced and nutritionally sound, inexpensive, and fit for human consumption. Ultimately, government, health, and school officials hope that, because good nutrition promotes health, and health affects learning, those students who are the recipients of sound school food programs will have a much more enjoyable and successful learning experience.

The majority of schools in the United States provide school lunches to students. Food is being prepared daily for large numbers of people. This food must be maintained and prepared in a way that will keep it from biological or chemical contamination or other toxic substances. A possible consequence of failing to provide students with quality food is illness in epidemic proportions.

The school dietician and the school district's food purchasing agent are the persons primarily responsible for the protection of the food. Longree has identified their responsibilities as:

1. Getting the most wholesome food for the money they have to spend.
2. Finding out whether or not the sources from which the food has been purchased are safe and sanitary and comply with all laws relative to food.
3. Ensuring that the food, when purchased, is in good condition, free from spoilage, filth, or other contamination and is safe for human consumption.
4. Ensuring that the storage area is cool, well ventilated, dry, and in the 50–60% range for relative humidity.
5. Protecting the food from invasion by rodents, insects and bacterial contamination. [1980, p. 211]

Highly perishable foods, such as fish, meat, poultry, dairy products, eggs, fruits, and vegetables, must be stored in a freezer or refrigerator.

Regardless of whether the storage area is dry or cold, it must be kept clean. This means that the dry storage area must be emptied of its contents and thoroughly cleansed periodically. In addition, daily cleaning activities, such as sweeping and mopping of the dry storage area, must occur. The cold storage area must be defrosted periodically and cleaned. Cleaning will also aid in minimizing odors. While cleaning of the storage area is taking place, an auxiliary storage area must be available. This area must also adequately protect the quality of the food.

The floor, walls, ceilings, equipment, and utensils in the food preparation area should be cleaned daily. They all should be constructed of material that is easily cleaned. Equipment and utensils should be made of materials that are durable, are of high sanitary quality, and are easily dismantled for cleaning.

The surfaces of the floor, walls, and ceilings must be kept in good repair; cracks, chips, or any other defects may harbor bacteria. These surfaces must be cleaned daily. Wood, galvanized steel, and iron are not materials that wear well; thus they are not recommended for use in constructing kitchen equipment or utensils.

Longree recommends that cleaning be thorough enough to eliminate contaminants and be done soon enough after lunch to prevent microbial buildup. Further, she reports the FDA recommendations for cleaning as these:

1. "Tableware shall be washed, rinsed, and sanitized after each use."
2. "To prevent cross-contamination, kitchenware and food-contact surfaces of equipment shall be washed, rinsed, and sanitized after each use and following any interruption of operations during which time contamination may have occurred."

Kitchens should be kept clean.

3. "Where equipment and utensils are used for preparation of potentially hazardous foods on a continuous or production line basis, utensils and the food-contact surfaces of equipment shall be washed, rinsed, and sanitized at intervals throughout the day on a schedule based on food temperature, type of food, and amount of food particle accumulation."

4. "The food-contact surfaces of grills, griddles, and similar cooking devices and the cavities and door seals of microwave ovens shall be cleaned at least once a day; except that this shall not apply to hot oil cooking equipment and hot oil filtering systems. The food-contact surfaces of all cooking equipment shall be kept free of encrusted grease deposits and other accumulated soil."

5. "Non-food-contact surfaces of equipment shall be cleaned as often as is necessary to keep the equipment free of accumulation of dust, dirt, food particles, and other debris." [1980, p. 265]

Explicit directions for cleaning various pieces of equipment should come with the equipment. All kitchen personnel should be familiar with how to clean each piece of kitchen equipment thoroughly.

The proper storage of equipment and utensils, once they are cleaned, is necessary to prevent them from being resoiled and possibly contaminated. The FDA reports in *Food Service Sanitation Manual* (1976) that cleaned and sanitized utensils be stored in a clean, dry location at least six inches above the floor. They should be protected from dust and other sources of contamination.

A school's kitchen and
cafeteria staff should be
aware of the importance
of cleanliness.

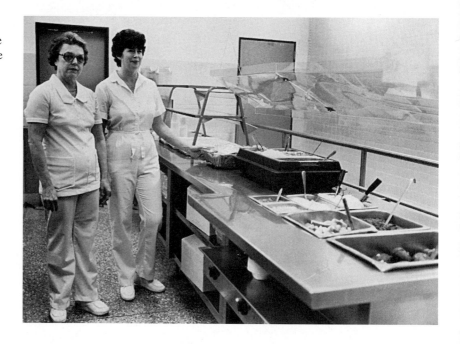

It is also suggested that utensils be air dried before being stored or be stored
in a self-draining position. Glasses and cups shall be stored inverted (Longree,
1980, p. 267).

Garbage cans and disposals must be cleaned daily. Mops should be laun-
dered and dried before being stored. Wet mops should not be stored, for they
serve as a potential reservoir for bacterial growth.

A school's kitchen and cafeteria staff is often culpable in the contamination of food, equipment, and utensils. With the potential for mass infection
so great in a school cafeteria, school administrators and health personnel must
make sure that anyone working in either the kitchen or the cafeteria is aware
of the importance of and necessity for cleanliness. Food service personnel
should be trained to practice proper hand washing and other personal cleanliness practices (such as wearing clean clothing; keeping skin, hair, and nails
clean; and so on).

The cafeteria should be spacious enough to accommodate the lunch period
that has the most students. It should be well ventilated and well lighted and
separate from the kitchen. There should be enough garbage cans in the cafeteria to adequately handle all of the trash that the largest lunch class might
have.

The cafeteria floor should be swept prior to the first lunch period and after
each subsequent period. After the last lunch period, the floor should be wet-
mopped and cleaned. The walls and ceiling should be cleaned on a periodic

Organization of School Health Programs

basis. The tables in the cafeteria must also be kept clean. To aid the cafeteria staff in keeping the room clean, teachers should supervise the lunchroom activities and ensure that proper table manners are displayed by the students. These teachers should also assist the cafeteria staff in seeing to it that the students properly dispose of all food waste.

SUMMARY

Students have a right to a healthful and safe school plant. Teachers, administrators, nurses, food service staff, and custodians have the responsibility of providing the student with a school that is healthful and safe. They do so by properly maintaining the school, promptly repairing any damage that may be hazardous to the students' safety and health, and checking the school daily for any condition that may not be in accordance with current health and safety standards.

REVIEW QUESTIONS

1. How does the maintenance of the school plant contribute to and support students' optimal health status?
2. Who are the persons in the school directly responsible for the protection of cafeteria food?
3. What are some of the steps that must be taken to ensure that the quality of the school's food is maintained at a high level?
4. What are some of the major considerations that must be addressed in order to adequately maintain a healthful school plant?

REFERENCES

Anderson, C. L., and W. H. Creswell, Jr. *School Health Practice.* St. Louis: C. V. Mosby, 1980.

Boles, H. W. *Step by Step to Better School Facilities.* New York: Holt, Rinehart & Winston, 1965.

Commission on School Buildings of the American Association of School Administrators. *Schools for America.* Washington, D.C.: The Association, 1965.

Cornacchia, H. J., L. K. Olsen, and C. J. Nickerson. *Health in Elementary Schools.* St. Louis, Mo.: Times/Mirror/Mosby, 1984.

Food and Drug Administration. *Food Service Sanitation Manual.* U.S. Department of HEW, Public Health Service. DHEW Pub. No. (FDA) 78–2081. Washington, D.C., 1976.

Jenne, F. H., and W. H. Greene. *Turner's School Health and Health Education,* 7th ed. St. Louis: C. V. Mosby, 1976.

Joint Committee on Health Problems in Education. *Healthful School Environment.* Washington, D.C.: National Education Association and the American Medical Association, 1969.

Longree, Karla. *Quantity Food Sanitation,* 3rd ed. New York: Wiley-Interscience, 1980.

Probart, C. K. "Issues Related to Radon in Schools." *Journal of School Health* 59:10 (December 1989); 441–443.

Public Health Service: Division of Environmental Engineering and Food Protection, General Engineering Branch and the Office of Education Division of State and Local School Systems, School Administration Branch. *Environmental Engineering for the School: A Manual of Recommended Practice* (PHS Pub. No. 856). Washington, D.C.: U.S. Department of HEW, 1961.

U.S. News & World Report. "A Nontoxic Childhood," March 4, 1991, pp. 56–60.

Emotional Climate

7

The provision of a healthful school environment requires that all aspects of the environment that affect the health, safety, and maximum functioning of the student be addressed. The purpose of this chapter is to address one of those aspects, the emotional climate. Emotional climate is defined as "that mood which characterizes the collective behavior and attitudes of teachers, administrators and students, and affects the students' emotional growth and development" (National Education Association and the American Medical Association, 1969, p. 15). It is hoped that upon completion of this chapter, the reader will have a better understanding of the relationship that exists between the emotional climate of the school and

1. The organization of a healthful school day.
2. The physical considerations of the school rooms.
3. Pupil-to-pupil relationships.
4. Teacher-to-pupil relationships.
5. Teacher-to-teacher relationships.
6. Administrative relationships to teachers and pupils.
7. Discipline.
8. Grading.
9. Grade placement.
10. Parental participation.

ORGANIZATION OF A HEALTHFUL SCHOOL DAY

The organization of the school day in a fashion that contributes to the health, the safety, and the ability of students to function to the best of their capacity with minimal environmental interference is in large part an administrative concern. Since the student is in school from three to eight hours each day, individual academic programs should be arranged so that the school experience is enjoyable to the student and so that assigned tasks can be performed with utmost efficiency. If not much thought and consideration are paid to the organization of the school day, it is quite likely that both students and teachers will be required to perform their daily tasks in an atmosphere of tension. Organization in this light can be seen to have an effect on the health and safety of the students and school personnel.

A healthful school environment contributes to students' emotional growth and development.

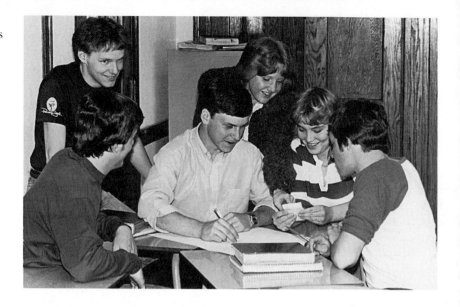

Although the organization of the school day is the responsibility primarily of the school administrator, it might best be shared by the teachers and some of the other school health team members. Some guiding considerations for these members are the social, emotional, physical, intellectual, and spiritual aspects of the students' development. When careful thought and consideration are given to the developmental characteristics of students, the students will be likely to appreciate and enjoy the school experience and develop a sense of purpose, confidence, and security.

Organizing the school day means addressing two major issues: (1) daily time allotment and (2) the length of the school year. Each of these features plays an important role in the provision of a healthful school environment.

Although it is seemingly a simple concern, trying to fit all of the necessary school activities into one school day can present administrators with sched-uling nightmares. The coordination of classes and teaching schedules is not a task that is accomplished quickly. The administrator should spend a great deal of time working with the various program coordinators in the school to ensure that the needs of each department (such as classroom space, staff, materials, and so on) are being met to the best of the school's ability. It also means that the administrator and advisors must be certain that the teacher's talents, skills, and interests are being utilized in the most efficient and beneficial manner.

Another scheduling issue has to do with the length of time the students and teachers will be required to spend in school and in the various classrooms each day. If student alertness varies throughout the length of the school day, and the demands of each academic subject are not given much attention, the result is likely to be a school day that is completely out of balance. Students may well find themselves trying to perform in an environment that is unnec-essarily demanding and one that is causing them a great deal of tension.

Organization of School Health Programs

In scheduling the school day, several questions related to health education arise:

1. What are the state requirements for health education?
2. How much total time is set aside for direct instruction?
3. Is the time block to be the same length each period the classes meet?
4. Is health instruction scheduled daily or once or twice a week?
5. Is the schedule flexible enough to vary the length of a class period in keeping with the nature of the lesson?
6. Does the schedule accommodate team teaching, mini-lessons, mini-courses and flexibility for innovative programs? [Willgoose, 1982, p. 87]

Responses to these questions will vary from state to state and will be dependent largely upon the particular state's view of the role of health instruction in the school. Following is an excerpt of a policy statement on health education, which was approved by the Virginia State Board of Education in 1975:

Elementary and secondary schools shall present a comprehensive health education program which focuses attention on problems related to alcohol and drug abuse, smoking and health, personal growth and personal health, nutrition, prevention and control of disease, physical fitness, accident prevention, personal and family survival, environmental health, mental health, and consumer education.

1. Elementary Schools. Since the early development of sound health attitudes, habits, and practices are important, time shall be provided at each grade level for health instruction.
2. Secondary Schools. At least 40 percent of the time for the required health and physical education program shall be devoted to health education. The remainder of the instructional time shall be devoted to physical education.
   a. Alternate Plan. A school division electing to offer a concentrated health instruction program may offer a semester of health education at both the eighth grade level and either the ninth or tenth grade level. Under this plan, the remainder of the instructional time at the eighth, ninth, and tenth grade levels shall be devoted to physical education. [State Department of Education, 1976, p. 3]

The second organizational issue has to do with the length of the school year. For years, in various places throughout the United States, there has been a push toward a 12-month school year. This pressure is generally a result of a desire to more effectively utilize school facilities. Much of what has been written about the length of the school year supports the current approach of having school interspersed with vacations for both students and teachers. Both teachers and students benefit from these vacations; however, it is not certain as to whether a two-month summer vacation is necessary. Further research into what constitutes the length of the most effective school year should be conducted.

Some other organizational concerns are: (1) What size group or class would be most conducive to learning? (2) Will student learning best occur in classrooms that are self-contained? (3) Does the school structure require that the programs be departmentalized? (4) Will it be more helpful to both students and teachers if some subjects are team taught? (National Education Association, 1969, pp. 17–20).

PHYSICAL CONSIDERATIONS OF SCHOOL ROOMS

The physical character of school rooms has a direct impact on the health, safety, and comfort of both students and teachers. As mentioned in Chapter 6, heating, ventilation, illumination, glare, noise, size, and color are aspects of the room that can have a direct effect on the comfort of the room's occupants and the emotional atmosphere of the room. No one likes working in a room that is either too hot or too cold, too stuffy, too poorly lighted, too noisy, too small, or too big. Also, the choice of color for the room affects the emotional well-being of both students and teachers. The color of a room should be selected so that it produces the desired emotional outcome. An appropriately colored room can aid greatly in providing an atmosphere in which students enjoy working and in which they feel safe and secure. To achieve this ideal atmosphere, it is generally recommended that for northern exposures, warm colors be used (such as yellow); for southern exposures, cool colors might be used (such as light blue); light pastels help in attaining the proper reflectance factor. For large areas, light colors are recommended (such as white or buff).

Other physical factors that contribute to the emotional setting of the classroom are:

1. The room should be clean and free of clutter and trash.
2. Bright, cheerful colors should be used throughout the room to contrast with the predominant room color. Some ways in which this might be accomplished are:
   a. Use bulletin boards that are colorful, cheerful, informative, motivating, and enable students to learn faster and retain the information for a longer time.
   b. Display projects, posters, essays, or artwork developed by the students.

Since a great deal of student and teacher school time is spent in the classroom, they should enjoy it. Working and residing in a room that is enjoyable can't help but enhance learning.

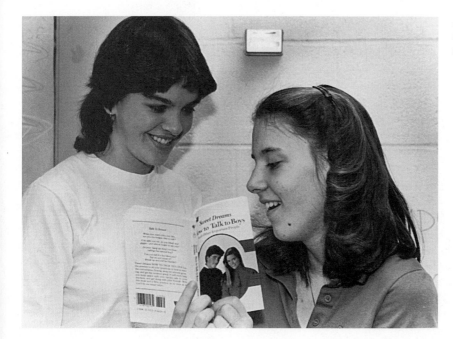

A healthful school environment encourages student interaction.

The classroom must be able to accommodate the largest class likely to inhabit it. It should be spacious enough to contain all the materials and equipment required for teaching. The furniture should be movable and, in some instances, adjustable. There should be enough seats so that each student has a place to sit and work. Seats should be comfortable and should support the growth needs of the student.

The room must also be kept in good repair. Chalkboards should be properly located in the classroom, should be in good condition, and should be cleaned regularly.

RELATIONSHIPS

Schools are responsible for more than just academics. The school, the family, and the community share the responsibility for aiding the student in acquiring appropriate attitudes about health matters. The attitudes that are developed by students govern their behavior. A concern, then, for teachers should be those factors that influence the students' acquisition of appropriate attitudes. The emotional climate of the school and classroom and the relationships that exist between teachers and teachers, pupils and pupils, and teachers and pupils are areas that must be considered.

Pupil-to-Pupil Relationships

Students share in the responsibility for the school atmosphere. When students are allowed and encouraged to interact with each other, a healthy emotional climate results. Under these circumstances, students learn to be more responsible for themselves, learn more efficient and more productive ways to cope, learn to work through cooperation, and develop the sense of security that comes from being a member of a group in which one is accepted and permitted to express his individuality. The student in this situation also learns to be more independent and develops a more positive self-concept. The more students are encouraged to interact with each other, the more they learn how to get along with other people. They also learn that people have differing needs, opinions, abilities, feelings, and interests.

In considering pupil-to-pupil interaction, the Virginia state departments of education and health write, "Pupils should be encouraged to participate in classroom and school improvement projects, and should be given their share of responsibility in planning for and maintaining desirable conditions within the classroom and throughout the school. Such practices provide a functional approach to learning and help develop a sense of pupil responsibility and pride for achieving and maintaining a safe, attractive, and healthful school environment" (State Department of Education, 1975, p. 11).

How students relate to other students depends upon their stage of development and how important they consider their peers to be. For example, the relationship that exists between elementary school students is different from the relationship that exists between senior high school students. For the elementary school students, their relationship with classmates is just beginning, as is their drive to establish themselves outside of their homes. Progressively, these relationships change shape as students get older. Around junior high school age, students become more assertive, and they collectively begin to inform the teacher what they are interested in and what they feel that they need.

Pupil-to-pupil relationships become increasingly important to the student in junior high school. These peer-group relations help them in their struggle to establish their identity. The school provides an opportunity for peer interaction by offering a full complement of extracurricular opportunities, from athletics to student government. These activities promote learning and aid the students in developing the skills that will be needed to become active, contributing community members.

In high school these relationships become a barometer of student success. Individual orientation is toward achievement. The spirit of competition becomes obvious in peer relationships. Through these competitive relationships, students learn the value of dependability and the meaning of commitment. More lasting relationships begin to take shape.

A school environment that is emotionally healthy is one in which these relationships are nourished. The long-term goal is to develop emotionally sound adults.

Organization of School Health Programs

Teacher-to-Pupil Relationships

The relationship that has perhaps the most profound influence on the emotional climate in the school is the interaction between teacher and pupil. The teacher is the person whom the child sees in school each day. The teacher, because of this unique advantage, can promote learning, assist the child in moving from dependence to independence, facilitate social adjustment, play a part in the validation of the student's self-concept, and provide an environment that encourages the child.

In their interactions with students, teachers must be concerned about consistent and equitable treatment. Teachers should strive to provide the pupil with an environment that is accepting of individual differences and one in which the pupil can work without fear of ridicule. This emotionally sound environment is influenced by the teacher's self-perception and by the teacher's ability to identify and communicate with students. It is further influenced by personal values, beliefs, concerns, and prejudices. Teachers who have been successful at providing an emotionally healthy environment for their pupils have the following characteristics:

1. They listen to students without passing judgment on what they are saying.
2. They show enthusiasm for the subject matter and for life.
3. They reward appropriate behavior.
4. They are supportive of students.
5. They maximize student assets.
6. They value their students.
7. They allow students to freely express themselves in class.
8. They train students to accept responsibility for their own behavior.
9. They make learning fun.
10. They are concerned about their students.
11. They deal with students and all other persons humanely.
12. They are not sarcastic or unduly harsh toward the students.
13. They accept and respect their students as fellow human beings.
14. They trust their students.
15. They encourage student participation in all classroom activities.
16. They get to know their students.
17. They nourish healthy competition between students.
18. They encourage student curiosity and questions.
19. They apply discipline firmly and fairly.
20. They provide guidance and counsel to students.
21. They have faith in their students.
22. They encourage students to do their best and enable them to recognize their assets.

Teachers who exude self-confidence and are able to motivate their students are more likely to be successful at providing their students with a healthy emotional environment than teachers not possessing these attributes. The teacher's personal appearance and physical status are important factors that influence the environment. They must be able to handle the daily demands of teaching. They must have an intact self-concept and must serve as role models for the students.

Teacher-to-Teacher Relationships

The relationship among teachers should be supportive. Teachers working cooperatively together to maintain wholesome classroom and school conditions will most likely have contented students.

Teacher-to-teacher relationships that result in a healthy emotional climate:

1. Are supportive of the teacher as an individual.
2. Provide freedom of expression and support the teacher's right to academic freedom.
3. Allow teachers to develop good human relationships with each other.
4. Allow teachers to work cooperatively with each other.
5. Provide teachers with encouragement.
6. Value teachers as persons.
7. Show faith in teachers.
8. Are supportive of a job well done and give recognition for effort.
9. Nourish self-confidence.
10. Provide teachers with counsel and advice.
11. Stress the communality of school problems.
12. Support teachers' experiments with new teaching methods.
13. Encourage the sharing of information as well as teaching strategies and techniques.
14. Include sharing responsibilities outside the classroom (such as lunchroom supervisory duty, bus duty, and so on).

The relationships between teachers may not always be healthy. When this occurs, teachers should be professional enough to leave their disagreements and differences out of the classroom. If they fail in this regard, it is likely that students will pick up on the disharmony. This may result in student discontent.

Administrative Relationships

Just as students are likely to pick up on teacher-to-teacher discord, they are also likely to be aware of administrator-teacher conflict and tension. For this reason, it is important that these persons put aside their professional or personal differences and together work toward establishing a healthy emotional climate in the school.

Positive relationships between administrators and teachers are likely to be felt in the various classrooms. In fact, positive relationships between administrators and teachers and all other school personnel will likely set off an emotional chain reaction, the impact of which will be felt throughout the school.

Teachers in a healthy relationship with their administrators are supportive of the administrator, keep the administrator up to date regarding classroom matters, and follow school policies and regulations. Administrators, on the other hand, might do the following:

1. Treat all teachers equally and fairly.
2. Support an adequate pay scale and raises for teachers.
3. Keep the lines of communication open between the central office and the classroom.
4. Give teachers curricular autonomy (within reason).
5. Provide teachers with the opportunity for in-service training regarding matters pertinent to their duties.
6. Provide teachers with a support network of counselors, nurses, custodians, and secretarial staff to assist them in their daily activities.
7. Clearly delimit the teachers' duties and responsibilities.
8. Ensure all teachers a fair workload.

Concerning the relationship between administrators and students, administrators should:

1. Ensure that the school programs are flexible and that they reflect what is currently known about a particular subject.
2. Ensure that the school's programs will reflect an understanding of the growth and development characteristics of students.
3. Provide students with well-trained teachers and guidance personnel.
4. Provide students with a wide array of extracurricular activities.
5. Provide students with a healthy social environment.

DISCIPLINE

Periodically, matters of control and discipline will arise. Handling these matters is primarily the responsibility of the teacher. Teachers should deal with these matters in a prudent, humane, and professional manner. The student's self-respect should not be damaged. In disciplining students, it is important that the teacher make sure that the student understands exactly why the reprimand is occurring. Discipline must always be dispensed in a consistent manner. Teachers should have a clear understanding of what is and is not an appropriate use of discipline. Administrators can help clarify this for teachers by providing them with guidelines.

GRADING

The grading of all students should be done in a fair and consistent manner. Grading methods should be clearly explained to students on the first day of class so that they know exactly what is expected of them. Students' grades are a private matter and should not be discussed with any other students. It has been recommended that teachers avoid using grades to make comparisons between students but that they be used as a measure of individual achievement.

Since all students do not have the same intellectual capacity for achievement, they cannot be expected to reach the same level at the same time (National Education Association, 1969, p. 85).

GRADE PLACEMENT

Ideally, school districts should present a comprehensive health instruction program for all students in grades K through 12. To avoid either duplication or omission of health instruction content, health classes should be comprised of only one grade level. When several grade levels are mixed together, it becomes difficult to schedule students for subsequent years in a way that ensures that content is not being duplicated, and to provide a balance in the curriculum between student needs and interests.

PARENTAL CONTRIBUTIONS

The parental contributions to the school's emotional climate may be summarized as follows:

1. There should be direct, positive parent–teacher communication and cooperation.
2. The parents should become active members of the school health team.
3. Parents should be supportive of the school health program.
4. Parents should encourage at home the health behaviors that are learned in the school.
5. Parents should follow up on suggested health services or remedial programs for their children as suggested by the school.
6. Parents should exercise good judgment when deciding whether or not they should send an ill child to school.

SUMMARY

There are many aspects of the school environment that affect the emotional and mental well-being and development of the students. Responsibility for providing an atmosphere that is conducive to student growth and development rests with the teachers and the school administrator. The interactions between these two groups will result in an emotional chain reaction that is likely to be felt in the classroom. All efforts should be made to enhance student-to-student interaction, as well as interaction among students, teachers, and administrators.

REVIEW QUESTIONS

1. How might the emotional climate of a school be characterized?
2. What effect do the interactional patterns between pupils; teachers; pupils and teachers; and administrators, teachers, and pupils have on the emotional climate of the school?

3. How does the physical character of school rooms impact on the health, safety, and comfort of students and teachers?
4. What contributions do parents make to the school's emotional climate?

REFERENCES

National Education Association and the American Medical Association. *Healthful School Environment.* Washington, D.C.: NEA, 1969.

Silbergelt, S., G. R. Koening, and R. W. Manderscheid. "Classroom Psychosocial Environment." *The Journal of Educational Research* **69**:4 (1975): 151–155.

State Department of Education. "School Health Education." Richmond: Department of Education, Division of Secondary Education, 1976.

State Department of Education and the State Department of Health. *Health Manual for Schools.* Richmond: Department of Education and Health, 1975.

Willgoose, C. E. *Health Teaching in Secondary Schools,* 3d ed. Philadelphia: W. B. Saunders, 1982.

PART

Services

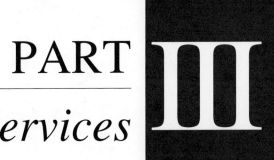

III

Health Appraisal

8

School personnel have many responsibilities, but health appraisal should be considered one of the most important. How can a student expect to profit from the school experience if some health problem impairs the learning potential? If health problems are corrected early in the student's school years, his or her ability to learn will be maximized.

Unfortunately, not all health problems are easily appraised in the school setting. However, there are some major types of health problems that can be observed and dealt with before the problem turns into a learning disability. The most basic form of health appraisal is teacher observation.

TEACHER OBSERVATION

The classroom teacher is in perhaps the most strategic position to observe any health problem or defect among students. Teacher observation is dependent upon many factors. First, the teacher must know the signs and symptoms of unusual conditions among students. Second, the teacher must be alert and responsible to individual needs. Third, the teacher must be willing to recognize and respect health differences among students. Finally, the teacher must listen to the child's complaints.

Referrals usually begin with the teacher. The teacher observes some health problem and refers the student to the school nurse. The advantage the teacher has is that he or she can compare the student with other students in the class, an opportunity that the parents do not have. Therefore, if the teacher recognizes variations from the norm, a student can get medical help before the problem gets out of hand. Indicators of possible medical problems can be found in Table 8.1.

SCREENING

Health screening is a useful tool in the appraisal of the overall health of students; however, the screening itself is but one step in a larger program. Screening should not be confused with a diagnostic procedure, for it merely provides ''a preliminary evaluation of the state of development or functioning of various body organs to uncover health problems not identified by observation of pupil appearance and behavior'' (Webster, 1980, p. 493).

Much of this chapter focuses on the various types of screenings commonly performed in the schools. It is important to point out that a successful screening program is not merely one by which those students in need of treatment are identified, but one that also ensures that necessary follow-up in the form of appropriate treatment is received (Webster, 1980, p. 494).

TABLE 8.1

Indicators of Potential Medical Problems

Indicators	Potential Problem Area
Sties or crusted lids	Eyes/vision
Inflamed eyes	
Crossed eyes	
Repeated headaches	
Squinting, frowning or scowling	
Protruding eyes	
Watery eyes	
Rubbing of eyes	
Excessive blinking	
Twitching of the lids	
Holding head to one side	
Discharge from ears	Ears/hearing
Earache	
Failure to hear questions	
Picking at the ears	
Turning the head to hear	
Talking in a monotone	
Inattention	
Anxious expression	
Excessive noisiness	
Persistent mouth breathing	Nose and throat
Frequent sore throat	
Recurrent colds	
Chronic nasal discharge	
Frequent nosebleed	
Nasal speech	
Frequent tonsilitis	
Nits on the hair	Skin and hair
Unusual pallor of face	
Eruptions or rashes	
Habitual scratching of scalp	
Uncleanness	
Excessive redness of skin	

TABLE 8.1 Continued

Indicators	Potential Problem Area
Uncleanness	Teeth/mouth
Gross visible caries	
Irregular teeth	
Stained teeth	
Gum boils	
Offensive breath	
Mouth habits such as thumb sucking	
Underweight—very thin	General condition and appearance
Overweight—very obese	
Does not appear healthy	
Tires easily	
Chronic fatigue	
Nausea or vomiting	
Faintness or dizziness	
Failure to gain regularly over three-month period	Growth
Unexplained rapid gain in weight	
Enlarged glands at side of neck	Glands
Enlarged thyroid	
Excessive breathlessness	Heart
Tires easily	
Any history of ''growing pains''	
Bluish lips	
Excessive pallor	
Asymmetry of shoulders and hips	Posture
Peculiarity of gait	
Obvious deformities of any type	
Anomalies of muscular development	
Overstudious, docile, and withdrawn	Behavior
Bullying, overaggressive, and domineering	
Unhappy and depressed	
Overexcitable; Uncontrollable emotions	
Stuttering or other forms of speech difficulty	

Reprinted by permission from National Education Association, Joint Committee on Health Problems in Education. *School Health Services.* Washington, D.C.: National Education Association and the American Medical Association, 1964, p. 41.

FIGURE 8.1

Model for health
screening program.

*Reprinted with permission
from Journal of School
Health.* Planning and
Implementing Health
Screening Programs. Vol.
50, No. 9, November 1980,
p. 493. Copyright, 1980.
American School Health
Association, Kent, OH
44240.

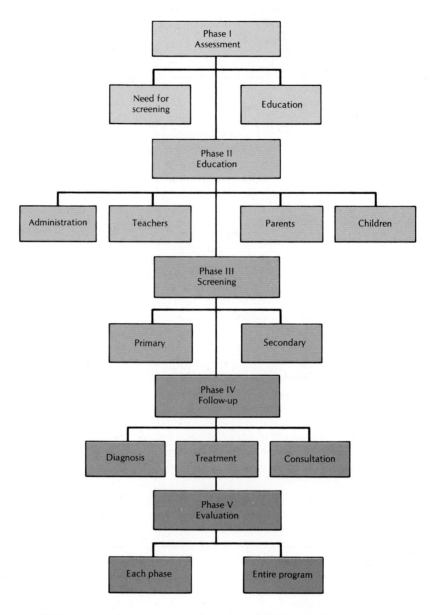

Webster developed a model for a successful screening program that can be employed in the schools. This model can be found in Figure 8.1. As can be seen from the figure, the screening process is a very intensive one, not merely a simple referral and follow-up.

School districts usually have policies that are directed at the types of screenings to be performed in the schools in that district. Most students participate in the district-required screenings; these screenings are usually held during a physical education class.

MEDICAL DEPARTMENT

RICHMOND PUBLIC SCHOOLS

TEACHER–NURSE REFERRAL FORM

Dear ______________________

The school nurse in each school is making an effort to assure that any student who appears to be having problems, whether physical or emotional, is given consideration and help.

Because of the important place you hold as an observer of students, we are asking you to cooperate with us and return these forms promptly to the nurse.

Please list any observations in the appearance and behavior of pupils in your class which seem to be a departure from good health. Such observations as poor posture, excessive fatness or thinness, listlessness, squinting eyes and "just seems under par" should be listed.

Thank you for your help.

Please return this form to the school nurse by ______________________
(Date)

1. Name of Student	Observations and Remarks
2.	
3.	
4.	
5.	
6.	
7.	
8.	
9.	
10.	

Nurse's Investigation: (Reserved for Nurse)

FIGURE 8.2
Teacher-nurse referral form.
Source: Richmond Public Schools, Richmond, Va.

Another type of screening is a screening that results from a teacher–nurse referral. In this case, a teacher notices a particular problem and refers the student to the school nurse. In some cases, teachers are asked to refer students whom they think might have some health problem. Figure 8.2 shows a letter and form used for such a referral. It is important to note that the teacher's role does not end after referral. The teacher must follow up to make sure an action has been taken. Follow-up is critical to the success of any referral. Referral and follow-up will be discussed later in the chapter.

It is important to first discuss the major types of health problems that can be detected early through proper screening. Once the health problems have been discussed, the specific screening procedures relative to the health problem will be presented.

VISION

Sight is one of the most precious and complex processes of the human body. With sight, we are able to interpret environmental events that include not only actions and stimuli from a variety of common sources, but also those events that occur within the classroom, such as lecturing, written work, and general classroom activities. The American Optometric Association has identified vision skills students need. These skills include (AOA, 1986):

- **Near Vision.** Ability to see clearly and comfortably at 13 to 16 inches, the distance at which school desk work should be done;
- **Distance Vision.** Ability to see clearly and comfortably at ten feet or more;
- **Binocular Coordination.** Ability to use the two eyes together;
- **Eye Movement Skills.** Ability to aim the eyes accurately, move them smoothly across a page and quickly and accurately from one object to another;
- **Peripheral Awareness.** Ability to be aware of things to the side while looking straight ahead;
- **Eye/Hand Coordination.** Ability to use the eyes and hands together.

When a student has a problem with one or more of these skills, learning potential is affected.

Before discussing visual problems and the procedures to be followed in detecting a possible vision problem, it is important to discuss the process of vision so that the reader can best understand the nature of visual disorders.

Physiology of Vision

The eye is a jelly-filled sphere with an outer layer of tough fibrous material called the sclera (Figure 8.3). The sclera is the ''white'' of the eye and is embedded in a protective layer of fat and muscle. At the front of the eyeball is the cornea, which is a transparent circular structure covered by a transparent protective skin called the conjunctiva.

Behind the cornea lies the iris, a thin, circular muscle usually colored blue, green, gray, brown, or a mixture of these colors, depending upon the amount of pigment present. The iris has the ability to constrict or dilate, and the opening resulting from this process is called the pupil. The pupil appears as the dark circle in the middle of the iris. A soft, transparent lens lies behind the pupil and is suspended by ligaments from a ring of ciliary muscles controlled by the autonomic nervous system. The ciliary muscles and ligaments allow the lens to bulge, thus shortening its focal length. This process is referred to as accommodation and is necessary in order to view objects less than or greater than 20 feet away. Constant adjustment of the muscle–ligament–lens systems allows us to see distant objects clearly one moment and refocus to see close objects equally well moments later.

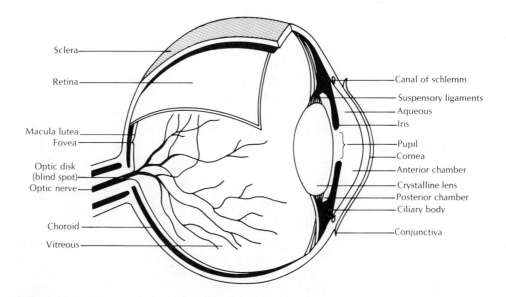

Sclera
Retina
Macula lutea
Fovea
Optic disk
(blind spot)
Optic nerve
Choroid
Vitreous

Canal of schlemm
Suspensory ligaments
Aqueous
Iris
Pupil
Cornea
Anterior chamber
Crystalline lens
Posterior chamber
Ciliary body
Conjunctiva

In front of the lens and iris lies a chamber that is filled with a watery jelly substance called the aqueous humor. The aqueous humor, together with the cornea, forms an additional lens system that cannot be adjusted. If it alters shape, which is possible during growth or old age, the adjustable lens within can compensate up to a point.

The main chamber of the eye, located behind the lens and aqueous humor, and comprising the bulk of the eye, is called the vitreous humor. This substance contributes to the firmness and shape of the eye.

Surrounding the vitreous humor is a structure called the sclera. Within the sclera lie two important, highly sophisticated structural systems called the choroid and the retina. The choroid contains blood vessels and is responsible for bringing nourishment to the structures inside the eye and carrying away metabolic wastes. Within the choroid is the retina, which contains important sensory cells called rods and cones. These structures are responsible for converting radiant energy into electrical energy, and for color perception. Each eye contains some 140 million rods and cones, with rods outnumbering cones approximately 15 to 1. Rods are most abundant around the sides of the eye, and cones are most abundant and increase in density toward the back of the eye; they are tightly packed in the area called the fovea.

The fovea is a small area of the retina, diametrically opposite to the pupil; it is the point at which the cones are connected to nerve fibers.

At the back of the eye is an area in which nerve fibers and blood vessels converge to form the optic nerve, which then is connected through intricate pathways to the brain. At the point where this nerve fiber–blood vessel system is connected to the retina, both rods and cones are missing; this point is referred to as the blind spot.

FIGURE 8.3

Anatomy of the human eye.
Copyrighted by the National Society to Prevent Blindness. Reprinted by permission.

Process of Vision

All of the structures mentioned previously are important to the process of vision and the clarity of vision. These structures are all dependent upon one another, and problems or defects in any one structure can lead to visual problems of varying degree.

The process of vision naturally begins with light. The light from environmental stimuli is called radiant energy and begins its travel into the eye as parallel light rays. These parallel light rays pass through the cornea, aqueous humor, and iris. The pupil will constrict, which allows fewer parallel light rays to pass through. The light rays then pass through the lens, which is responsible for refracting or bending the light rays so that they can come to a point on the retina.

Once the refracted light rays come to a point on the retina, the rods and, more specifically, the cones, acting as light receptors, convert the radiant energy into electrical energy; this electrical energy or impulse is carried by the optic nerve to the occipital lobe of the brain, where it is perceived as an image.

The process is extremely sophisticated and not totally understood by medical science. However, it is important to note that the brain is responsible for transcribing the impulse into a meaningful or recognizable form, and the eye acts much like a camera, in that it regulates the amount of light entering it and transforms one type of energy into another.

Most of the time, this process of refracting light, transforming radiant energy into electrical energy, and interpreting the impulse is adequate for a person to see. However, there are many kinds of problems, especially prevalent among school-age students, that can influence the quality of vision, thus influencing their ability to learn.

Common Visual Problems

The most common visual problems affecting the school-age student are those that are involved with the refraction of light. As mentioned earlier, the lens is responsible for the refraction or bending of the light so that it can come to a point on the retina. If there is some problem with the lens or with the ciliary muscles or ligaments that regulate the size of the lens, or if the eyeball is too small or too large, the individual could have what is termed a refractive error.

Refractive Errors

When light rays refract and come to a normal point on the retina, the process is called emmetropia. Emmetropia is not necessarily normal vision; it is just a term used to indicate the fact that light rays are refracting and coming to a point in the normal manner (Figure 8.4).

There are two common refractive errors in which the refracted light comes to a point before the retina and after the retina. These are termed myopia and hyperopia, respectively.

Organization of School Health Programs

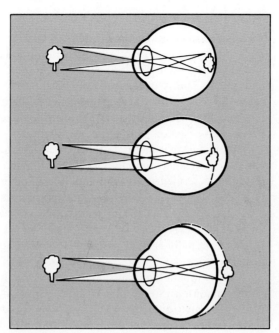

FIGURE 8.4

Refractive errors. Top: eye, with normal vision, in which image of object is focused on retina. Center: eye with myopia (nearsightedness), in which image falls in front of retina. Bottom: eye with hyperopia (farsightedness), in which image falls behind the retina. Dotted lines show where the focus is in relation to retina. *Source: American Medical Association;* How Are Your Eyes? *(Chicago: American Medical Association, 1977) p. 7.*

Myopia is a condition wherein light rays refract through the lens and focus at a point in front of the retina (Figure 8.4). A person with this condition is classified as myopic or nearsighted. This simply means that the individual sees objects that are close more clearly than objects at a distance.

In most cases, the cause of myopia is that the eyeball has grown somewhat larger than normal. This causes the focal length of the eye to be too great; therefore, the light rays focus in front of the retina. Normally, myopia is not a major visual problem and can be treated with corrective lenses. A defect in the lens can also cause myopia, but this is not normally the case.

Hyperopia is a condition wherein light rays refract through the lens and focus at a point behind the retina. This condition is also termed farsightedness. It simply means that an individual can see objects at a distance more clearly than objects that are close.

Hyperopia is a far more common visual disturbance than myopia among young school-age students. This is largely due to the fact that the eyeball is still growing until about age nine. As the eyeball grows, the degree of hyperopia will decrease. This concept will become clearer when visual acuity is discussed later.

It should be pointed out that if a severe case of hyperopia is present, corrective lenses can be used to decrease the condition somewhat and aid in bringing visual acuity to a normal level.

Other common visual problems affecting students are those that are not related to refraction of light, but to muscle problems or irregular curvatures in certain eye structures. The two most common of these problems are strabismus and astigmatism.

Strabismus

Within or around each eyeball are six muscles called extraocular muscles. These muscles are normally in perfect coordination and result in both eyes moving in the same direction at the same time. They are responsible for the individual's ability to focus on an object or event with *both* eyes and to perceive the event in a singular manner, excluding extraneous stimuli, stimuli that would be admitted if one eye were focused on one point and the other eye were focused on another point (Figure 8.5).

If for some reason, the extraocular muscles are not in perfect coordination, one of the eyes may tend to point in a different direction from the other. This condition is termed strabismus and, like all other visual problems, it can vary in degree. The most severe type of strabismus is the condition in which both eyes face inward, thus giving a cross-eyed appearance.

Strabismus is a serious condition and must be treated as soon as possible. It is an extremely critical impairment to learning and perception of environmental events.

The treatment for strabismus largely depends upon the extent and severity of the condition. Some mild cases of strabismus can be treated by simply placing a patch over the good eye, thus forcing the weak eye muscles to strengthen and come into alignment. In more severe conditions, corrective lenses and surgery might be indicated. But again, it is important that treatment begin as soon as medically possible. If treatment is delayed, the individual will begin to suppress the image in the weak eye, resulting in a further complication called lazy eye, or amblyopia.

An individual with amblyopia has suppressed the image in the weak eye to the point that the only visual stimuli perceived and interpreted are those stimuli coming into the good eye. It must be noted that in most cases there is nothing wrong physiologically with the weak eye. The muscles are simply weak or not in alignment, thus confusing the individual and impairing the quality of perception of stimuli.

Amblyopia is an extremely serious condition, because if suppression continues, the individual can lose the sight in the weak eye. Obviously, if there is nothing wrong with the eyeball as such, the condition becomes a psychological one, and the event of continuous suppression becomes almost impossible to treat. However, if strabismus is treated early enough, amblyopia will not result.

Astigmatism

Astigmatism is a common visual disorder; it occurs most frequently when there is an irregular curvature of the cornea or lens or both. This irregular curvature will project a blurred image on the retina. Like all other visual disorders, the degree of severity varies. If individuals suffering from severe astigmatism are not treated, their learning and activities can certainly be affected.

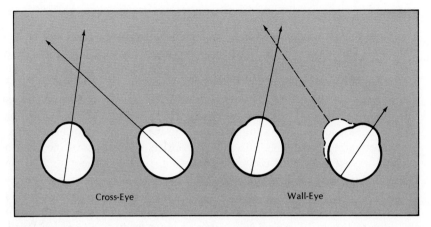

Cross-Eye   Wall-Eye

FIGURE 8.5
Ocular muscle balance problems.
Source: American Medical Association, How Are Your Eyes? *(Chicago: American Medical Association, 1977) p. 9.*

Most of the time, astigmatism is treated with corrective lenses that will enhance the capability of projecting a clear image on the retina. With the continued sophistication of optics, the problem of treating astigmatism is constantly becoming easier.

Other Visual Disorders

There are a variety of visual problems that are not related to refraction of light, extraocular muscle problems, or irregular curvatures of eye structures. The other problems center around color perceptual problems and common infections of the eye.

Color Perceptual Visual Problems

Color perceptual visual problems usually means that an individual has problems perceiving one or more of the three basic colors: blue, green, or red. The vast majority of color perceptual problems are hereditary and affect mainly males. For example, approximately 2 percent of all males cannot perceive the color red and are red-color blind, and 6 percent cannot perceive the color green so are green-color blind, while only one female in 1250 has some problem perceiving red–green colors.

The perception of color has nothing to do with clarity of vision, but it can be a problem when educational activities involve relationships to color. It is also a problem from a safety standpoint. Such situations as reacting to traffic signals, doing electrical work, or engaging in other activities in which color relationships are established can become life-threatening events if colors are not perceived correctly.

There is no medical treatment for color-perception problems. The only thing that can be done is to establish associations between such things as placement and color. For example, in a traffic signal, the top light is the red one.

Infections of the eye

There are three common infections that occur in the eyes. These are blepharitis, sties, and conjunctivitis. Blepharitis is characterized by a crusting at the base of the eyelashes. The eyelashes may begin to fall out, and the eyelid edges may appear reddened. The student may complain of a burning sensation and eye fatigue. Blepharitis is for the most part a chronic condition and can be associated with both sties and conjunctivitis. In addition, chronic infections with staphylococcus play an important role in the occurrence of blepharitis.

The treatment of blepharitis usually consists of removal of the crusting through the use of a moist cotton-tipped swab. If the condition persists, then chemotherapy may be used.

A sty is caused by a staphylococcus organism and is an infection of the glands of the eyelid. It usually appears as a tender, red raised area close to the edge of the eyelid. Often a swelling may appear in the area surrounding the raised area.

The treatment for sties usually consists of the application of hot-water compresses three to four times a day. In more serious cases, antibiotic drops or ointments may be prescribed by a physician. When sties continually recur, a physician should definitely be consulted, which means that a student must be referred, since this may indicate a more serious condition.

Conjunctivitis is a swelling of the protective skin located under the eyelids. Some discharge might occur, and this discharge could cause the lids to stick together, especially in the morning. Some types of conjunctivitis are contagious. For example, viral conjunctivitis may be transmitted through swimming-pool water. In most cases, simple treatment with antibiotics will reduce the inflammation. It should be noted that sound eye hygiene, such as not sharing towels and using disposable tissues, will significantly reduce one's risk of contracting the contagious form of conjunctivitis. As with blepharitis and sties, if conjunctivitis becomes a regular condition, the student must be referred and a physician consulted.

Signs and Symptoms of Visual Difficulty

School personnel, especially teachers, should be aware of the common signs and symptoms of some visual difficulty. The most common signs lie primarily in three observable areas: behavior, appearance, and complaints.

The most common behaviors indicating possible visual trouble include the following:

1. Attempts to brush away a blur.
2. Rubbing the eyes frequently.
3. Frequently frowning.
4. Shutting or covering eyes frequently.
5. Thrusting head forward when looking at near or distant objects.
6. Having difficulty in reading or in other work requiring close use of the eyes.

Organization of School Health Programs

7. Blinking more than usual.
8. Frequent crying or irritability when doing close work.
9. Stumbling or tripping over small objects.
10. Holding books or small objects close to eyes.
11. Being unable to participate in games requiring distant vision.
12. Being unduly sensitive to light. [Provided courtesy of the National Society to Prevent Blindness]

Some of these signs or symptoms are difficult to identify, and that is why teacher observation is so critical. The appearance of the eyes is also an indicator of possible visual problems. The following definitely indicate vision problems:

1. Red-rimmed, encrusted, or swollen lids.
2. Recurring sties.
3. Inflamed or watery eyes.
4. Crossed eyes.
5. Constant oscillation of eyes. [Provided courtesy of the National Society to Prevent Blindness]

Complaints by the student may be one of the best indicators of possible vision problems. However, a teacher or other school personnel are more likely to suspect a vision problem through behavior or appearance than complaints. Some common student complaints that might indicate a vision problem include:

1. Inability to see well.
2. Dizziness following close work.
3. Headaches following close work.
4. Nausea following close work.
5. Blurred or double vision. [Provided courtesy of the National Society to Prevent Blindness]

The appearance of one or more of the preceding symptoms is grounds for referral of the student for a visual screening.

Visual Acuity

Clinically, visual acuity is usually determined by use of the Snellen charts viewed at a distance of 20 feet. The individual being tested reads aloud the smallest line he or she can distinguish. The results are expressed as a fraction. The numerator of the fraction is 20, the distance at which the subject reads the chart. The denominator is the greatest distance from the chart at which an individual with normal vision can read the smallest line. Normal visual acuity is 20/20; a subject with 20/15 visual acuity has better than normal vision, and one with 20/100 visual acuity has subnormal vision.

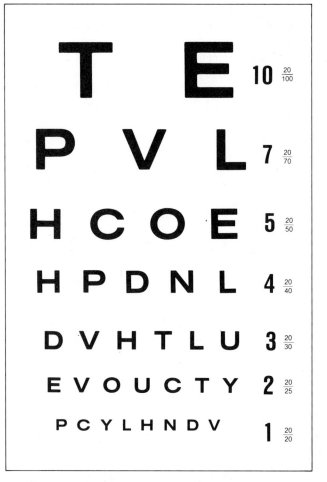

VISUAL SCREENING

Visual screening is really a simple process that can be easily performed within the school environment. The most common instruments used for vision screening are the Snellen chart and the various electronic vision screeners. Vision screening should be performed annually through elementary school and every two years after elementary school. Naturally, vision screening can be done on a referral basis anytime during the students' school experience.

Snellen Chart

The Snellen chart is a large, rectangular chart that contains letters of various sizes. The letters on the chart correlate to the visual acuity level of the individual. Figure 8.6 is an example of a Snellen chart.

A well-lit room is necessary for use of the Snellen chart. The chart is hung on a wall and a line is drawn 20 feet from the chart. A student who is to be screened stands on the line and is given a card. The individual performing the

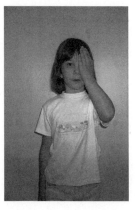

A student participating in a visual screening using the Snellen chart.

Organization of School Health Programs

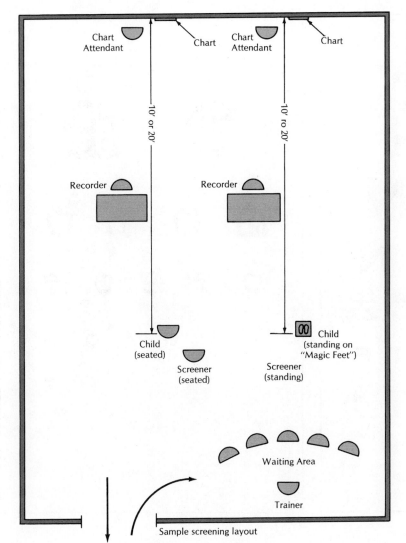

FIGURE 8.7
Proper vision screening environment.
Copyrighted by the National Society to Prevent Blindness. Reprinted by permission.

screening will ask the student to place the 3 × 5-inch card over the right eye and will point to a line of the Snellen chart. The student will then verbalize what he or she sees on the line, normally letters. The screener then replicates this process while the student holds the card over the left eye and again while the student is able to look at the chart with both eyes (Figure 8.7).

The basis for referral is if the student misses one more than half the letters or symbols on the 20/30 Snellen line. This indicates that there might be some visual problem and that it is necessary for the student to see a specialist for further testing.

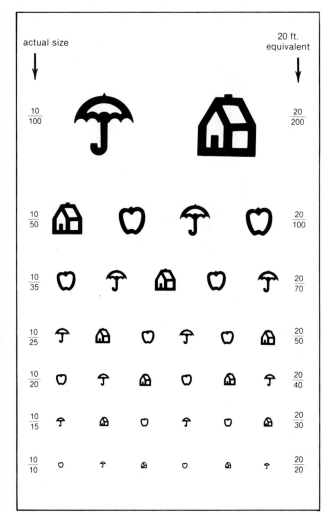

| LETTER CHART FOR 20 FEET | Faye symbol chart |

Snellen letter chart

FIGURE 8.8

Variations of the Snellen chart.

Copyrighted by the National Society to Prevent Blindness. Reprinted by permission.

Variations of the Snellen Chart

Figure 8.8 shows variations of the Snellen chart that are available. There is a need for a variety of forms, since in some cases we are screening students who cannot read and must identify in which direction the letter "E" is pointing (tumbling E Snellen chart).

Use of Glasses

If a student wears corrective lenses, then he or she should be screened wearing the glasses. It should already be apparent from the glasses that there is some visual problem and that some attempt is being made to correct it. Not allowing the student to wear the glasses would probably result in an unnecessary referral.

Organization of School Health Programs

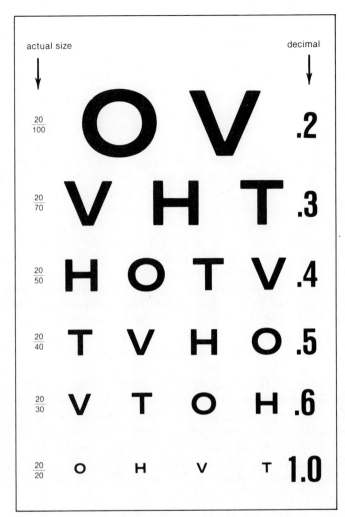

actual size

decimal

$\frac{20}{100}$	O V .2
$\frac{20}{70}$	V H T .3
$\frac{20}{50}$	H O T V .4
$\frac{20}{40}$	T V H O .5
$\frac{20}{30}$	V T O H .6
$\frac{20}{20}$	O H V T 1.0

SYMBOL CHART FOR 20 FEET

The HOTV or matching symbol test

Snellen E chart

Disadvantages of the Snellen Chart

FIGURE 8.8
Continued.

The Snellen chart is a sound and commonly used vision screening device, but it does have some minor disadvantages. First, it does not screen for astigmatism. Unless the student mentions that the letters are blurred, the screener may not refer, since the student is reading the letters correctly. Second, there is no color-perception test incorporated into the Snellen chart; therefore, it would be impossible to identify a possible color perceptual visual problem.

It should be pointed out that the Snellen chart screening is effective enough to result in the referring of over 80 percent of the students with some visual problems. In addition, the Snellen chart is very inexpensive, and there is no need for the hiring of specially trained personnel to perform the screening.

OTHER VISUAL SCREENING INSTRUMENTS

Electronic Screeners

There are a variety of electronic screening instruments available for use in visual screening. The Titmus Vision Tester is a popular type of screener and is used in schools, by ophthalmologists and optometrists, and even in the visual examination for obtaining a driver's license.

The electronic screener works on the same principle as the Snellen chart. The major difference is that in the electronic screener the visual stimuli are reproduced on a plate that is inserted into the screener. The individual being screened looks into the instrument and reads the letter he or she sees. The person performing the screening has a sheet in front of him, which shows exactly what the individual is seeing. When the individual misses some of the letters, the screener checks them off on the sheet. The basis for referral is the same as that with the regular Snellen screening.

In addition to screening for possible visual acuity problems, the electronic screeners include plates for color-perception screening. These plates are called pseudoisochromatic plates. When the plates are inserted, the individual sees a circle or a series of colored circles with a letter or number in the middle. If there are no color perceptual problems, the individual should be able to see the number or letter through the colors.

Other types of plates, such as the ocular muscle balance tests, which test the quality of the extraocular muscles, can also be inserted into the electronic screeners. Unlike using the Snellen chart for screening, all that is necessary for the electronic screener is a table to hold the portable instrument and a chair for the student. The main disadvantage of the electronic screener is the expense of the equipment. During a time when school budgets are being closely examined, administrators might not feel there is a need for sophisticated equipment.

A variety of other specific types of tests can be performed during the screening processes. Some of these other tests include the ocular muscle balance test and the convergence-near-point test. These tests are simple to conduct and could be done in almost any setting.

The Ocular Muscle Balance Test (Screen Test)

The Ocular Muscle Balance Test is a test for determining the coordination of the eyes at the reading distance of 13 to 15 inches.

This test can be done by holding a pencil about 14 inches directly in front of the pupil's eyes and have him or her look fixedly at it. Cover one eye with a 3 × 5-inch card and shift the card quickly from one eye to the other. Note whether the uncovered eye moves to find the pencil point. If there is a

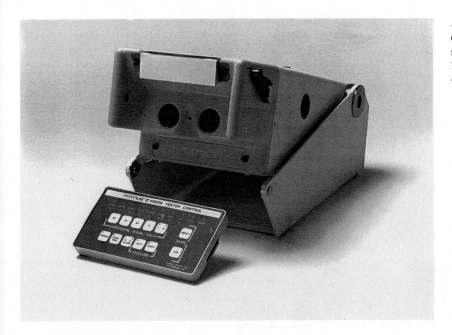

An example of an
electronic vision
screener.
*Titmus Optical Inc.,
Petersburg, Va.*

noticeable movement, refer the child for further examination. Some of the
conditions causing lack of coordination include:

1. One eye muscle stronger than its opposing muscle.
2. Faulty attachment of muscles to the eyeball.
3. Inequality of the refraction of the eyes.
4. Undeveloped fusion sense.

The practical significance of ocular muscle imbalance is that it makes it difficult for the child to maintain fusion. Fusion is impossible if the eyes are in
a state of constant imbalance.

This test should be given to all pupils having any difficulty in reading or
in other close work, if their visual acuity is normal.

The Convergence-Near-Point Test

This test is simple and is done by having the student focus on a point, such
as the top of a pencil, 13 inches straight in front and slightly below the plane
of the eyes; then have him or her follow the point as it is gradually moved
toward the top of the nose. Both eyes should converge equally until the point
reaches a distance of not more than 3 inches from the eyes. Marked failure, 5
inches or more, is an indication of convergence insufficiency. It warrants recommendation for further examination.

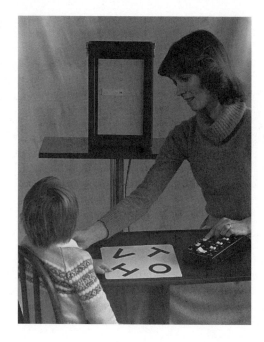

The HOTV screening procedure is a popular screening device. *Source: Good-Lite Company.*

This test determines the ability of the child to converge his or her eyes equally while fixing them on a common point. Its practical significance is that it determines the ability to easily obtain a visual image of a common point with each eye simultaneously when performing the close tasks, such as reading, writing, or fine mechanical operations.

It has been mentioned many times that the end result of screening is referral, not diagnosis. Therefore, when a visual referral is indicated, it is important that the referrals be to the right person. In most cases, the referral is to an ophthalmologist. An ophthalmologist is a physician who specializes in disorders and diseases of the eye. Many school districts refer to an optometrist. An optometrist holds a Doctor of Optometry degree from a college of optometry and is mainly concerned with diagnosing refractive errors and prescribing glasses if necessary. Many optometrists can identify other types of disorders besides refractive errors and prescribe glasses if necessary.

If indicated, the ophthalmologist can prescribe drugs or conduct surgery. The optometrist can do neither. In addition, the optometrist often must refer clients to the ophthalmologist, which can increase the expense for the visual evaluation.

HEARING

Like vision, hearing is an extremely complex process and is strongly correlated with the ability to learn. Since hearing problems are common disorders of students, it is important for the school health personnel to be aware of the major problems associated with this sense.

Organization of School Health Programs

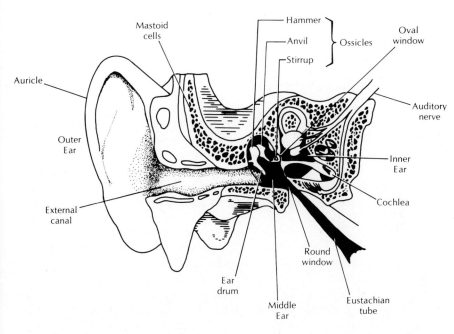

FIGURE 8.9

Anatomy of the human ear.

Source: J. Friedman, "Teacher Awareness of Hearing Disorders," in R. Haslam and P. Valletutti, Medical Problems in the Classroom *(Austin: Pro-Ed, Inc., 1975).*

Before discussing the major types of hearing problems affecting students, a brief discussion of the physiology of hearing will be presented.

Physiology of Hearing

The part of the ear most visible is the *auricle.* The auricle is a flap of skin-covered cartilage, which guards the entrance to a narrow tube called the outer ear. Within the outer ear lies a hollow chamber called the middle ear, and the coiled tubes and canals of the inner ear. (See Figure 8.9.)

The three major structures just mentioned and the smaller structures, all necessary for hearing, are shown in Figure 8.9. The process of hearing begins when sound waves fall on the outer ear and are deflected into the auditory canal. The auditory canal is protected by hairs and a wax secretion. The sound waves then reach the tympanic membrane (eardrum), which in turn vibrates in response to a wide range of frequencies. Its movements are transmitted across the chamber of the middle ear by three linked ossicles, or tiny bones, called the malleus (hammer), incus (anvil), and stapes (stirrup). These three tiny bones are suspended from the roof of the chamber by small muscles and ligaments.

The stapes, which is the bone farthest from the eardrum, vibrates with the same frequency as the eardrum but with a force more than 20 times greater. This vibration is then transmitted to fluid filling the cochlea in the inner ear.

The cochlea is a spiral chamber in the solid bone of the skull and is divided into a number of smaller chambers. The most notable of the smaller chambers is the organ of Corti. The organ of Corti responds to different frequencies of sound waves transmitted through the fluid and generates nerve impulses accordingly. The more than 30,000 fibers of the auditory nerve pick up these impulses and relay them to the brain for interpretation as either meaningful patterns of sound, such as speech or music, or meaningless and possibly disturbing noise.

Common Hearing Problems

The most common hearing problems of students are those that are caused by infection. Usually the infections result from the common cold, upper respiratory infections, or tonsil infections. The most common type of infection is termed otitis media, or middle ear infection. Otitis media is characterized by the secretion of mucus and pus from infected mucous membranes of the middle ear. If the condition is untreated, swelling and earache result. If it is still left untreated, a much more severe infection called mastoiditis can result.

Deafness

There are two types of deafness that can occur not only among students but among the general population as well. These two types are conductive deafness and sensory deafness. Conductive deafness is the most common type of deafness occurring among students and it usually does not result in a total loss of hearing. Instead, there is lessened ability to perceive sound intensity, which results in hearing losses in the low frequencies. The most common cause of conductive deafness is some impairment to the cochlea.

Sensory deafness is a term used when there is some hearing impairment as a result of the specific hair cells of the cochlea becoming damaged or not functioning properly. Again, the term *deafness* is misleading, because in this case, generally the student is not clinically deaf but rather has trouble hearing sound in the high or middle frequencies.

Finally, the accumulation of wax in the outer ear may cause some temporary loss of hearing. Simple removal of this wax by a physician will generally help to restore hearing.

Indicators of Hearing Problems

There are many indicators of possible hearing problems that can and should be noticed by a teacher or other school personnel. Table 8.2 outlines the potential problem areas and indicators of hearing problems. A student exhibiting any of these signs should be referred immediately to the school nurse.

Hearing Screening

Screening for hearing problems is an important responsibility of the schools and should be performed annually during the elementary school years and every two years after that. There are a variety of ways to do this, but the most popular, scientifically sound, and above all, accurate screening test is accomplished by using a puretone audiometer.

There are two tests that can be performed by using the puretone audiometer. The first test is called the sweep test. The sweep test is accomplished by setting the decibel (db) dial at 25 db and setting the frequency at 6000 hertz, or cycles per second. The decibel level remains constant, but the fre-

TABLE 8.2

Indicators of Possible Hearing Problems

1. Recurring otitis media (ear infection) or upper respiratory infections
2. Mouth breathing
3. Draining ears
4. Earaches
5. Frequent request to repeat things
6. Turning one side of head toward speaker
7. Talking either too loudly or too softly
8. Indistinct speech (slurring and omission of sounds)
9. Watching the lips of the speaker
10. Inattentive to classroom discussion
11. Frequently makes mistakes in following directions or taking dictation
12. Tends to isolate self, is passive and may tire easily
13. Sudden failure following severe illness

Reprinted by permission from National Association of School Nurses, Inc. Englewood, Colorado, 1984.

quency sweeps through different cycles per second. The most common cycles per second used are 6000, 4000, 2000, 1000, 500, and 250 Hz. If a student fails to hear two or more of the sounds at the different cycles per second, he or she is given the sweep test again. If two or more sounds are again missed, then the student is administered the threshold test. The primary reason for administering the sweep test again if two or more sounds are missed is to reduce the number of false referrals.

The threshold test is also performed using the puretone audiometer. In order to conduct this test, the decibel level is set at 30 db and the student is tested at frequencies from 500 Hz to the highest, 6000 Hz. If a student misses two or more sounds at 30 db or one sound at 35 db, the student is referred for a full diagnostic hearing evaluation by specialized medical personnel. Table 8.3 shows probable handicap and needs with respect to hearing level deficits.

Audiometry provides specific information relating to hearing potential. Another hearing screening that can be performed is *tympanometry,* which provides a way to determine conductive hearing loss and what conditions might be causing the loss (Micro Audiometrics, 1991). Tympanometry tests for impedance to determine if anything is impeding sound from passing through the tympanic membrane and ossicles, and inhibiting sound waves from stimulating nerves required for hearing (Micro Audiometrics, 1991).

A tympanometry screening is noninvasive and takes only three seconds to perform. During the screening a probe is placed in the ear and a seal is made. The tympanometry screening instrument measures the size of the outer

TABLE 8.3

Hearing Levels and Associated Probable Handicap and Needs

Hearing Level* ANSI 1969	Probable Handicap and Needs
26 to 40 dB Mild loss	Has difficulty hearing faint or distant speech; needs favorable seating and may benefit from lip-reading instruction.
41 to 55 dB Moderate loss	Understands conversational speech within 5 feet; needs hearing aid, auditory training, lip-reading, favorable seating, and speech conversation.
56 to 70 dB Moderately severe loss	Conversation must be loud to be understood, great difficulty in group and classroom discussion; needs all of above plus language therapy, and perhaps a special class for hard of hearing.
71 to 90 dB Severe loss	May hear a loud voice near the ear, may identify environmental noises, may distinguish vowels but not consonants; needs special education for deaf children with emphasis on speech, auditory training, and language; may enter regular classes at a later time.
More than 90 dB Profound loss	May hear some loud sounds, does not rely on hearing as primary channel for communication; needs special class or school for the deaf; some of these children eventually enter regular high schools.

*Average of hearing levels for 500, 1000, and 2000 Hz.
Adapted from: Davis H., and Silverman, D., *Hearing and Deafness,* 3rd Ed., Holt, Rinehart & Winston, New York, 1970; and Goodman, A. C., *Reference Zero Levels for Puretone Audiometers,* Mexico Audiological Series, Vol. 4, Rept. 7, 1966.
Reprinted by permission from National Association of School Nurses, Inc. Englewood, Colorado, 1984.

canal, introduces a low frequency tone and changes the air pressure in the canal. The resulting graph displayed reveals if anything is impeding sound.

A hearing screening should consist of both audiometry and tympanometry. The results of both provide a clear picture of the hearing mechanism.

HEIGHT AND WEIGHT

Height and weight screening is perhaps the most difficult type of screening that is performed in the schools. It is not difficult in terms of technique, but it is difficult in terms of deciding upon a basis for referral. Since students, for a variety of reasons, grow and develop physically at different rates, it is difficult to determine if a student is deviating from a "normal" pattern (Figures

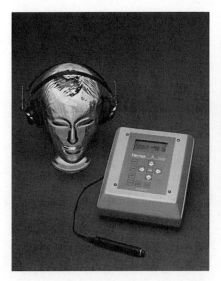

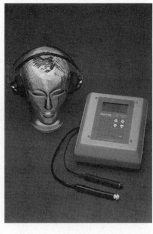

An example of a puretone audiometer. (Earscan ™ Microprocessor Puretone Audiometer).

An audiometer with tympanometry features. (Earscan ™ Acoustic Impedance MP Audiometer with data output).

8.10 and 8.11). Therefore, it is important to use a screening instrument sensitive enough to discriminate between the wide range of normal physical growth and development patterns as well as the range of possibly abnormal growth and development patterns.

The simple height and weight tables popularly published are fine for a cursory evaluation, but in order to detect a possible growth and development problem, a more specific instrument should be used. Such a grid or tool allows for a cumulative evaluation of the student; it is easy to see when a student deviates from a normal pattern.

In order to use such a grid several different measurements are necessary. First, a height and weight measurement is taken and then plotted. Second, a body (physique) type is determined. Third, the child's age is recorded. Finally, all of these measurements are cumulatively used to determine the growth and development curve of the child. The resulting curve is compared to ''normal'' curve, and if it deviates significantly, the student is referred for further examination.

These grids are somewhat complicated and it is important for yearly measurements to be taken, but it does provide for an accurate appraisal of the wide range of growth and development patterns.

Finally, most height- and weight-recording also allows for recording immunizations, health records, and comments of the school personnel. Thus, the school not only has a record of growth and development patterns, but a record of the child's health status in general.

The most sophisticated method of growth and development screening was developed in 1980 by Professor Milo Zachmann, University of Zurich, Switzerland, in conjunction with Serono Laboratories, Inc. The system is called Theoretical Growth Evaluation (TGE) and provides a fast and accurate

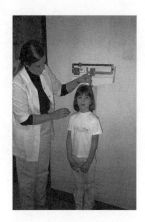

Accurate height and weight measurements are a part of the ongoing growth and development screening.

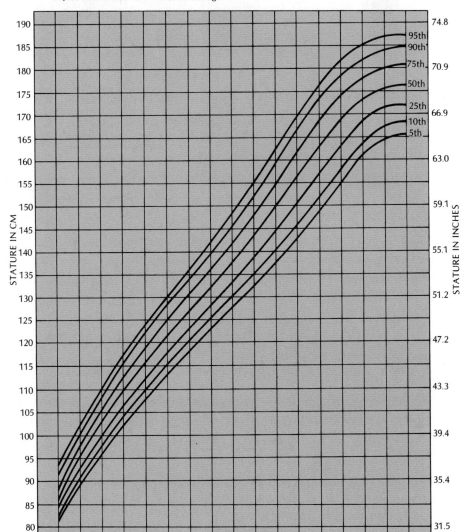

INSTRUCTIONS FOR PLOTTING HEIGHT:
1. SIDEA. Boys
2. Use washable marker.
3. Plot age in years on horizontal line;
   plot height in centimeters or inches on vertical line.
4. Take note of 5th and 95th percentile lines.
5. Just wash marker off chart and use again.

FIGURE 8.10

Height and weight, boys 2 to 18 years, NCHS percentiles.
Source: Reprinted with permission of National Center for Health Statistics.

Organization of School Health Programs

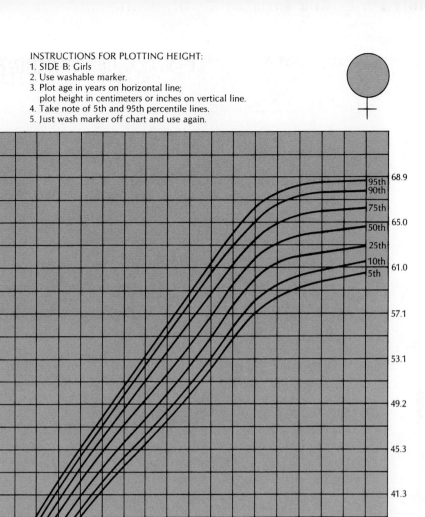

INSTRUCTIONS FOR PLOTTING HEIGHT:
1. SIDE B: Girls
2. Use washable marker.
3. Plot age in years on horizontal line;
   plot height in centimeters or inches on vertical line.
4. Take note of 5th and 95th percentile lines.
5. Just wash marker off chart and use again.

AGE IN YEARS

FIGURE 8.11

Height and weight, girls 2 to 18 years, NCHS percentiles.
Source: Reprinted with permission of National Center for Health Statistics.

Blood pressure screening is an important and often neglected screening.

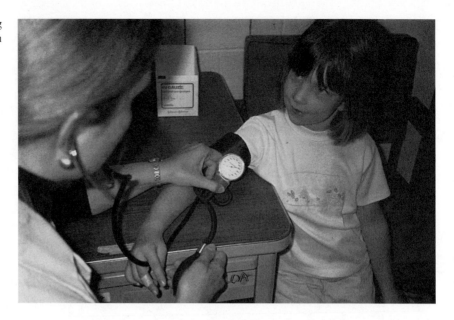

analysis of bone age using the methodologies of both Tanner and Greulich-Pyle. In addition to bone age determinations, TGE also predicts final adult height and screens for possible growth disorders.

In 1981, collaborative studies with four major medical centers were conducted to test the accuracy of TGE's computer analysis of bone age assessments. The results were statistically identical and prove great accuracy in the bone age evaluations, the computer analysis of height predictions, and possible explanations of abnormal growth patterns.

TGE may be conducted for any child age three and above. The average referral age of a child with an abnormal growth pattern is nine years. An ideal time to identify children with growth problems is as soon above age three as possible, or by the age of five, when they receive physical examinations upon entering school. The earlier a child is identified as having an abnormal growth pattern, the sooner therapy may be initiated and the full benefit of therapy can be obtained.

In the United States, there are approximately 3.6 million children (birth to thirteen years of age) who are above the 95th percentile or below the 5th percentile in growth and development.

BLOOD PRESSURE

Screening for blood pressure problems is a relatively new concept in the school setting. The main reason for this is that it is very difficult to develop normal parameters for what a child's blood pressure should be. The use of the normal adult ranges of 100–140 mm Hg systolic and 60–90 mm Hg diastolic would be too great for children and would almost certainly indicate some early blood pressure problem.

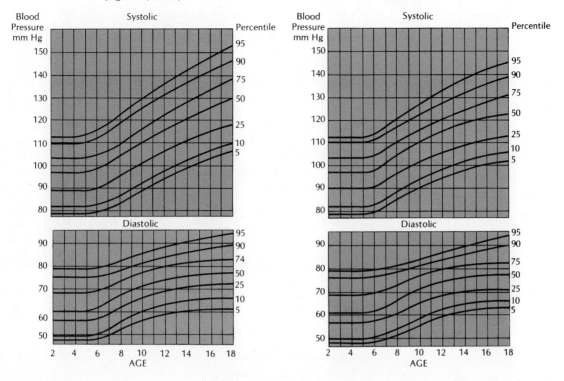

Percentiles of Blood Pressure Measurement in Boys
(Right arm, seated)

Percentiles of Blood Pressure Measurement in Girls
(Right arm, seated)

For years concerned school personnel and health professionals have stated that it is important to screen for blood pressure; only now it is becoming more of a reality. The main reason for this is that high blood pressure is a major heart disease risk factor. This is important, since it is now generally accepted that the prevention of heart disease begins in childhood. Children and adolescents with hypertension are almost always asymptomatic, so detection depends on detection of possible abnormal blood pressure. Blood pressure should be taken annually.

Blood pressure is simply a measure of the pressure of blood against the arterial wall. It is measured with an instrument called a sphygmomanometer. The sphygmomanometer measures the blood pressure in millimeters of mercury (mm Hg). The following procedures should be used when conducting a blood pressure screening.

"The examining area should be quiet. The child should be reassured, and sufficient time should be allowed for recovery from apprehension or recent activity. The student should be seated comfortably and the right arm should be supported at mid-chest level. The largest cuff that will snugly fit the child's arm should be selected. Not only should the inflatable bladder width cover most of the arm, but its length should encircle the entire arm without overlapping. The cuff is then rapidly inflated to about 30 mm Hg above the point at

FIGURE 8.12

Percentiles of blood pressure measurement in boys and girls.
Source: Reprinted with permission of National Center for Health Statistics.

Cholesterol screening is becoming a more common screening procedure.

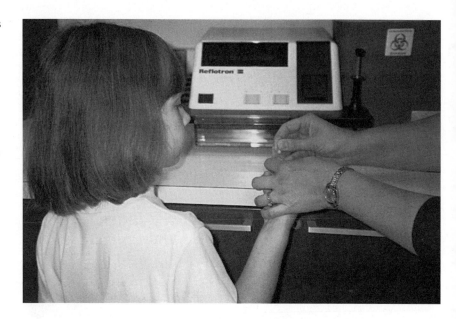

which the radial pulse disappears. It is then slowly deflated while auscultation (listening for pulse) is performed over the brachial artery. As the cuff is deflated, onset of a clear tapping sound corresponds to systolic blood pressure; with further deflation, muffling of the tapping corresponds to diastolic blood pressure'' (Weidman, 1979, p. 213).

Taking blood pressure is simple and painless. The blood pressure levels in Figure 8.12 represent the average systolic and diastolic pressures of various age groups at rest. Referring students between the ages of 6 and 16 is determined by systolic or diastolic readings 10 percent above average. It is important to note that this does not indicate hypertension. If a student does present a blood pressure over the 10 percent figure, a number of different readings should be taken, since many variables can cause a one-time elevation of blood pressure. ''Measurements between the 90th and 95th percentile on repeated measurement can be considered borderline hypertensive, perhaps at a higher risk of later development of sustained hypertension'' (Weidman, 1979, p. 213).

CHOLESTEROL SCREENING

Coronary heart disease is the leading cause of death in the United States. Atherosclerotic coronary artery disease, the most common form of heart disease, refers to a build-up of a fatty substance (atheroma) in the coronary arteries that provide the heart muscle with blood.

A major risk factor for the development of atherosclerotic coronary artery disease is a diet high in saturated fat and cholesterol. This fatty build-up in coronary arteries begins in childhood. Because the dangers of high cholesterol are so well publicized it has become a common practice for adults to test their

Organization of School Health Programs

cholesterol level. However, it is relatively uncommon for the cholesterol levels of children to be known which does present a problem since, according to studies by Davidson, about 10 percent of children 9 to 10 years of age have blood cholesterol levels exceeding the upper limit advised for adults (Davidson, 1989). As a result there has been some concern that not enough is being done to determine children's cholesterol levels.

Determining cholesterol levels can be a very simple procedure. The simplest procedure involves using a unit called a Boehringer Mannheim Reflotron or Reflotron for short. The Reflotron provides results within three minutes, is a reliable measure of cholesterol and inexpensive (generally less than $2.00 per test).

During a cholesterol screening the school nurse or other health professional obtains a one- to two-drop sample of blood using a lancet and pricking the student's finger. This small blood sample is then analyzed by the Reflotron and provides almost immediate feedback as to the student's cholesterol level.

Once the screening is complete, parents are notified about the results of the screening test—naturally if the results indicate a high cholesterol level, a referral is necessary for a retest to verify that a problem might exist.

The most common problem associated with cholesterol screenings is some students' anxiety to getting their finger pricked with the lancet. Students should never be forced to have this procedure done. If the screener cannot talk the student out of his or her anxiety, it is best to make a notation to screen that student at some point in the near future.

A second problem involves the potential for possibly using a dirty lancet. If the lancet doesn't get thrown away immediately after use, there is the potential that the screener might use the dirty lancet to prick the next student's finger. Therefore, it is important that protocol be developed stating that the lancet should be thrown away immediately after pricking the finger before getting the blood sample.

Because modern technology has made cholesterol screening economical and time efficient, it is expected that more and more school districts will provide this screening for students. It is comforting to know that the schools are in a position to not only help prevent heart disease through education but also identify those students who are at risk because of high cholesterol.

POSTURE

Kyphosis, lordosis, and scoliosis are common posture abnormalities seen in the school-age child. All of these conditions are deformities of the musculo-skeletal system, and in severe instances they can be crippling. Kyphosis is a disorder that results in a round-back deformity and usually occurs in the 11- to 16-year-old age group. Lordosis is a swayback disorder also seen in this age group. The most common and severe of the posture abnormalities is scoliosis. Scoliosis is a lateral curvature, side to side, of the spine, and is most commonly observed in the 12- to 16-year-old age group, occurring more frequently in females than in males—approximately an 8:1 ratio. The incidence

School nurses are a valuable resource for conducting posture screenings.

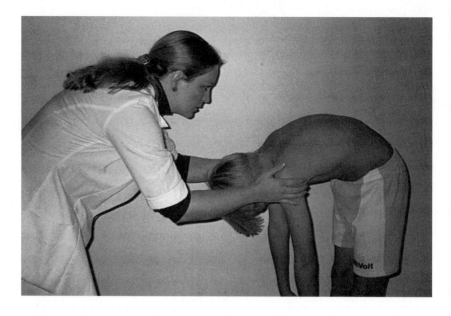

of scoliosis in the 12- to 16-age group is estimated to be 4.5 percent (Wallace, 1977, pp. 619–620). The student with scoliosis will have one scapula (shoulder blade) more prominent than the other as well as one shoulder or hip higher than the other.

The cause of scoliosis is unknown. If scoliosis is discovered early before growth is complete, nonsurgical treatment can be applied with extremely successful results. The treatment of scoliosis depends upon the extent of the curvature, the location of the curvature, and the age of the student. An X ray of the spine is used to measure curves. Curves of 20 to 44 degrees are usually managed by use of a special brace. Curves of 45 degrees and above need surgical correction. Ideally, the earlier a brace is applied, the better is the chance of correcting the condition and without surgery. For example, a student of 16 or older with a 40- to 50-degree curve is unlikely to benefit by a brace because growth is probably almost complete.

Screening for scoliosis can be a very simple procedure. Since a shirt or blouse must be removed for screening, physical education classes provide an ideal setting for screenings. However, whether entire classes are screened or individual students are screened in the nurse's office, it is important that the person conducting the screening be experienced and capable of identifying the following conditions:

1. Shoulders not level or even.
2. Obvious spinal curvatures.
3. Ribs prominent on one side.
4. Increased swayback.
5. Increased round back.
6. Unequal hip prominence.
7. Arm to body space unequal. [Wallace, 1977, pp. 619–620]

Organization of School Health Programs

Students who exhibit one or more of the preceding signs are referred for further posture evaluation.

HEALTH EXAMINATIONS

The appraisal of a student's overall level of health can be made best through a comprehensive health examination. This examination must be performed by a physician. Some of the key features of a comprehensive health examination include a health history and a physical evaluation.

The health history provides useful medical information to the physician. This history should include biographical information, history of illnesses, description of any present illness, family medical history, psychological and social developmental information, and any other information deemed necessary by the physician.

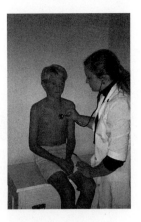

Simple physical examinations should be included as a part of a school screening program.

The physical evaluation includes a clinical physical examination. This exam normally includes an assessment and evaluation of the following: the skin; head, skull, face; eyes; ears; nose, mouth, throat; neck; chest; cardiovascular system; respiratory system; gastrointestinal and excretory systems; and musculoskeletal system. It also should include a neurological evaluation.

In most cases this exam is done in a physician's office. The health examination is necessary for two reasons. First, this exam will help to identify any health problems; second, it will generate baseline data on the student and can be used for comparison later. A comprehensive health examination should be done before a student enters school and about every three to four years thereafter.

Other types of health examinations include a periodic health examination and a referral health examination. The periodic health examination is less intensive than the comprehensive health examination but should be conducted in essentially the same manner. Results of the periodic health examination can be compared with the results of the previous comprehensive health examinations. The referral health examination is just what the name implies, that is, a health examination that is done as a result of a health referral.

DENTAL HEALTH SCREENINGS

By age 17, 94 percent of children and youth experience dental health problems requiring medical intervention (McCormack, 1990). Dental health screenings provide major benefits, but can be very expensive, since they require the services of dentists, dental hygienists, or both. In some areas of the United States, dental health screenings in the school, like many other screenings, are performed by public health dentists. If this is the case, the cost to the school or district is minimal.

Students participating in a dental health screening should be screened for the following:

1. Dental caries: decayed, missing, and filled teeth and surfaces
2. Condition of the gingivae (gums)
3. Debris and calculus on the teeth

4. Need for periodontal treatment
5. Orthodontic needs
6. Any conditions needing immediate attention, such as those likely to cause pain or infection
7. Any oral disorders or abnormalities, e.g., enamel defects such as opacities, pigmentation or hypoplasia or lesions that might be precancerous. [Rebich et al., 1982, pp. 50–53]

A complete dental screening and recording of findings when performed by an experienced team can take as little as 5 to 8 minutes per student (Rebich et al., 1982, p. 51).

Since large numbers of students will be referred after a dental health screening, some districts and schools have eliminated them and concentrate on dental health education programs for their students. Despite large numbers of referrals it is important for students to participate in a dental health screening. The benefits derived from such a screening should far outweigh the costs. Dental health education should not be considered a substitute for dental health screenings but rather a complement to the screenings.

Finally, with the increasing use of dental sealants on teeth it is likely that less youth will experience such problems as dental caries. Sealants literally seal the tooth, making the development of caries more difficult. In the near future, it is likely that application of sealants will be a part of dental health screenings.

HEALTH OF THE FEET

An often ignored area in discussions of screening is the health of the feet. It is an important area to discuss, since 85 percent of the girls and 65 percent of the boys in high school have foot defects by the time they graduate. These problems start very early in life, especially between the ages of two and six. It is during this time that the bony structures of the feet are soft and incomplete, and if certain conditions occur, these bones can become misshapened and weak.

Nearly all defects and deformities of the feet could have been prevented if students had worn both shoes and hosiery that fit properly and were of the correct type, especially during formative years. Some basic guidelines to follow in selecting the correct type of shoes and socks include the following:

1. A shoe should have a flexible sole. It should provide adequate support under the arch and fit snugly but not tightly around the heel.
2. To eliminate the pressure on toes caused by tight socks, a sock that is one-half inch longer than the longest toes should be worn.
3. Socks should be capable of keeping the feet dry under conditions of heat, cold, dampness, and perspiration induced by extreme activity.
4. Bulky socks, especially in tight-fitting shoes, tend to produce irritations that frequently result in calluses, corns, or blisters.

5. Shoes and socks should be examined frequently to be sure that the student's foot has not outgrown either. [American Podiatric Medical Association]

School personnel should keep in mind the preceding five points and cover podiatry units in the classroom so that students themselves are aware of the importance of proper footwear. This information should be made available to parents so that they can select proper footwear for their children.

HEALTH RECORDS

A student health record provides the school with important physical, mental, and social information about the student. The record provides a good document for following a student's physical, mental, and social development over time and helps to identify any deviation from his or her normal status or progress.

There are many standard health record forms available that have been developed specifically for use in schools. The health record form or card selected for use should have substantial space available for recording parental information, observations of teachers, findings of health examinations, screenings of test results, reports or findings from intellectual or psychological evaluations, as well as space available for any other important information regarding a particular student.

The health record should be considered as important a document as a student's school records. Therefore, the health record should follow a student from school to school or district to district just as academic records do.

The information in the health record must be objective, not subjective. Objective information is clear and less likely to be misinterpreted. Subjective information can be easily misinterpreted. Therefore, it is important that written policies and procedures be developed that specifically state who is able to record information in the health records, how the information is to be recorded, when information is to be recorded, and who has access to the health record. It is imperative that the policies stress confidentiality.

REFERRAL AND FOLLOW-UP

Obviously, the health appraisal activities discussed throughout this chapter are critical to the success of the health services component of the school health program. Not only is the appraisal component important, but the quality of the referral and follow-up processes is also critical.

The referral process is usually initiated in one of two ways. First, during the screening process, a particular student is found to have some potential health problem and is referred to the family physician or school nurse. Second, a teacher makes an observation that a student might have a health problem and refers the student to the school nurse. The first instance, in a sense, is a simple referral, since some screening measure has singled out a student. The second instance, however, is a bit more complicated.

Usually when a teacher notices some possible health problem, he or she will note the name of the student on a preprinted form and send this form to the school nurse. The nurse can then conduct an independent screening or, if necessary, refer the student immediately.

Regardless of the process used, as soon as a referral begins, several conferences need to be organized. These conferences include conferences between the teacher and the nurse, the parent and the nurse, and the student and the nurse.

Teacher–Nurse Conference

The purpose of the teacher–nurse conference is to coordinate the health and educational needs of the student and to exchange information about the health of the student, formally or informally. Some key conference points include:

1. Schedule conferences periodically throughout the school year. In secondary schools, the teacher's planning period may be a good time.
2. Prepare a list of problems or items that need discussing. List of health problems should not be distributed at random.
3. For known cases of handicapping conditions, a conference should be scheduled at the start of the school year to discuss any modifications of the classroom that may be necessary.
4. The teacher should be encouraged to keep a record of his or her observations of children who cause concern.
5. Extensive planning should be done for children, such as diabetics and epileptics, who might need special assistance quickly.
6. A time should be scheduled when the persons involved will not be interrupted. [Vincent, 1976, pp. 37–39]

Parent–Nurse Conference

The purpose of the parent–nurse conference is to clarify goals or actions, to monitor progress that may have occurred with respect to a particular health problem, and to recommend follow-up procedures for a health problem that has been identified. Some suggestions for successful parent–nurse conferences include the following points:

1. The conference may be held at school or in the home.
2. Prepare for the conference by reviewing health records, results of screening procedures, conferences with appropriate school personnel, and other agencies if necessary.
3. Encourage parental conversation by the use of open-ended questions that do not suggest or limit the answer, such as "How do you feel about this problem?" and "Tell me about it."
4. Repeat questionable statements so that everyone understands what each is trying to tell the other.

Organization of School Health Programs

5. Use simple, easy-to-understand language.
6. Assist the family in identifying and using community, state, and local services and resources if this need is indicated. [Vincent, 1976, pp. 37–39]

Student–Nurse Conference

The purposes of student–nurse conferences are to provide an opportunity for the student to discuss his or her other health concerns, to help the student make a responsible decision, and to obtain up-to-date information on the health status of the individual. Some suggestions for successful student–nurse conferences include the following points:

1. Schedule an initial conference with all new students entering the school.
2. Each student from K through 12 should have a health conference during the year.
3. Accept the student's statement as a valid report on how he [or she] feels at present. The primary child often becomes ''ill'' under pressure. Family changes can also initiate ''illnesses.''
4. Try to identify factors that may be affecting the individual—for instance, the frequency of visits to the health room.
5. Involve the student in the management of his [or her] problem, providing him [or her] with possible alternatives and avenues of assistance.
6. Use open-ended questions that do not suggest or limit the answers. [Vincent, 1976, pp. 37–39]

Finally, it is important to note that even though a student is referred for further medical evaluation, the whole referral process does not end at that point. It is easy for a student to get lost in a referral process or through ''red tape.'' Therefore, it is important for all school personnel to follow up on the referral. This follow-up procedure is not necessarily complicated, and in its pure form, might be simply asking a question of someone about the student. However, notations in the student's medical record or health form should include room for comments regarding follow-up from referrals.

SUMMARY

Health appraisal is considered by some school health professionals to be the most important aspect of health services in the school setting. As can be seen by the information presented in this chapter, there are many important and comprehensive activities necessary to carry out the process of health appraisal.

School personnel have a responsibility to detect possible health problems. The detection of possible health problems should be one of the major goals of the health appraisal component of the school health program. Through employing the activities covered in this chapter, this goal can be achieved.

REVIEW QUESTIONS

1. What is the main purpose of teacher observation?
2. Describe several vision disorders and the probable effect these disorders will have on student performance.
3. Describe several types of vision screening instruments.
4. What are the major indicators of potential hearing problems?
5. Describe other health screenings that can be performed in the school setting besides vision and hearing.
6. Discuss the major components to referral and follow-up.
7. Identify conditions that may be indicators of potential health problems.

REFERENCES

American Optometric Association (AOA).*Your School-Age Child's Eyes.* St. Louis: American Optometric Association, 1986.

Cass, R., and P. Kaplan. ''Middle Ear Disease and Learning Problems: A School System's Approach to Early Detection.'' *Journal of School Health* **49:**10 (December 1979), 557–559.

Davidson, D. M., B. J. Bradley, S. M. Landry, C. A. Iftner, and S. M. Brambett. ''School Based Cholesterol Screening.'' *Journal of Pediatric Health Care,* **3:**1 (Jan/Feb, 1989).

''Mail-in Height-Prediction Service Spots Potential Shrimps and Bean Poles.'' *Medical World News* (December 6, 1982), 47–48.

McCormack-Brown, K., E. M. Vitello, R. J. McDermott, and C. E. Richardson. ''Development of the Dental Health Assessment Profile.'' *Journal of School Health* **60:**9 (November, 1990), 455–458.

Micro Audiometrics. *Tympanometry and Hearing.* South Daytona: Florida. Micro Audiometrics, 1991.

Miller, D., and C. Lever. ''Scoliosis Screening: An Approach Used in the School.'' *Journal of School Health* **52:**2 (February 1982), 98–102.

National Society to Prevent Blindness. *Vision Screening of Children.* New York: National Society to Prevent Blindness, 1979.

Rebich, T., J. Kumar, B. Brustman, and E. Green. ''The Need for Dental Health Screening and Referral Program.'' *Journal of School Health* **52:**1 (January 1982), 50–53.

Serono Laboratories. *Experts in Children's Growth Disorders Stress the Value of Computerized Growth Evaluation.* New York: Serono Laboratories, 1982.

U.S. Department of Health, Education, and Welfare. *Vision Screening of Children.* Washington, D.C.: USDHEW, 1971.

Vargo, S. W. ''Auditory Screening in the Schools—Failure or Success?'' *Journal of School Health* **50:**1 (January 1980), 32–34.

Vincent, E. *The School Health Program: A Guide to Responsibilities.* Dover: Delaware Department of Public Instruction, 1976.

Wallace, A. ''A Scoliosis Screening Program.'' *Journal of School Health* **47:**10 (December 1977), 619–620.

Webster, K. ''Planning and Implementing Health Screening Programs.'' *Journal of School Health* **50:**9 (November 1980), 493–495.

Weidman, W. H. ''High Blood Pressure and the School-Age Child.'' *Journal of School Health* **49:**4 (April 1979), 213–214.

Communicable Disease Control

9

T he fact that the school health program is an extension of the public health program has been stressed throughout the entire text. It is sometimes difficult to separate responsibilities where the health of students is concerned, since the school health program and the public health program share the responsibilities.

Communicable disease control is an area where the overlapping of responsibilities is most noticeable. The simple fact that children are grouped together in a school setting provides an easy mode of transmission for many communicable diseases. This grouping in many cases poses a serious public health problem. Identifying diseases in a school setting and sending a student home constitute a form of disease control. This aids public health efforts in controlling the spread of communicable diseases.

This chapter will focus on the facts concerning the various organisms responsible for communicable diseases, a discussion of the body barriers to disease, a description of the infectious disease process, and recommended school policies in relation to communicable diseases. These are all important points for school personnel to understand so that their role in both intervention and prevention can be maximized.

PATHOGENS

A pathogen is a disease-causing organism. Several other terms are used to describe various organisms, including *agents, microorganisms,* and *germs.* However, not all agents, microorganisms, and germs cause disease. *Pathogen* is a term that exclusively means ''disease-causing.''

There are six major types of pathogens. These include bacteria, viruses, fungi, protozoans, parasitic worms (metazoans), and rickettsia. Each form of pathogen has unique characteristics that cause specific responses from the human body when the body is invaded by it (Tables 9.1 and 9.2).

Bacteria

Bacteria are microscopic single-celled plants capable of producing different types of infections. *Bacteria* and *disease* often are thought of as being synonymous terms. However, of the thousands of different kinds of bacteria, only about 100 are pathogenic, or disease-causing to humans. As a matter of fact, certain types of bacteria are important and aid the individual. For example, we have indigenous microbiota in our large intestine, which aid in the digestive process. Any disruption of these bacteria can cause serious consequences. This relationship, where we depend upon bacteria and the bacteria depend on us for survival, is symbiosis, a term commonly used in ecology.

Table 9.1

Major Pathogen Groups

Illustrative Plate	Group and Size Scale	Description	Examples of Diseases Caused	Mode of Action
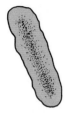	Viruses (10 to 250 nanometers*)	Minute, submicroscopic particles composed of nucleic acids and protein; intracellular parasites	Rabies, polio, yellow fever, colds, influenza	Disrupt protein synthesis of cells, sometimes kill cells
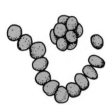	Rickettsia (less than 1 micrometer*)	Small bacteria always associated with insects and other arthropods	Typhus fever; Rocky Mountain spotted fever; Q-fever	Interfere with metabolism of host cells; all are intracellular parasites
	Bacteria (1 to 10 micrometers)	Single-celled, plantlike; abundant in the biosphere; secrete disease-causing toxins; are commonly found in a rod, spiral, or spherical shape	Tuberculosis, syphilis, pneumonia, scarlet fever, boils, meningitis	Produce toxins and enzymes that destroy cells or interfere with their function

*A nanometer is one billionth of a meter; a micrometer is one millionth of a meter; a meter is 39.37 inches.
Reprinted by permission from Jones, Shainberg, and Byer, *Dimensions* (New York: Harper & Row, 1979), p. 416.

Most bacteria come in one of three shapes: round, spiral, and rodlike. Cocci are round bacteria, while bacillus bacteria appear as rod-shaped when viewed under a microscope. Bacteria invade the body through many different portals. The common portals of entry include the lungs, skin, nose, urinary tract, or mouth.

Once bacteria invade the body, they can localize in specific areas or organs of the body or, in some cases, they can be disseminated throughout the body. Once inside the body, most bacteria proliferate in the intestine. Proliferation means that the bacteria find a suitable environment for dividing through the process called binary fission—one cell simply becoming two, two becoming four, and so on—until the division process is stopped. Inflammation can be a response of the human body to a bacterial invasion.

Major Pathogen Groups

Illustrative Plate	Group and Size Scale	Description	Examples of Diseases Caused	Mode of Action
	Fungi (a few micrometers to several inches)	Single-celled or multicelled plantlike organisms; consist of threadlike fibers and reproductive spores, molds	Athlete's foot; most commonly diseases of the skin, hair, nails, and lungs	Release enzymes that digest cells
	Protozoa (a few to 250 micrometers)	Microscopic animals; each is single-celled	Malaria, amebic dysentery, and African sleeping sickness	Release enzymes and toxins that destroy cells or interfere with their functions
	Parasitic worms (1/32 inch to 20 to 30 feet)	Multicellular animals; common types are round or flat	Pinworm, trichinosis, tapeworms,	Release toxins; compete for foods; block digestive tract and blood and lymph vessels

Even though the types of bacteria are structurally similar, they will destroy human cells and tissues in different ways. For example, the most virulent bacterium, called *Clostridium botulin,* secretes exotoxins, which are lethal poisons. These exotoxins can kill human cells upon release, or they can impair the basic processes of the cells. Another example of a virulent bacterium is staphylococcus. Staphylococci are capable of producing certain enzymes or catalysts that can act upon connective tissue. The range of bacterial infection varies, depending upon the type of bacteria, the common areas of proliferation, and whether or not the bacteria secrete exotoxins or specific enzymes capable of destroying human tissue.

There is a wide range of diseases associated with bacterial infections. Some of these diseases are staphylococcal infections, meningitis, enteric

TABLE 9.2

Childhood Diseases

Disease	Pathogen	Incubation Period	Common Symptoms
Poliomyelitis (polio)	Poliovirus types 1, 2, and 3	Usually about 7–12 days	Fever, headache, stiff back and neck, gastrointestinal disorder, often followed by paralysis
Infectious parotitis (mumps)	Paramyxovirus	12–26 days	Fever, swelling and tenderness of the parotid glands (near the ears) and other salivary glands
Rubella (3-day or German measles)	Rubella virus	14–21 days	Fever, malaise, swelling of lymph nodes, blotchy rash spreading from face to trunk*
Rubella (10-day measles)	Measles virus	8–13 days	Fever, conjunctivitis, cold-type symptoms, bronchitis, blotchy rash that spreads from face all over skin
Varicella (chickenpox)	Varicelia-zoster virus	2–3 weeks	Fever, malaise, widespread eruptions of the skin and mucous membranes, appearing first on the face and trunk
Pertussis (whooping cough)	*Hemophilus pertussis* bacterium	7–14 days	Early, mild nighttime cough; late, severe spasmodic cough, followed by loud whoop and expulsion of a thick, clear mucus

*If acquired by a woman in the early months of pregnancy, rubella may be passed on to the fetus, who may suffer retardation, deafness, cardiac defects, and other serious complications.
Reprinted by permission from *Health Today*. New York: Macmillan Publishing Co. 1983, pg. 424.

bacterial infections, gonorrhea, syphilis, tetanus, botulism, diphtheria, whooping cough, plaque, tularemia, typhoid fever, brucellosis, leprosy, and tuberculosis. Naturally, some of these infections are more serious and devastating than others, and not all will be seen in the school setting, owing to specific laws regarding immunization for the school-age child.

The more common bacterial diseases frequently observed in the school setting include staphylococcal infections and streptococcal infections. Both of these infections have the potential for becoming serious.

Staphylococcus bacteria are spherical microorganisms that usually appear in irregularly shaped clusters. Various strains of staph cause such disorders as boils, food poisoning, and certain types of pneumonia. Both the skin and internal organs are vulnerable to staph infection.

The principal symptom of staph infection is the appearance of a pus-filled skin infection, which may take the form of a boil or abscess. Pus draining from the infected area is a prime source of contagion. Once the pus is gone, there is no danger of infection spreading. The most serious situation is when the pathogens infect the lungs, causing staphylococcal pneumonia, or when the pathogens are carried by the bloodstream to other body organs.

Streptococci are spherical-shaped pathogens that form chains rather than clusters. Among the strep pathogens, the most important in human disease are the hemolytic streptococci, which produce a substance that destroys red blood cells. These pathogenic agents are responsible for streptococcal sore throat, scarlet fever, rheumatic fever, and streptococcal pneumonia.

For most bacterial infections, antibiotics are the treatment drugs of choice. The antibiotics will destroy the bacteria and, in most cases, give the infected person an excellent prospect of recovery. Normal body defenses, which will be discussed later, are also important in recovery from bacterial infections.

A bacterial disease that has received much publicity in recent years is Lyme disease. Lyme disease is caused by a spirochete that is commonly carried on a certain species of deer tick. If an infected deer tick attaches itself to a human for a period of time, millions of spirochetes are transferred to the person and the potential result is a case of Lyme disease.

Lyme disease has received much attention because it is an enigmatic disease. Its symptoms mimic other diseases and, as a result, Lyme disease often goes undiagnosed or misdiagnosed. Most commonly reported are typical flu-like symptoms and a rash that usually appears within a few weeks after being bitten by the infected tick.

Lyme disease can become particularly dangerous if it progresses beyond the flulike symptoms and rash. Neurological problems, cardiac disorders, and chronic arthritis are serious complications of untreated Lyme disease. Early medical intervention which includes use of antibiotics is recommended.

As with most communicable diseases there is a strong prevention component. Lyme disease prevention includes knowing where the disease is likely to occur geographically and what a person living in a high-risk area should do.

The highest incidence of Lyme disease is reported in Connecticut, Rhode Island, New York, Georgia, New Jersey, Wisconsin, and Pennsylvania. While these states do represent a variety of climates and areas, it is important to note that wherever the deer tick thrives so does the potential for Lyme disease. Since the bacteria-causing Lyme disease can be carried on migratory birds, it is possible that more and more states will be reporting cases of Lyme disease.

The personal health behaviors most important in protecting oneself from Lyme disease include (University of California, 1990):

1. When walking through wooded areas or fields, wear a long-sleeved shirt with buttoned cuffs. The shirt should be tucked into pants and the pant legs should be tucked into socks or boots.

2. Light-colored fabrics should be worn so that ticks can be easily spotted.
3. Insect repellent should be sprayed on pants, socks, and shoes.
4. When walking or hiking stay near the center of trails.
5. Check occasionally for ticks when standing or walking through underbrush or wooded areas.
6. Always check your entire body after being outdoors. Have someone look at your back and head if possible.

Finally, the classroom teacher and school nurse are in strategic positions to help prevent Lyme disease. Both must educate students as to what Lyme disease is, especially if living in a high-risk area. Also, information about Lyme disease should be distributed to parents as well so that they can in turn make sure that they and their children take the proper precautions.

Viruses

Viruses are perhaps the most complex, dangerous, and medically baffling form of pathogen. Viral infections can range from the common cold to acquired immune deficiency syndrome (AIDS). Simply, viruses are particles of genetic material (DNA or RNA) with a protein coat. Once a virus invades a specific cell, it proliferates inside the host cell, utilizing the genetic material inside the cell for its own purposes. The virus cannot replicate by itself as the bacteria can; therefore, it must become a parasite on the host cell if it is to replicate.

Viruses are the smallest of all pathogens. Further, scientists are not really sure if a virus is living or dead, since it has properties of both states. Recently, viruses have been linked to all forms of diseases that have an unknown etiology, such as cancer.

Since the virus is somewhat disguised, it is difficult for medical doctors to determine the type of infection. This is why people are often told, ''You have a virus.'' This is no simple blood test for a virus, which at times makes it impossible to determine the etiology of the disease unless it is a very common form of viral infection, such as measles or chicken pox.

The most common viral infections seen in the school setting include the common cold, influenza, and infectious mononucleosis. All of these diseases are potentially serious.

The most common viral infection of the upper respiratory tract is the common cold. One reason that the common cold is so common is that the pathogen involved can be any one of more than 100 different types of viruses. These viruses are easily spread through direct contact or via droplets expelled from the nose or mouth by coughing and sneezing.

The infection may be confined to the mucous membranes of the nose, or it may affect the throat or larynx too. Coughing, sneezing, itchy or sore throat, and general malaise are the most common symptoms. Usually these symptoms do not persist longer than one week.

Influenza is much more severe than the common cold. Influenza is characterized by sudden fever, coughing, headache, chills, and prostration. Most students will recover in about two to seven days. The great public health danger posed by influenza stems from the characteristic swift spread of the infection, the nearly universal susceptibility to it, and the variety and number of the viral pathogens that cause it.

Infectious mononucleosis is caused by the Epstein–Barr virus. This disease usually strikes children and young adults, sometimes in epidemic outbreaks. Along with such common symptoms of viral infection as sore throat and fever, mononucleosis is characterized by general fatigue, swollen lymph glands, and a high lymphocyte count. In children, the symptoms of mononucleosis can be so mild as to pass unnoticed. The principal immediate danger for young adults is the possibility of rupturing the swollen spleen. Because of this, treatment initially centers around keeping the victim as inactive as possible.

Herpes infections are caused by two kinds of herpes viruses, properly labeled type I and type II. Most people harbor type I viruses, which lie dormant in the body after an initial childhood infection. Emotional stress will trigger a recurrence of infection. Most recurrences take the form of cold sores on the lips or canker sores in the mouth. These usually disappear within 10 days.

Type II, a more serious infection, is normally transmitted venerally; the symptoms include small, painful blisters, usually in the genital area, sometimes accompanied by fever. Like type I, the virus may subside and recur periodically.

Acquired immune deficiency syndrome (AIDS) is perhaps the most publicized viral infection in recent years. Since AIDS is so serious and has such a well-defined prevention protocol, we have decided to provide an expanded discussion on AIDS in Chapter 13.

For the most part, treatment for viruses depends mainly upon the host's ability to destroy the virus through natural methods. At the present time, there is no antiviral chemical, like an antibiotic, that can be administered to the patient to reduce the viral infection. It is primarily because of this that certain viral infections are deadly. Unless the host has the ability to reduce the infection through natural methods, the consequences can be quite severe.

With many viral infections, once the body fights the infection, the individual can maintain immunity to the infection. This means that if that virus is introduced into the system again, the body will react against it, so that physiologically, it is unable to proliferate. However, the immune system does vary with each individual.

One of the most promising recent discoveries for fighting viruses is called *interferon,* a chemical released from virally infected cells. Interferon will not protect the cell being invaded, but there is evidence that it will protect surrounding cells from being invaded by the viruses. However, until discoveries like interferon are perfected and widely and successfully used in treatment, the physician is limited to basically treating symptoms of a viral infection and not the attacking virus itself.

Fungi

Fungi are classified as plants that lack chlorophyll. Fungal infections are very common and, for the most part, are not particularly dangerous. Most fungi live on the skin and only occasionally cause minor discomfort. Other types of fungi are found in the oral cavity and the digestive system, where they can live with the normal bacterial flora without being destroyed. Most fungi have a limited ability to cause disease; however, fungi may produce serious localized or systemic infections in individuals who are susceptible. The two major factors that predispose individuals to systemic fungal infections are a disturbance in the normal bacterial flora and an impaired immunologic defense.

There are types of fungal infections that can be quite serious; these are called primary disseminated fungal infections. With these infections, the proliferation and action of the fungi are not on the external parts of the body, such as with athlete's foot; instead, the fungi proliferate on the inside of the body in specialized areas such as the lungs. This type of fungal infection can stay localized in one spot, with the host displaying mild symptoms such as a rash and fever; or it can be released from a single area, to become a systemic infection that affects other organs of the body. Although it must be mentioned that systemic fungal infections are rare, they do occur and can be a serious, if not fatal, condition.

The treatment of localized, external fungal infections is primarily topical. Many of these topical treatments are available over the counter. The systemic form of fungal infection requires intensive medical therapy.

Athlete's foot is a common name for fungal infection of the foot. The infection agents are various kinds of fungi that reproduce by forming spores; they can also infect the scalp, the skin in general, and the toenails. Athlete's foot is marked by scaled or cracked skin between the toes or by blisters. Ringworm looks the same except it also has a round, raised appearance. Both skin infections can spread to other parts of the body. Students can be exposed to pathogens by contact with the infected skin or with contaminated clothing or surfaces. Fungicides applied to the affected area usually eradicate the infection.

Coccidioidomycosis and histoplasmosis have the potential of being very dangerous fungal infections. Coccidioidomycosis is endemic to the Southwest and begins with the inhalation of a spore found in certain parts of the desert. Histoplasmosis is endemic to the eastern and central United States and also begins with the inhalation of a spore, usually found in soil around chicken houses, in caves harboring bats, and in soils with high organic content. In most cases, the infection is characterized by an acute attack of influenzalike symptoms, which occur after an incubation period of from one to four weeks. More rarely, the infection will spread progressively through the body. This progressive, systemic form of the disease is usually fatal.

Organization of School Health Programs

Protozoans

Protozoans are animal pathogens that are simple, one-celled organisms. Protozoans usually require a fairly specific mode of transmission before infecting a human being. The usual modes of transmission include insects such as the mosquito or vehicles such as food and water. Once inside the human, protozoans undergo very complex changes as a part of their life cycles. Often the life cycle of the protozoan is carried out on another living creature such as the mosquito.

It is unlikely that school personnel in the United States will be directly exposed to a student with a protozoan infection. The two most important protozoan infections in humans are malaria and amebic dysentery. In the case of malaria, a student most likely would have had to have visited a Third World country, including parts of Africa, Asia, Central America, and South America. They also would have had to have been bitten by a certain type of mosquito. If preventive measures are taken, there is little chance that any American, even one who visits other parts of the world, will contact malaria.

Amebic dysentery is a protozoan infection of the intestinal tract. The life cycle of the protozoan includes several phases, and the human can become infected by ingesting contaminated food and water. The result of this ingestion can be ulcers and symptoms of inflammation of the colon.

Metazoans (Parasitic Worms)

Metazoans are animal pathogens of which there are three groups: roundworms, tapeworms, and flukes. The classification of the various types of worms is based on specific characteristics such as segmented bodies (tapeworm), unsegmented bodies (roundworms), and possession of one or more sucking discs (flukes). The most common types of metazoan infection found in the United States and ones that school personnel are likely to encounter include ascariasis (roundworm) and enterobiasis (pinworm).

Ascaris is a large roundworm, similar in size to an earthworm. This roundworm lives in the intestinal tract of the human being and discharges eggs in the feces. Humans become infected with roundworm through ingesting material contaminated with Ascaris eggs. Once ingested, the worms hatch in the intestinal tract, and small larval forms of the worm burrow through the intestinal wall into the circulatory system. Then they are carried by the blood and are filtered out by various organs. The larval forms that are carried by the circulatory system to the lungs lodge in the alveolar walls and then migrate to the bronchi, where they are coughed up and swallowed. After being swallowed, they go into the small intestine, where they grow to maturity.

The Ascaris infection depends upon a simple process of ingestion, elimination, and reingestion. Many medications are available to kill the adult Ascaris and the various forms of Ascaris. However, in massive infestation, adult worms living in the small intestine can migrate upward and be coughed up, or they may even pass out the nose. In some cases, they may block the bile ducts or the appendix.

Pinworms are small roundworms that are frequently found in children; the infection usually spreads throughout a family. The elimination–ingestion–elimination cycle also applies to pinworm infections. However, the life cycle of the pinworm is not nearly as complex as that of Ascaris. The pinworms stay in the colon and at times, usually in the evening, migrate out of the colon to the anus and deposit their eggs on the perianal skin. This is usually done while the individual is asleep. The main symptoms of pinworm infection are anal and perianal itching.

Poor hygiene habits are responsible for humans getting both Ascaris and Enterobius infections. However, it should be noted that adults might not be aware if children have washed their hands, especially after bowel movements, and through contact with the hands of the child, the eggs may pass from one person to another.

The best method for dealing with ascariasis and enterobiasis is prevention. Education about the organisms and good hygiene habits should literally eliminate one's risk of infection. However, the medications available for eliminating both organisms are extremely effective.

Tapeworms and flukes are also metazoans; however, infections of either form are rare in the United States. In the case of the tapeworm, humans become infected by eating the flesh of an infected animal that contains the larval form of the parasite. Most commonly, these foods are pork, beef, and, on occasion, fish. Flukes are mainly found in Asia and are really of no concern in the United States.

Rickettsia

Rickettsia are very small intracellular pathogens that are structurally somewhere between a bacteria and a virus. Most often, rickettsia are included as a part of discussions about bacteria. Rickettsia are pathogens carried by insects and are transmitted to human beings by insect bites. The organisms multiply in cells of the small blood vessels. The blood vessels can in turn become swollen, which can lead to the formation of blood clots.

Rickettsial infection usually causes a high fever and a skin rash. The most common types of rickettsial infections seen in the United States are typhus and Rocky Mountain spotted fever. Most of the rickettsia are sensitive to antibiotics.

ARTHROPOD INFECTIONS

Scabies and lice are two common skin infestations that are not related to pathogens but are actually insects. Lice are classified as ectoparasites and are usually of three forms: head louse, body louse, and pubic or crab louse. All forms are similar in that they are small, flat, and wingless, and the male is generally smaller than the female.

Both lice and scabies are transmitted through personal contact and by objects such as combs, clothing, and bed linen. Since lice and scabies are contagious, such social acts as holding hands can spread an infestation.

Lice

The most pressing complaint of lice infestation is itching. The main reason for the itching is that nits (lice eggs) are attached by the lice to hair shafts or clothing. The nits are readily visible to the naked eye. Infected areas resulting from scratching are common. Diagnosis of lice infestation is made by identifying the insect and the nits.

Head and pubic lice can be identified on the infected individual. Nits appear as whitish structures, which are usually attached to hair shafts.

Scabies

Scabies are highly contagious and result in skin lesions. A complicated lesion consists of burrows, solid elevation on the skin, and blisters. Severe itching usually accompanies the disorder. Scabies are most often transmitted by close personal contact with infested individuals.

Once scabies is present in an individual, it spreads rapidly. The primary symptom for diagnostic purposes is intense itching, which worsens at night after the bed is warmed by the patient's body heat. A severe itch that persists for weeks or months, often coupled with similar eruptions among people who are close contacts, should arouse suspicion of the presence of scabies.

Treatment for both lice and scabies is simple. The medication is an antiparasitic medicated shampoo, cream, or lotion, such as Kwell. If the treatment is applied in accordance with a physician's orders, an individual suffering from either infestation should see results immediately.

INFECTION AND THE INFECTIOUS DISEASE PROCESS

Infection is a term that is used to denote any invasion of body tissue by pathogens that can damage body tissue in some way. The symptoms of an infection include not only the damage caused directly by the pathogen or by the toxins it generates, but also the often severe reactions of body tissue to invasion. An infection unrelated to other health problems is called a primary infection. When illnesses or injuries predispose the body to invasion by a pathogen, the resulting disorder is termed a secondary infection. For example, pneumonia is a primary infection when contracted by an otherwise healthy person, but it is a secondary infection when contracted by a bedridden patient whose immunity has been lowered by a different debilitating disease.

Infections are either acute or chronic in development and local, focal, or systemic in impact. Acute infections develop rapidly and usually result in high fever and severe sickness. Chronic infections develop slowly and exhibit symptoms that generally are milder and are restricted to one area of the body.

In a local infection, such as a boil, the infectious agent is restricted to one area of the body. Usually more serious in impact are focal infections, such as abscesses, in the course of which the pathogens themselves move from the initial site of the infection to other parts of the body. In systemic infections, the pathogens are transported throughout the body via the circulatory system.

All infections develop in a process that can be broken down into three phases: (1) transmission of the pathogen from a source to a host and invasion of the host's body by the pathogen, (2) the carrying out of the life cycle of the pathogen inside the host's body and the body's reaction to it, and (3) the pathogen's exit from the body.

Humans and animals are the ultimate source, or reservoir, of nearly all pathogens. Human reservoirs usually exhibit symptoms of the infections caused by the pathogen they harbor. Less frequently, human reservoirs will be carriers—individuals who harbor a pathogen without exhibiting clinical symptoms. There are three types of carriers: (1) healthy carriers, who have never contracted the disease caused by the pathogen they carry; (2) incubatory carriers, who have the disease in its early stage, before any symptoms are apparent; and (3) chronic carriers, who have recovered from the disease but still carry the pathogen. Because they seem to be uninfected, carriers pose a difficult disease control problem.

Pathogens spread from sources to new hosts in a variety of ways. These ways are called *modes of transmission.* Modes of transmission are termed either direct or indirect. Direct transmission from reservoir to host can occur through body contact or through droplets released from the mouth or nose of an infected person. Indirect transmission takes many forms. Pathogens may be ingested with food or water, or they may be inhaled. Inanimate objects provide another mode of transmission for the spread of pathogens—for example, a glass used by an infected person. Finally, other organisms, usually animals or insects, may carry a pathogen mechanically (on the exterior of the body) or biologically (if at least part of the pathogen's life cycle transpires within the body of the insect).

Once transmitted from a reservoir, the pathogen must be "caught" by the host. In order to infect body tissue, the pathogen must find or create a way of entering the host's body. Obvious candidates for the invasion routes are the body orifices: nose, mouth, urogenital tract, eyes, and ears. Other openings are provided by breaks in the skin such as cuts and abrasions. A few pathogens create their own openings by directly attaching to the skin.

Upon gaining access to the body tissue, a pathogen leads a parasitic existence in order to live and reproduce. As the pathogens multiply, sometimes producing toxins, they damage cells or prevent normal cell functions, thus producing disease. Typically, such disease has four stages:

1. Incubation—the time period between the host's exposure to the pathogen and the onset of clinical symptoms. Incubation periods can range from a few hours to several months.

2. Prodromal stage—early signs of a disease, such as a scratchy throat or runny nose, appear. Since these symptoms are typically minor, the infected person often does not ascribe them to illness of any significance.

3. Acute stage—the disease is fully manifest and the body defenses have swung into action. Since it is during this stage that the host pathogen is at its peak, the symptoms are usually worse.

4. Convalescence—the time period when the body's defenses have successfully fought off the pathogen and the individual is recovering from the disease. It should be noted that particularly serious infections or secondary infections that strike an already weakened person can result in death rather than convalescence.

In most cases, the infectious disease cycle ends with the elimination of the pathogen. For some diseases, recurrent attacks may arise, since the pathogen can lie dormant in the body and increase its numbers when an individual is in a weakened state.

During the acute and convalescent stages of an infection, the body often tries to flush out the pathogen. Pus, mucus, vomitus, blood, or other fluids are discharged. These fluids serve to transport many pathogens out of the body. Other pathogens are expelled in coughs and sneezes, and pathogens that settle in the intestinal tract are excreted in feces or urine.

BODY DEFENSES AGAINST INFECTION

The human body has several lines of defense against pathogen invasion. Unless weakened by injury, illness, or congenital defects, these defenses can cope with almost all infections. The three major body defenses against infection are epithelial defenses, inflammation, and immunity.

Before a pathogen can attack body tissue, it must reach the barrier posed by the body's epithelial defenses—the layers of skin and mucous membrane that sheathe the vulnerable inner parts of the body. A pathogen that succeeds in penetrating the epithelial barrier and establishes itself in body tissue triggers the body's second line of defense, the inflammatory process. The inflammation we see at the site of an infection actually stems from the body's attack on a pathogen, not vice versa.

Inflammation provides an effective defense against most local infections, but it is too limited a mechanism to deal with particularly virulent and fast-spreading pathogens. Against these more serious threats, the body's most important defense mechanism is the immune system. Since immunity simply means "resistance to infection," both inflammation and the epithelial barrier can be viewed as a part of the body's immune system.

TABLE 9.3

Natural and Artificial Immunity

	How Acquired	How Immunity Is Produced	Advantages	Disadvantages
Natural				
Active	Contraction of disease	Organisms act as antigens and stimulate body to produce specific antibodies to destroy the antigens.	Long-lasting immunity. Specific antibodies last a long time and body's ability to produce certain antibodies is now easier.	Discomfort and disadvantages of the disease
Passive	Mother passes specific antibodies through placenta to developing child.	Child possesses specific antibodies for certain antigens he or she may acquire.	Newborn child is born with immunity for certain diseases. Helps protect child against diseases at first.	The immunity is not long lasting.
Artificial				
Active	Vaccination with killed or attenuated organisms	Killed or attenuated organisms stimulate production of antibodies. The antibodies protect the body against actual organisms that may enter.	No discomfort and disadvantages of the disease and longer-lasting than artificial passive (months to years)	Not as long-lasting compared to natural active
Passive	Injection of antiserum or antitoxin	Person receives specific antibodies, therefore is immediately immune to certain diseases.	Immediate immunity. Good if person has been exposed to a disease or already has a disease	Immunity not as long-lasting as artificial active. Usually gives 4 to 6 weeks' immunity

T. R. Langford, *Integrated Science for Health Students,* 2nd edition, 1979. Reprinted by permission of Reston Publishing Company, a Prentice-Hall Company.

Immunity refers to a complex system by which the body defends itself against particular types of pathogens. Unlike the epithelial barrier and the inflammatory process, which defend body tissue against all foreign invaders, the immune system sets up specific defenses against specific pathogens, regardless of how they enter the body or where they spread within it.

Immunity to an infectious disease can be either natural or acquired. Natural immunity means an inherent lack of susceptibility to a disease. Some pathogens simply cannot survive in the bodies of certain individuals (Table 9.3).

Organization of School Health Programs

TABLE 9.4

Immunization Schedule for Children

Age	Vaccination	How Administered
2 months	DTP*	Injection
	Poliomyelitis	By mouth
4 months	DTP	Injection
	Poliomyelitis	By mouth
6 months	DTP	Injection
15 months	Measles	Injection
	Mumps	
	German measles (rubella)	
1ᵈ years	DTP	Injection
	Poliomyelitis	By mouth
24 months	HBV**	Injection
4–6 years	DTP	Injection
	Poliomyelitis	By mouth
14–16 years	DT***	Injection

*DTP Diphtheria, tetanus, and pertussis (whooping cough) vaccine

**HBV Hemophilus B vaccine. Designed to protect child against spinal meningitis.

***DT Diphtheria and tetanus vaccine

Acquired immunity is a more complex phenomenon, based on the body's ability to recognize the presence of a particular pathogen and produce agents that will destroy or neutralize it. Among the white blood cells that rush to an infection site during inflammation are lymphocytes. Once exposed to any pathogen lymphocytes retain the ability to recognize that pathogen if and when it reappears in the body. Upon its reappearance, lymphocytes produce antibodies—chemical agents whose sole function is to destroy the specific pathogen recognized by the sensitized lymphocytes.

This cycle of exposure–sensitization–reexposure–recognition–reaction is called active acquired immunity. It is acquired because it comes about only after exposure to a pathogen; it is active because the body manufactures its own antibodies. Active immunity can be acquired either naturally (from an actual case of the disease) or artificially (from vaccines). New vaccines can be composed of four types of substances: (1) killed pathogens, (2) live but attenuated (weakened) pathogens, (3) pathogens of a disease closely related to but less severe than that for which immunity is desired and (4) toxoids or nonpoisonous duplicates of the toxins produced by pathogenic bacteria. Whatever its composition, a vaccine is designed to provoke the body's immune system into producing antibodies against a specific pathogen without actually causing the disease associated with that pathogen. Table 9.4 shows an immunization schedule for children.

In addition to active immunity, the body can acquire passive immunity by receiving antibodies from an outside source. Like active immunity, the passive variety can be acquired either naturally or artificially. Naturally acquired passive immunity occurs in the womb, when antibodies pass through the placenta from a mother's blood to that of her unborn child. This process can be duplicated artificially by injecting a serum containing antibodies into the bloodstream.

MEDICAL INTERVENTION AND PREVENTION

In addition to the body's defense against disease, there is medical intervention, which consists of specific treatment for pathogen-related diseases. The treatments are usually in the form of medications, which are either preventive or directly treatment-oriented.

Prophylactic medications are directed at protecting the body from infection by keeping blood levels of the medication sufficiently high to protect a person who is quite susceptible to an infection. Treatment intervention is the administering of medications that act directly on the pathogen involved. Antibiotics are examples of treatment medications, whereas tetrabutaline and aminophylline are examples of prophylactic medication. However, it must be noted that the most effective way to fight off any infection is through natural body processes and through prevention of exposure to pathogens.

Education is the best method of prevention and has been appropriately termed *primary prevention*. Education about pathogens and the infectious disease process is critical to the comprehensive health education curriculum. Students need to be aware of the major pathogens and the preventive measures necessary to reduce their risk of infection.

A large part of the prevention process involves sound personal health practices and an understanding of one's own body in order to recognize susceptibility or a disease process that is in operation. It is through comprehensive health education in K through 12 that primary prevention will be most effective.

CONTROL OF COMMUNICABLE DISEASES

When large segments of the population, especially students, are susceptible to a particular pathogen, prevention may not be as effective. However, when a disease outbreak occurs good health habits are still useful to preventing more severe reactions to the infectious disease process.

There are several ways to control communicable diseases, that is, to minimize the spread of the disease. The more extreme ways include quarantine and closure of premises. Naturally these control measures are used only if absolutely necessary.

The more practical control measures include isolation and disinfection and hospitalization. Isolation should be encouraged if a student is highly contagious. This simply means keeping the student home until he or she is fully recovered and not infectious. The difficulty in isolation, at least in a school setting, is in the area of effectiveness.

With some diseases, an individual is most contagious during the incubation or prodromal (early signs of a disease) states. If that is the case, probably no one will recognize the disease in time; thus, by the time the disease is diagnosed, many susceptible students will have already come into contact with the infected student. At that point, isolation is of little value from a control standpoint, but it may still be important for individual recovery.

Disinfection is an important control measure when the mode of transmission of the disease is an indirect one. Public health rules and regulations exist for disinfection and should be followed closely. In addition, the physician making a diagnosis is aware of the disinfection process and can advise both school and parents.

Finally, control procedures vary with each communicable disease. For a more specific description of control measures for specific diseases, it is important to consult with a local, county, or state health department or refer to the latest edition of *Control of Communicable Diseases in Man,* published by the American Public Health Association.

Generally, schools are not closed as a result of a communicable disease outbreak except in the event of an emergency and even then only after the approval of the Department of Public Health. Students infected with a disease that is reportable should not be permitted to attend school. If isolation for the student has been recommended, the student should not be permitted to reenter school until written documentation on the child's state of health is obtained.

School personnel need to be aware of the most common signs and symptoms of communicable diseases. A communicable disease may be suspected when a combination of any two or more of these symptoms are present: headache, watery and inflamed eyes and nose, cough, elevated temperature, skin eruptions, sore throat, vomiting, and diarrhea. If a communicable disease is suspected, the following procedures are in order:

1. For the benefit of the sick child and others at school, separate him [or her] from school associates in the place designated for this purpose.
2. Notify the parents and arrange for the child to be sent home as soon as possible.
3. Make him [or her] as comfortable as possible.
4. Keep him [or her] under close observation, in order to note any changes in his [or her] condition.
5. Do not attempt to make a diagnosis. Do not give any medications. Water may be given if desired.
6. A child with a known or suspected communicable disease should not be sent home in a conveyance with other children. [State Department of Education, State Department of Health, Commonwealth of Virginia, 1980]

SUMMARY

The best method for controlling communicable disease is prevention. In order to prevent the spread of disease, it is imperative that school personnel have some knowledge of the major pathogens causing communicable disease, the major modes of transmission, and the infectious disease process in general. Once the main concepts regarding communicable disease control are understood by school personnel, each person in the school environment must take an active role in both prevention and control process.

REVIEW QUESTIONS

1. Discuss the differences among the major pathogens.
2. Identify examples of diseases associated with each major pathogen.
3. Describe the infectious disease process.
4. Why is it important for school personnel to have an understanding of communicable diseases and the infectious disease process?
5. Discuss the major concepts associated with medical intervention and prevention of communicable diseases.
6. What is Lyme disease? How can it be prevented?

REFERENCES

American Public Health Association. *Control of Communicable Diseases in Man,* 15th ed. Washington, D.C.: American Public Health Association, 1990.

Taylor, J. M., and W. S. Taylor. *Communicable Diseases and Young Children in Group Settings.* Boston: Little, Brown and Co., 1989.

University of California. *The Wellness Encyclopedia.* Boston: Houghton Mifflin Company, 1991.

Counseling and Interpretation

10

Counseling is one of the most important aspects of school health services and yet one of the areas that is most often neglected. Perhaps one of the most important reasons that counseling and interpretation of test results are neglected in the school setting is that school personnel, including teachers, are unsure of what counseling encompasses. In addition, it is often difficult to decide which students need counseling.

In many people's minds, counseling is a process that is involved only when psychological and emotional problems arise and the individual is in need of intensive psychological care. Most counseling is not of this type, especially in the schools. However, school personnel may be the first professionals to notice a possible problem—intellectual, psychological, or emotional—that might indicate that a student needs some counseling.

There is a wide range of topics that must be covered under the topic of counseling and interpretation. First, it is important that school professionals be aware of the various tests, both intelligence and personality, that can be used in school settings and the advantages and disadvantages of such tests. Second, it is important that school professionals be aware of the importance of techniques involved in counseling students. Finally, it is important that school professionals know the potential indicators of psychiatric disturbances in students so that the proper referrals can be made.

TESTING

Both intelligence and personality tests are commonly performed in the school setting. It is hoped that the tests are standardized, reliable, and valid. *Standardized* means the test has established norms. *Reliability* refers to a measurement that insures consistency—the test can be used with a variety of populations, and the investigator can be assured that the results are accurate. The *validity* of a test simply means that the test measures what the user wants it to measure.

Function of Tests

Some authorities believe that the primary use of standardized tests in counseling is to provide information to students about themselves that is helpful in resolving decisions and problems that confront them. However, since students are not knowledgeable about the information tests can provide, the counselor must know how they can contribute to self-analysis and self-understanding. To achieve these purposes, the counselor must have clearly in mind the functions tests serve. Some of the more important uses of the tests are:

1. To provide diagnostic information prior to counseling. . . .
2. To provide information that aids in determining the applicability of particular counseling methods, tools, or techniques and to provide information for treatment planning. . . .
3. To provide information to [students] about their attributes and to clarify self-conceptions. . . .
4. To predict the probabilities of success in an occupation or an educational or training program. . . .
5. To help students arrive at appropriate educational and vocational decisions. . . .
6. To stimulate interest in career planning. . . .
7. To facilitate student conversation and exploration in counseling. . . . [Blackham, 1977, pp. 100–101]

Intelligence Testing

The intelligence tests used today are direct descendants of the original Binet scales. Intelligence tests are designed for use in a wide variety of situations and are validated against relatively broad criteria (Anastasi, 1976, p. 230). The end result of responding to items in an intelligence test is a single score, which represents the individual's general intelligence level. The system of scoring the intelligence test is based on the individual's performance. This performance is reflected in a score or IQ, and this score is compared with the scores of other individuals in various age groups.

Because so many intelligence tests are validated against measures of academic achievement, they are often designated as a test of scholastic aptitude. Intelligence tests are frequently employed as preliminary screening instruments, to be followed by tests of special aptitudes. This practice is especially prevalent in the testing of normal adolescents or adults for educational and vocational counseling, in personnel selection, and for similar purposes. Another common use of general intelligence tests is in clinical testing, especially in the identification and classification of the mentally retarded. [Anastasi, 1976, p. 230]

In the words of Johnson and Magrab (1978, p. 214):

Perhaps the area the psychologist is most frequently asked to assess is that of intellectual development. General intelligence tests often serve as an excellent screening basis for further evaluation of the strengths and weaknesses of the child's learning abilities. It is not necessarily the overall level of the child's intellectual development that is of most interest, but rather the pattern of functioning that he [or she] demonstrates on the intelligence test. With this as a framework, there are several other points to consider before discussing the most frequently used tests and their relative usefulness.

Intelligence develops in a continuous pattern with age. Intelligence tests measure the current status of a given child with respect to the norms of that child's [age] group. Intelligence quotient (IQ) represents the relationship between a child's mental age (MA) and his [or her] chronological age (CA).

Mental age actually refers to a normal or average score on an intelligence test. In addition, this score is compared with age norm test scores. For example, if a ten-year-old student performs as well on an intelligence test as the average ten-year-old, he or she is said to have an MA of 10. CA refers to the actual age in years of the student taking the intelligence test. The actual IQ score is a relatively ambiguous type of score. Johnson and Magrab (1978, p. 214) succinctly address this point by stating the following:

> Although IQ scores are expressed in points, it is important to understand that there is little difference between IQ scores that are only several points apart. The real differences lie in the pattern by which the scores were obtained. In terms of looking at the total IQ score, it is best to view it as more general than a point score. Broader classification systems have been developed for this purpose. The following categories are from the Stanford-Binet Intelligence Scale for children functioning at an average level or above.

Near genius	140
Very superior	130–139
Superior	120–129
Above average	110–119
Average or normal	90–109

The Stanford-Binet and Wechsler scales are perhaps the most commonly used intelligence tests. The student taking the Stanford-Binet test is faced with a variety of tasks, including block design, picture arrangement, and object assembly. As the test progresses, the tasks become more and more verbal in nature. One of the major criticisms of the Stanford-Binet test is that it relies too heavily upon the subject's verbal ability and fails to measure other aspects of intelligence.

The Wechsler Intelligence Scale for Children (WISC-R) was developed in an attempt to improve on the Stanford-Binet test. The WISC-R measures a broader range of abilities than does the Stanford-Binet and provides separate IQ scores for performance and verbal skills. According to Johnson and Magrab (1978, p. 217), the test ". . . is designed to provide a full-scale IQ score as well as a separate verbal IQ score and a performance IQ score. The test is composed of six verbal subtests and six performance subtests that correspond to different areas of mental and physical functioning." Such functions as long-range memory or information, immediate auditory memory, language development, and arithmetic reasoning are considered in the verbal section. Visual organization and sequencing, visual attention to detail, spatial relations, eye–hand coordination, and visual memory are included in the performance subtest.

Johnson and Magrab (p. 217) further state that the WISC-R ". . . is most useful in beginning to pinpoint specific strengths and weaknesses of a child. Noting whether there is a discrepancy between a child's verbal and performance (non-verbal) IQ score is a first step in delineating specific problems.''

Personality Testing

Personality can simply be defined as mental habits, that is, the common sequences of behaviors, responses, and so on that are perceived by others. The use of inventories to examine personality has certainly attracted much attention in psychiatry and psychology. There are various methods for examining personality. One of the measures widely accepted by psychologists and psychiatrists is projective testing.

Projective Techniques

Projective tests focus on the unconscious in terms of conflicts, predispositions, and needs. The two most common types of projective techniques are the Rorschach inkblot test and the Thematic Apperception Test (TAT). Both these tests are referred to as projective personality tests. Evaluation of these tests is only to be done by certified professionals.

The Rorschach test consists of a series of 10 inkblot cards. The individual participating in the test is asked what he or she sees in each of the inkblot cards. There is no time limit. Once the description of what is seen is accomplished, the person is then asked to explain what led to the impression. Once this explanation is made, it gives the counselor some indication of potential personality problems.

The TAT is a projective technique in which pictures are presented to the client and the client is asked to imagine a story behind each of the pictures. The pictures in the TAT are much more obvious than the Rorschach inkblots. Most of the pictures are of individuals reacting to or involved in some solitary activity. Although somewhat ambiguous, the pictures contain enough information to help identify or guide a person's associations in a particular direction. The basic assumption underlying the interpretation of the TAT is that the stories people tell reflect their internal needs as well as their perception of external pressures.

The biggest criticism of the projective techniques of testing is that they lack reliability because they place too much emphasis on the interpretive skills of the evaluator. Studies have shown that several psychiatrists working from the same Rorschach results can arrive at completely different conclusions. In addition, studies have failed to prove that projective tests are truly valid instruments that measure what they are supposed to measure.

Objective Techniques

Because of the criticisms of the projective types of tests, many professionals prefer to use more objective types of personality inventories. These inventories measure distinct personality traits rather than deep internal needs and unconscious desires. Another advantage of using objective inventories is that the role of the professional as interpreter is greatly reduced, thus making the inventory result more reliable.

The most well-known personality inventory is the MMPI, or Minnesota Multiphasic Personality Inventory. This inventory consists of over 550 statements to which a person responds *true, false,* or *cannot say.* The test has included several subscales and can be a tremendous aid in diagnosing psychiatric disorders.

Regardless of what type of test is utilized, either projective or objective, the information provided from these tests should be used only in conjunction with other information in order to make some type of diagnosis. It *should not* be used exclusively as a tool in diagnosis. As with intelligence tests, it is imperative that, before using personality tests in a school setting, a thorough review of the limitations of the test be made.

Test Interpretation

In addition to reviewing the limitations of any intelligence or personality test used in a school setting, it is important that a responsible, highly trained, certified professional interpret the test results—professionals such as certified and licensed counselors, clinical psychologists, psychiatrists, and psychometrists. Unless authorized and certified personnel interpret test results, misrepresentation might occur. The implications of misrepresentation could affect the child's life in an extremely negative manner.

According to Blackham (1977, p. 106), "test interpretation involved two basic tasks: (1) determining the meaning of the results and (2) interpreting the meaning ascribed to the results in a way that is most useful to the student and the student's parents and, if necessary, school personnel."

It is important to note that test results are not mutually exclusive items that are all-encompassing. Any and all test results must be interpreted in light of and in conjunction with other pieces of information, including observation. Most important of all is the point that the interpretation of tests must be done by a qualified professional.

An important concept in both intelligence testing and personality testing is that some type of educational intervention might be necessary. The intervention can take the form of new or modified programs where different methodology is employed so the student can learn better. Alternatively, in the case of problems involving the personality, a change of environment may be called for, in order to reduce the stress that is influencing the problem. Intervention is important, but the role of prevention, especially in the area of personality problems, is of utmost importance. It certainly has major implications for school personnel, who are concerned with creating an educational environment where positive mental health (including both intelligence and personality) can be attained.

COUNSELING AS PREVENTION

The teacher is again in a strategic position to notice potential problems involving both intelligence and personality. However, it is important that school personnel be aware of individual differences and not label differences as problems. Many psychologists feel that the most common obstacle to knowing and understanding another person is simply a lack of interest in and appreciation of individual differences. Thus, it is extremely important that school personnel be interested in students and develop ways to appreciate individual differences. This can be done through using counseling as a form of primary, secondary, and tertiary prevention.

Litwack et al. (1980, p. 246) succinctly described primary prevention as

> the activities necessary to change structures and practices before the problems arise, thereby preventing the problems from developing. An example of a . . . problem calling for primary prevention might be the recognition that the development of a personal sense of worth and productivity can become an immense problem. It is important for school personnel to create an environment whereby students can experience a sense of personal worth and productivity before major problems result.

Secondary prevention focuses on the role of the health or psychological counselor. This type of prevention assumes that a minor problem exists; the counselor intervenes before the problem begins to affect the student's life. Secondary prevention implies that the intervention will be short, and the student will be able to resolve conflicts fairly quickly (Litwack et al., 1980, p. 26).

Tertiary prevention is more concerned with "treating a problem in a direct manner." The most common type of tertiary prevention is one-to-one or group counseling for emotional problems. Often this entails social skill-building programs for students. Tertiary prevention is usually the last attempt to correct a situation before a major problem occurs, in which long-term treatment is required (Litwack et al., 1980, p. 246).

The importance of creating an environment that will promote positive mental health among students cannot be underestimated. The creation of this kind of an environment depends heavily upon the actions and roles of school personnel in various types of prevention.

CRITERIA FOR SOUND MENTAL HEALTH

In order to identify students who might be having academic problems, it is important that the school have a mechanism for monitoring the student's learning capacity. This process is rather simple, for it relies heavily upon letter grades that the student receives. Any sudden change in a pattern of grades indicates that a potential problem exists, and the student should be referred for academic counseling. Grades can be fairly good indicators of progress and general intellectual functioning in the school setting.

It is much more difficult to identify students who are having adjustment problems. Unless the actions of a student are extremely noticeable, school personnel might never be aware that a particular student is experiencing an adjustment problem. There is no simple checklist for school personnel that will help in identifying students with potential adjustment or personality problems. However, if school personnel are aware of the characteristics of a healthy personality, they will have a type of barometer by which to evaluate students.

Maslow (1968, p. 157) developed a list of points, which are related to "Characteristics of a Healthy Personality." Nine of these points are particularly important for school health personnel to watch for in students.

1. Sound perception of reality.
2. Increased acceptance of self and others.
3. Increased spontaneity in actions.
4. Ability to focus on problems.
5. Desire for privacy.
6. Desire for autonomy.
7. Increased identity with human species.
8. Increased democratic character structure.
9. Creativity. [Maslow, 1968, p. 157]

Although not all students will display all nine characteristics, these are some criteria for observational evaluation. Naturally, students will possess these characteristics in varying degrees. It is important for school personnel to note to what degree a particular student possesses a characteristic. If it is obvious that certain characteristics are considerably lacking, the teacher might want to incorporate activities that would strengthen that particular characteristic.

Carl Rogers has made a monumental impact in the field of psychology. His methods with respect to counseling are used internationally. Rogers pointed out seven characteristics of what he terms "fully functioning" persons. These seven points include:

1. Adverse to facades.
2. Adverse to oughts.
3. Movement away from "meeting others' expectations."
4. Movement toward self-direction.
5. Movement toward accepting themselves.
6. Movement toward being open to their experiences.
7. Movement toward acceptance. [Rogers, 1961, pp. 167–180, as adapted by Litwack, 1980, p. 57]

The main advantage of Rogers' characteristics is that they tend to show movement in a direction. School personnel can identify movement in a positive or negative direction more easily than with some of the characteristics developed by Maslow. If both sets of characteristics are understood and used, school personnel can at least have a better grasp of what to look for in students, in order to refer them to the proper sources if significant deviations are noted. In addition, these lists help to identify the environmental influences that could be created, modified, or eliminated in order to aid students in developing both sets of characteristics.

TEACHER AWARENESS OF COMMON EMOTIONAL PROBLEMS

In addition to knowing and understanding the characteristics of a healthy personality or fully functioning person, it is important that teachers be aware of the indicators of common emotional problems among students. These indicators are immediate cause for referral and should be treated as such. Rodriguez and Fernandopulle (in Haslam and Valletutti, 1975, pp. 306–315) developed a list of such indicators; they are divided into mild and severe categories.

Preschool and Kindergarten

Mild
1. Poor motor coordination, as manifested by clumsiness in holding, carrying, or throwing objects.
2. Constant dropping of articles.
3. Walking as though the child has two "left feet."
4. General awkwardness in movement.
5. Persistent speech problems, particularly stammering, especially when excited, angry, or under other stress.
6. Constant loss of certain words while speaking.
7. Repetition of adjectives, verbs, nouns, and pronouns, when the child is under duress or even spontaneously.
8. Excessive timidity.
9. Persistent fears due to monsters, fire engines, and "spookies."
10. Perpetual problems with food idiosyncrasies, such as excessive eating, attempts at starvation, constant vomiting, eating nonedible food.
11. Aberration of bowel or bladder function, such as constant wetting, diarrhea or constipation.
12. Constant temper tantrums and infantile crying.
13. Total lack of interest in other children, ranging from complete isolation to a controlling position where the child will communicate with others only if others acquiesce to his [or her] wishes.

Severe
1. Excessive lethargy or hyperactivity.
2. Noncommunicative or demonstrating little or no speech.
3. Constant evacuation of the bowels without the existence of an infectious process.
4. Facial tics.

Organization of School Health Programs

5. Ritualism and repetitive acts.
6. Impulsive, destructive behavior.

Elementary School

Mild
1. Anxiety and oversensitivity.
2. Lack of attentiveness and apparent disinterest in learning.
3. Lying, stealing, temper outbursts, inappropriate social behavior.
4. Inability to do things for himself [or herself].
5. Difficulties and rivalries with peers.
6. Moodiness, withdrawal, few friends, isolation.

Severe
1. Extreme withdrawal, apathy, depression, grief, self-destruction.
2. Complete failure to learn.
3. Stuttering.
4. Sexual exhibitionism or sexual assaults on others.
5. Extreme somatic complaints.

Junior High and High School

Mild
1. Apprehension, fears, and guilt.
2. Constant preoccupation with sex.
3. Diminishing grades.
4. Inability to substitute or postpone satisfaction.
5. Defiant, negative, impulsive, or withdrawn behavior.
6. Extreme frequency of somatic complaints.
7. Extreme difficulties in learning.

Severe
1. Complete withdrawal.
2. School performance obviously retarded.
3. Acts of delinquency, asceticism, ritualism.
4. Overconformity.
5. Persistent anxiety, resulting in phobias.
6. Recurrent hypochondriasis.
7. Sexual aberrations. [Adapted from A. Rodriguez and G. Fernandopulle. "Teacher Awareness of Common Psychiatric Disorders in Children." In R. Haslam and R. Valletutti, *Medical Problems in the Classroom,* Austin: Pro-ed, Inc., 1975, pp. 306–315.]

It should be noted that many of the characteristics in the "mild" category do appear to be common types of behaviors displayed by students in the different age groups. The important point to remember is that, when the behavior is consistent, it might be an indicator of an emotional problem; it is only through referral that one would know if the behavior is normal. Also important for school personnel to note is whether the behavior in any way interferes with the student's life, both personal and academic. If it does, school personnel should take steps to get the student to appropriate referral services.

THE ROLE OF TEACHERS AND ADMINISTRATORS IN PROVIDING FOR POSITIVE MENTAL HEALTH

The role of teachers and other school personnel in providing for positive mental health has been stressed throughout this chapter. The overall efforts of teachers and other school personnel should be directed at fostering positive mental health and providing successful experiences for students, in order to avoid initiating negative self-concepts in them. Crisci (1978, p. 552) points out that this fostering of positive experiences is important because once students have developed negative feelings about themselves, it is very difficult to instill in them a positive self-concept.

Teachers and other school personnel can be effective in promoting positive mental health in two major areas: effectiveness training and counseling. Each of these areas will be examined separately.

Effectiveness Training

Several points are important for teachers to recognize when it comes to teacher effectiveness. First, a relationship of mutual respect can be established between teacher and students. This mutual respect can certainly lead to a beginning point for positive student mental health and for a belief on the part of teachers that they are effective. Second, "it is important to remember that it is the quality of the teacher–learner relationship that is viewed as the most critical component of teaching—far more critical than the subjects taught or the person teaching" (Crisci, 1978, p. 552).

An important approach to positive mental health in the school setting is for the teacher to work at developing the kinds of communication skills needed to establish quality relationships with students. Crisci (1978, p. 552) calls this "teacher effectiveness training" and goes on to say that:

> much of the emphasis in TET deals with developing the kinds of communication skills teachers need to establish a quality relationship with their students. They learn to listen attentively and speak in nonthreatening ways. Concepts such as respect for students' needs, effective education, and freedom to learn are integrated into the TET . . . program. Constructive conflict resolution is taught, wherein nobody is a winner or loser.

In addition to TET, teachers can maximize the effectiveness of the parent–teacher conference by allowing the student to participate in the conference. Crisci points out several reasons to include students in parent–teacher conferences. Teachers really have to "know" their students in order to talk to the student and parents together. Second, students are actually involved in the process by which decisions are made about them. Third, inclusion of students in the parent–teacher conferences can only enhance teacher effectiveness in the eyes of both students and parents, thus helping to create an optimal environment for positive mental health.

Counseling

School personnel are in a strategic position to counsel students. Naturally, we would not expect teachers to double as counselors, but if teachers are aware of the basic principles of counseling, perhaps they can help students before problems become serious. If a teacher is effective and can create a trusting environment, chances are the student actually will trust the teacher; then the teacher, in general conversation, can counsel the student much in the same way a professional, licensed counselor would. The following discussion of the basic principles of counseling and some counseling strategies certainly *do not* qualify a teacher to do counseling, but if a teacher knows some of these techniques, he or she can be more effective as a teacher and an observer of school health needs.

Litwack et al. (1980, pp. 25–28) state six points that are important to counseling and are appropriately called basic principles of counseling. These points include:

1. There is no simple, correct, or right way to counsel. . . .
2. Individuals have inner resources to help themselves.
3. Start where counselees are and accept them as they are. . . .
4. Each human being must be respected and potentialities for growth recognized. . . .
5. [Counselors] are not to moralize, preach, or impose their own values, the values of the institution, or those of the society upon counselees. . . .
6. The key to successful or effective counseling is nonevaluative listening.

If teachers and other school personnel are involved in counseling, it would benefit them to remember these six major points so that errors in judgment and communication will not occur.

Cormier et al. (1984, p. 23) state that there are many purposes for establishing what they term *core* or *facilitative* conditions for counseling. Some of these purposes—which are actually a combination of traits and behaviors that should be considered characteristic of school health counselors—include the following:

1. To establish a rapport.
2. To show understanding and support.
3. To clarify problems.
4. To communicate a willingness to work with the student.
5. To communicate interest in the student as a person.

6. To communicate acceptance of the student.
7. To communicate caring to the student.

One way to realize the foregoing purposes would be to start first by giving the student nonverbal cues of warmth. According to Cormier (1984, p. 30), the following behaviors should give the student a feeling of warmth:

1. Speak in a soft, soothing voice.
2. Facial expression should be smiling, interested.
3. Posture should be relaxed, leaning toward the student.
4. Look directly into the student's eyes.
5. Make sure gestures are open and welcoming.
6. Keep a close physical proximity.

The basic principles of counseling and the necessary counselor traits are extremely important and certainly help to create a favorable environment for communication. However, it is also important to know how to counsel, that is, to know the types of responses the counselor should exhibit during the counseling process. Counseling is not an easy task, and knowing how to respond to a student is as important as the basic principles and counselor traits. Blackham (1977, pp. 213–221) has identified 14 separate counselor responses that help exploration, understanding, and problem solving.

Blackham's* 14 counselor responses include attending, paraphrasing, reflecting, clarifying, perception checking, leading, summarizing, supporting, approving, confronting, interpreting, informing, instructing in appropriate behavior, and assigning tasks and contracting.

> An attending response has three important characteristics: (1) the counselor establishes contact by looking at the client as he or she talks, conveying interest by maintaining a relaxed and attentive posture; (2) the counselor uses natural gestures to convey the intended message; and (3) the counselor uses verbal statements that relate to, encourage, and reinforce the feelings the student wants to relate. [p. 213]

Paraphrasing is a response in which the counselor tries to restate the student's statement in fewer words. Paraphrasing helps in the counseling process by conveying to the student an attempt to understand what is being stated by the student. Similar to paraphrasing is reflecting. This means that the counselor attempts to state in different words the essential ideas or feelings the student has expressed. A paraphrase would restate more precisely what the student has said, whereas reflecting mirrors in different words the central ideas a student has tried to express (Blackham, 1977, p. 214).

Clarification is a counselor response in which the counselor tries to clarify what the student is attempting to express. Sometimes a student's message is vague or confused; therefore, it is important that the counselor clarify in a simple response what the student is trying to express.

*From *Counseling: Theory, Process, and Practice* by Garth Blackham. © 1977 by J. Wadsworth Publishing Company, Inc. Adapted with permission of the publisher.

Organization of School Health Programs

Perception checking is a response that asks the client to correct or verify the counselor's perception of what he or she has heard. "When a perception check is used, the counselor restates (paraphrases) what is heard, asks for confirmation, and permits the student to correct inaccuracies in the counselor's statement" (Blackham, 1977, p. 215).

Leading is a response in which the counselor encourages the student to talk about some facet of self or experience. According to Blackham (p. 216):

> there are two kinds of leads: indirect and direct. An indirect lead invites students to express their feelings, opinions, or thoughts within certain broad parameters. A direct lead provides more specific direction by inviting the student to clarify, illustrate, or elaborate on a particular theme.

Summarizing is a response that allows the counselor to tie together ideas and feelings expressed by a student. A supporting response is one in which the student is able to understand that his or her behavior or feelings are not unusual. An approving response is made by a counselor so that the student will feel that the counselor agrees with the student's ideas, feelings, or behavior.

A confronting counselor response is a statement "that conveys an honest and constructive reaction about some facet of the student's behavior or some element of the immediate situation" (Blackham, 1977, p. 218). This type of response faces clients with behavior that they prefer not to examine. One must be aware that this type of response can create a threatening situation. Therefore, even though this counselor response is mentioned here, it is not always important or advisable for teachers to employ this type of response, especially if the teacher feels that the response will create a particularly threatening situation for the student.

> An interpretation is a counselor statement that denotes a relationship between two or more events, thoughts, or feelings the student has expressed or experienced. The events that are the subject of the interpretation are usually related in some cause–effect way. The chief purpose of an interpretation is to help the student become more aware of and learn to exercise more control over some facet of behavior. [Blackham, 1977, p. 219]

An informing response is simply a counselor response directed at providing specific information that a student has requested that will help the student in the counseling process. Instructing in appropriate behavior is similar to informing. This response aids the student in learning behavior that is appropriate to specific situations (Blackham, 1977, p. 221).

Assigning tasks and contracting is a response that allows the counselor to assign the student specific activities in which the student should participate. It is hoped that the activities aid in resolving the problem or potential problem. The contracting phase of this response allows the student to feel committed to carrying out the tasks assigned.

All of the counselor responses are important and should be used only if the teacher or other school personnel conducting counseling understand fully what is involved in the various responses. The most important thing to remember is that if the teacher does not feel qualified to help the student in counseling, the student should be referred to someone who can carry out effective counseling.

The point to understanding the basic principles of counseling, the traits that facilitate counseling, and the proper responses for counseling is to aid the student in solving personal problems. The problem-solving process is succinctly described by Egan (1985) and adapted by Blackham (1977, pp. 126–129).

1. Help the client state his [or her] problems clearly and in a form that is workable and solvable. . . .
2. Establish problem priorities and work first on the problem that has the highest priority. . . .
3. Establish counseling goals that can be achieved. . . .
4. Analyze the means by which established goals can be achieved. . . .
5. Assist the client in selecting the best available means to achieve identified goals. . . .
6. Implement and evaluate means chosen to attain identified goals. . . .

It is important to mention that these six parts to the problem-solving process can be carried out effectively if the school personnel understand the basic principles, traits, and appropriate responses for counseling.

Generally, the teacher as counselor will help the student in solving problems. However, in some cases the teacher will help the student in making some voluntary adaptation in behavior when the student perceives a particular behavior as a threat to his or her health—physically, mentally, or socially. When discussing behavior change, it is imperative that Carl Rogers' six points relative to therapeutic ingredients promoting behavior change be discussed. Rogers' (1967) six points, as summarized by Blackham (1977, p. 117), include:

1. Two people, a teacher (counselor) and student, are in psychological contact.
2. The student is experiencing a state of anxiety, distress, or incongruence.
3. The teacher is genuine in relating to the student.
4. The teacher feels or exhibits unconditional positive regard for the student.
5. The teacher exhibits empathetic understanding of the student's frame of reference and conveys the understanding to the student.
6. The teacher succeeds in communicating empathetic understanding and unconditional positive regard to the student.

These six therapeutic ingredients are important as responses to the student. They are a starting point in developing a counseling relationship that will result in voluntary adaptations of behavior.

The modification of behavior does not end with Rogers' therapeutic in-gredients. Cormier et al. (1984, p. 285) identified six major points to modify behavior by regulating response consequences. These points include:

1. Remove antecedents associated with behavior to be modified.
2. Alter or change antecedents in order to make it difficult to display behavior.
3. Arrange antecedents so that behavior will be performed at a certain time and place.
4. Alter time–place sequence.
5. Build long pauses into time–place sequence.
6. Evaluate the effects of the stimulus–control strategy maintaining records of change in target behavior.

Attempts at modifying behaviors should only be done by skilled persons. In the process of health education, voluntary adaptations of behavior are some-times the end result; in that case, the preceding six points should be a part of the health education process and not necessarily a part of a counseling relationship.

SUMMARY

This chapter has covered a wide variety of topics relating to counseling and interpretation and the role of school personnel in this process. The importance, and especially the limitations, of both intelligence and personality testing have been explored. Also, the roles of the various school personnel in testing and test interpretation have been discussed.

The indicators of potential psychiatric disturbances have been presented and discussed. Finally, the major points in promoting teacher effectiveness in counseling have been presented and discussed. It must be reemphasized that counseling is an art, not just a method of communication. The points men-tioned in this chapter are not made in an effort to provide a how-to approach for school personnel, but rather are offered as goals and criteria for those who are doing counseling or thinking about doing counseling. These personnel should consider all the various facets to this complex process.

Students seeking further information about counseling would benefit by reading the following books:

*   Blackham, G. *Counseling: Theory, Process, and Practice.* Belmont, CA: Wadsworth, 1977.
*   Litwack, L., J. Litwack, and M. Ballou. *Health Counseling.* New York: Appleton-Century-Crofts, 1980.

REVIEW QUESTIONS

1. Discuss the usefulness of intelligence and personality tests.
2. Discuss some of the important functions of intelligence and person-ality tests.

3. Discuss how counseling can be considered as prevention.
4. List the important criteria for the development of sound mental health.
5. List some of the indicators of emotional problems of school-age students.
6. List and describe Blackham's fourteen counselor responses.
7. List the important elements for promoting behavior change.

REFERENCES

Anastasi, A. *Psychological Testing,* 4th ed. New York: Macmillan Publishing Company, 1976.

Blackham, G. J. *Counseling: Theory, Process, and Practice.* Belmont, CA: Wadsworth, 1977.

————, and A. Silberman. *Modification of Child and Adolescent Behavior,* 2nd ed. Belmont, CA: Wadsworth, 1975.

Cormier, L., W. Cormier, and R. Weisser. *Interviewing and Helping Skills for Health Professionals.* Monterey, Ca.: Wadsworth Health Sciences Division, 1984.

Crisci, P. ''Role of Teachers and Administrators in Providing for Positive Mental Health.'' *Journal of School Health* **48**:9 (November 1978).

Egan, G. *The Skilled Helper: A Model for Systematic Helping and Interpersonal Relating.* Monterey, Ca.: Brooks/Cole, 1985.

Gordon, T. *Teacher Effectiveness Training.* New York: Peter H. Wyden, 1974.

Hamrin, S. A., and B. Paulsen. *Counseling Adolescents.* Chicago: Science Research Associates, 1950.

Haslam, R., and R. Valletutti. *Medical Problems in the Classroom.* Austin: Pro-ed, Inc., 1985.

Johnson, R., and P. Magrab. *Developmental Disorders.* Austin: Pro-ed, Inc., 1978.

Litwack, L., J. Litwack, and M. Ballou. *Health Counseling.* New York: Appleton-Century-Crofts, 1980.

Maslow, A. H. *Motivation and Personality.* New York: Harper & Row, 1954.

————. *Toward a Psychology of Being,* 2nd ed. New York: Van Nostrand Reinhold, 1968.

Rodriguez, A., and G. Fernandopulle. ''Teacher Awareness of Common Psychiatric Disorders in Children.'' In Haslam, R., and R. Valletutti, *Medical Problems in the Classroom.* Austin: Pro-ed, Inc., 1975.

Rogers, C. *Client-Centered Therapy.* Boston: Houghton Mifflin, 1951.

————. *Counseling and Psychotherapy.* Boston: Houghton Mifflin, 1942.

————. *On Becoming a Person.* Boston: Houghton Mifflin, 1961.

————. ''The Conditions of Change from a Client-Centered Viewpoint.'' In Berenson, B. G., and R. R. Carkhuff (eds.), *Sources of Gain in Counseling and Psychotherapy.* New York: Holt, Rinehart and Winston, 1967.

Safety and Emergency Care

11

A ccidents are the leading cause of death for children 5 to 14 years of age.

Historically, nonmotor vehicle accidents have accounted for the highest mortality in this age group. However, reduction in death rates for nonmotor accidents and the increase in death rates for motor vehicle accidents have resulted in nearly equal numbers of deaths from these two causes since 1970. Fire and drowning are the two major causes of deaths from nonmotor vehicle accidents [USDHHS, 1982, p. 16]

It would seem on the surface that there is little that one can do to prevent accidents. After all, it is thought that the word *accident* actually means something that was not planned to happen and just did. But more and more evidence is pointing out that most accidents are indeed preventable; therefore, it is important that school personnel recognize their role in accident prevention and, if accidents do occur, their responsibility in providing aid to the injured.

Officially, an accident is defined as ''an unplanned act or event resulting in injury or death to persons or damage to property'' (Mroz, 1978, p. 1). An event must result in injury or property damage before it can be properly classified as an accident. A more appropriate definition of accident, which certainly has implications for school personnel, was developed by Licht and defines an accident as ''a sequence of sudden, unplanned events which has the potential for producing personal injury or property damage.'' This definition can be broken down into the following four major components: several events; sudden occurrences; unplanned events; potential for producing personal injury or property damage (Mroz, 1978, p. 3).

Accidents resulting in death are, in order of frequency of occurrence, motor vehicle accidents, falls, drowning, fires, and burns. In the 15- to 24-year-old age group, motor vehicle accidents are still the leading cause of death, followed by drowning; but poisoning is number three and deaths related to firearm accidents are number four.

Accidents can be classified into five major classes. These classes do not reflect the type of accident that occurs but rather describe the place the accident occurs. The five classes include traffic accidents, home accidents, school accidents, work accidents, and public accidents (Mroz, 1978, p. 6).

More than 6000 school-age children are killed in accidents every year in the United States. Over half of these accidents could have been prevented. According to Mroz, ''most of the school-related deaths are caused by accidents while the children move to and from school, whether on foot or by bicycle, automobile, or school bus'' (p. 6). In order to prevent accidents in the school setting as well as all settings, safety must be incorporated into all activities and programs, including parts of the school curriculum.

SAFETY

Safety, by definition, is ''the prevention of accidents and the mitigation of personal injury or property damage which may result from accidents'' (Mroz, 1978, p. 7). Examining this definition further, it can be seen that safety has two components. First, safety is accident prevention; second, safety is accident mitigation, or an altering of the events that lead to an accident (Mroz, 1978, p. 8).

The first step in developing a safety component to the school health program is to understand the nature and causes of accidents. It is in this way that program activities and responsibilities can focus on the causes of the problems. Accident causes can be classified under the following three major headings: human failures, environmental hazards, and defective agents (Mroz, 1978, p. 10).

Human failures include such factors as emotions, attitudes, personality traits, and habits. There four factors are responsible for approximately 80 percent of accidents. All of these human factors have accompanying behavioral responses that can be the first part of the sequence of events leading up to an accident. Such things as temper outbursts, which might include throwing objects or pushing, can result in an accident. Also, recognizing a potential hazard and not doing anything about it because of a poor attitude might also result in an accident.

Environmental hazards are the cause of approximately 15 percent of all accidents. Natural environmental hazards such as rain, snow, wind, and other phenomena cannot be controlled. The human response to these environmental hazards, however, can be controlled somewhat through safety programs. Such man-made environmental hazards as disorderly situations or improperly stored materials can be controlled through a sound philosophy of safety and written policies that focus on these hazards.

Finally, defective agents such as faulty mechanical structures can also be controlled through a comprehensive safety program. Even though these types of hazards account for only 5 percent of accidents, they are probably the most preventable cause of accidents.

The prevention of accidents extends far beyond simply removing hazards from the environment or addressing the human factors involved in an accident. The prevention of accidents relies upon a comprehensive safety program that is a strong and critical component of the overall school health program. However, before such a component can be developed, it is important that a committee or members of the school health team involved in the development of such a program develop a philosophy for the safety program and establish written policies.

PHILOSOPHY, WRITTEN POLICIES, AND SCHOOL RESPONSIBILITIES

As mentioned in Chapter 3, a philosophy is a series of beliefs that are felt to be true. Individuals have philosophies concerning many things, but the important thing is that the members of the school health team agree on a series of statements that they feel to be true with respect to safety and the role of safety in the school health program.

For practical purposes, the first step in developing a safety philosophy for a school or school district is to examine existing philosophies. Florio, Alles, and Stafford (1979, pp. 62–64) developed a safety charter for children and youth, which includes many salient points that should be included in a school safety philosophy. This charter is as follows:

> Children and youth are the nation's most valuable asset. They are wholesome and eager; they possess great vigor; they are adventurous. At the same time they are ingenious and mischievous. Most of all, they have faith and trust in adults whenever and wherever their safety is involved. This fact places a tremendous responsibility upon us all to provide:

For every child a dwelling-place safe. . . .

I. A home that assures freedom to live, work, and play safely; an environment with progressively reduced physical hazards; and a family program of continuous guidance that develops confidence and ability to protect one's self and others. All children and youth need:
   1. A home built, equipped, and maintained for safe living.
   2. A home where there is an atmosphere of acceptance of each individual—where sympathy, understanding, love, and affection promote the mental and emotional health essential to the development of desirable attitudes and practices of safe living.
   3. A home where parents and children alike assume their individual responsibilities for safe behavior in all situations.
   4. A home where the family practices safe living at all times.

II. For every child education for safety and protection against accidents to which modern conditions subject him. A school that recognizes ever-changing needs; progressively reduces physical hazards; and educates for safe living through instruction, example, and participation. All children and youth need:
   1. A school that provides and maintains a safe environment—buildings, grounds, equipment, supplies, machinery, heating, and lighting.
   2. A school that bases its education for safe living on continuous research, local and national.
   3. A school that uses a 24-hour-a-day accident reporting system as one factor in planning and evaluating its instruction in safe living.

4. A school where guidance, supervision, and instruction are geared to personal responsibility for one's safety and that of others, and where due emphasis is given to proper knowledge, skills, attitudes, and habits.
5. A school that provides, in all its activities, opportunities for pupils to develop the ability to make adjustments for safe living, both present and future.
6. A school that permits democratic participation of children and adults in planning and enforcing rules and regulations designed for safe living.
7. A school that reflects a philosophy which emphasizes educational experiences for youthful participants and which substitutes an increasing sense of personal responsibility for restrictive and supervisory measures imposed by others.
8. A school that facilitates interaction with the community for better safety.

III. For every child a community which recognizes and plans for his [and her] needs, protects him [and her] against physical dangers—provides him [and her] with safe and wholesome places for play and recreation. A community where all agencies and organizations, through individual and cooperative effort, develop a program of action that meets conditions affecting the safety of youth.
All children and youth need:
1. A community that provides for the safety of its citizens.
2. A community, rural or urban, that provides for and encourages safe living on the streets and highways, on the job, in recreation, and at home.
3. A community that considers the safe route to and from school, church, playground, and other youth centers in its planning.
4. A community with adequate regulations and enforcement for traffic, transportation, building, and fire safety.
5. A community that accepts its responsibility for appropriate leadership and supervision of group functions.
6. A community wherein safe and reasonable recreation programs are provided for children and youth, under adult guidance and supervision competent to assist children and youth in making appropriate social adjustments.

We, as educational leaders, recognizing that conservation of life depends upon the safety education of our children and recognizing that every individual has the right to contribute to safe living for all Americans, do hereby pledge ourselves to do all that is within our power to meet these needs of children and youth. [A. E. Florio, W. F. Alles, and G. T. Stafford. *Safety Education.* New York: McGraw-Hill, 1979]

Once a philosophy for a safety component of the school health program is developed, it is then important that objectives be developed that will reflect

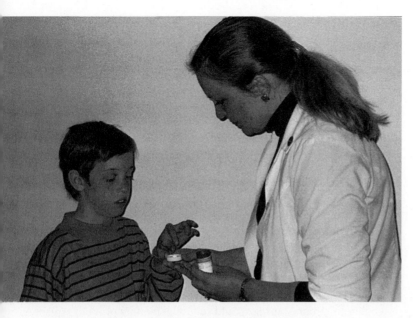

Administration of medication to pupils must be based on specific written policies.

the major components of the philosophy. The objectives should be statements that deal directly with the prevention of accidents. Most importantly, the objectives should reflect the philosophy and be measurable—the evaluation component of the program will assess directly whether or not the objectives have been met.

After the objectives have been developed and approved, it is then critical that written policies be developed. These policies should outline the responsibilities of school personnel in helping to reach the objectives. The written policies should be clearly stated and should be written in considerable detail. The policies should then be interpreted to all persons affected so that each person understands exactly what his or her responsibilities are with respect to preventing accidents.

As an example of specific written policies, the following policies focus on administering medications by school personnel:

1. The administration of medication to pupils shall be done only in exceptional circumstances wherein the child's health may be jeopardized without it.
2. Pupils requiring medications at school shall be identified by parents and/or physician to the school nurse, teachers, and other school personnel. Students observed by school personnel self-administering unauthorized medications should be reported to their parents.
3. After identification, the school nurse or properly appointed representative for the school shall make a home contract to identify the type, dosage, and purpose of said medication.
4. Written statements shall be required of:
    a. The family physician, who shall indicate the necessity of said medication being given to the child during school hours;

b. The parents, who shall request and authorize the designated school personnel to give said medication in the dosage to be prescribed by the physician and thereby releasing school personnel from liability should reactions result from the medications.

5. The physician shall then be requested by the parents to prescribe duplicate bottles of said medication, if it is necessary that it be given during school hours. One bottle will be kept at home and the other at school under the care of school authorities. Both bottles shall contain the name and telephone number of the pharmacy, the pupil's identification, name of the physician, and dosage of the drug to be given. Taking the dosage shall be supervised by the school nurse or other designated school personnel at a time conforming with the physician's indicated dosage schedule.

6. It is advisable to have in the principal's or school nurse's office a list of pupils needing medication during school hours, including type of medication, when given, and dose. This list should be reviewed periodically.

7. Under no circumstances should school personnel provide aspirin or any other patent medicine or nostrum to students.

If the school hopes to enlist the support of parents in the enforcement of this policy it will be necessary to interpret the rationale of the policy to them. Where parents do not understand the need for such procedures it is extremely difficult to secure their cooperation. [Minnesota State School Health Council, "State School Health Council Recommends Medication Policy," pp. 224–228]

As one can readily see, the development of written policies will take a considerable amount of time. The example of written policies regarding administering medications is just one of many areas in which written policies must be developed.

In addition to the individual responsibilities of faculty and staff, it is important that each school district establish administrative procedures for handling emergencies. The policies should be developed with input from the local medical and dental societies, local health department, and parents' organizations. The following represents an outline of some responsibilities that should be incorporated into policy form (Commonwealth of Virginia, 1980, p. 17).

1. Responsibilities that should be recognized:
    a. School authorities are responsible for providing first aid and emergency treatment until the parent or representative (physician) arrives to assume responsibility.
    b. Parents are responsible for keeping ill children at home and should be responsible for providing transportation home for children who become ill at school.

2. When a child becomes ill or suffers an accident, parents and the school principal should be notified immediately. Get in touch with the child's physician. If medically indigent, get in touch with the local health department or appropriate social services agency.

3. In serious cases where immediate medical attention is needed, call physician; otherwise, contact parents first and they will call their physician.

4. For each child, a card that is brought up to date each year should be readily available. It should contain:
   a. Home and business address and telephone number of parents or guardian. Name, address, and telephone number of a friend who can be contacted in an emergency when the parent is not available.
   b. Signed permission from parent or guardian authorizing medical or dental care, with first and second choice of physician or dentist to be contacted in emergencies.
   c. Any drug sensitivity or serious chronic condition in the child.

5. At least one person who is trained in first aid should be available in the school at all times.

It is important that an evaluation of the safety program be developed. The evaluation should not be done at the end of the school year, but rather should be an ongoing process so that any revisions can be made at important times in the school year. The evaluation should be based on the objectives developed and should include some evaluation of the written policies, which is the mechanism to reach the objectives.

Before one can develop a safety program or component, it is important to know what the major accident-related problems are at a particular school. Therefore, the safety program must develop a data base that will provide information on the major environmental hazards, as well as the types and frequency of accidents that occur at the school. These data can provide important information so that the program objectives, written policies, and evaluation will focus on the needs of the school and not just on general concerns that may or may not relate to a particular school.

PREPARATIONS FOR HANDLING EMERGENCIES, ACCIDENTS, AND ILLNESS

It is nice to think that through comprehensive safety, all accidents can be prevented. In theory it is true, but in reality, due primarily to human failures, it is unlikely. Therefore, it is important that, if accidents do occur, school personnel be in a position to provide emergency care to the injured.

Before examining some of the major factors related to emergency care, it must be noted that students and school personnel should check their state laws or district regulations to see just what they are legally required to do or *not* to do in emergency situations. Not all states have the same regulations; therefore, it is imperative that school personnel understand the legal aspects of emergency in their particular situations.

There are a variety of types of emergency care that can be employed in various situations. These types of emergencies vary according to the skill level of the person rendering aid to the injured person. What is considered primary, of course, is providing what is termed *first aid.* According to the American Red Cross, first aid is the immediate care given to a person who has been injured or has suddenly become ill. This definition includes the provision of care until proper medical help can be obtained.

Emergency care can go beyond the immediate care given to an injured person. Hurt (1975, pp. 2–4) identified five conceptual positions for the provision of emergency care: basic emergency care, medical self-help, lay medical, medical corps, and medical emergency care.

Basic emergency care is simply procedures, based upon the latest medical information, that are taught by the American Red Cross for providing aid to the injured. These procedures will provide immediate and temporary care until the services of a physician can be obtained. Individuals must be trained in the procedures required for basic emergency care.

Medical self-help includes basic emergency care and, in addition, continued care in the event of major disasters. The major difference between basic emergency care and medical self-help lies in the area of continued care. The continued care might require additional skills that are not included as a part of basic emergency care training. Therefore, medical self-help must be learned in addition to basic emergency care.

Lay medical emergency care consists of basic emergency care and, in addition, continued care in the home environment. Since continued care is in the home environment, lay medical emergency care is more related to emergency care in family situations than in school settings. Included in this category of emergency care is the administration of minor drugs or analgesics such as aspirin. Naturally, it is assumed that the person administering the medications is educated enough to know what to administer and in what situations certain medications can be administered. Much of lay medical care really relies on good judgment and, since families are involved, there are few legal ramifications if, in using one's own judgment, something transpires that increases the severity of the injury.

The fourth conceptual position is that of medical corpsperson. Medical corpspeople are used in the armed forces and, since their training is so extensive, they are permitted to go far beyond basic emergency procedure and administer powerful medications and, in certain situations, conduct minor surgery. It must be noted that these procedures would only be performed in a military setting, where these men and women are trained specifically to address common injuries, especially those that occur in war situations.

The last conceptual position is termed medical emergency care. This category includes the most highly skilled person to provide medical care, the physician. This position essentially involves the physician in an emergency setting, such as a hospital.

School personnel at times may be confused about the conceptual position best suited to them. Naturally, the nurse is highly skilled, but in most cases, state laws limit the extent of the nurse's emergency care. Therefore, the most important and relevant position for all school personnel to adopt is the first, which is to provide basic emergency care to the injured. It is highly recommended that all school personnel be trained in basic first aid and emergency care. At a minimum, one person so trained should be available whenever children are legally on school property.

In the first edition of this text we identified numerous medical emergencies and procedures to be followed in dealing with such emergencies. Because of the potential to aggravate an emergency by nontrained individuals applying specific procedures, we elected not to present procedures. We would like to reemphasize that all school personnel be trained in first aid and CPR (cardiopulmonary resuscitation).

Emergencies and 911

Every member of the school health team as well as students themselves must be aware of the 911 system. Simply, in most communities, 911 is the telephone number for emergency medical services as well as the number for summoning police and fire fighting services. The most common protocol for operation of this system involves the 911 call being received by an emergency communications center in a community. A trained person receiving the call gets the necessary information from the caller and then immediately dispatches appropriate emergency assistance.

A trained 911 telecommunicator is available 24 hours a day, 7 days a week including holidays. The number should be used only for attempts to save a life, to report a fire, or to report or prevent a crime. The number should not be used to discuss business questions, general information, or nonemergency calls.

The 911 system works effectively in communities and because it is so well designed and integrated, many lives each year are saved. Information regarding 911 should be incorporated into all facets of the school health program.

LEGAL ASPECTS OF EMERGENCY CARE

As mentioned previously, it is important for school personnel to be informed of state laws regarding the provision of emergency care. These laws can exist at any level, including state, county, or local levels. Violations of these laws can result in serious legal infractions, which can certainly affect both the individual teacher and the district.

Legally, the basis for liability resulting from providing emergency care rests in the area of negligence. Negligence is a result of school personnel violating legal responsibilities. According to Trubitt (in Hurt, 1975, p. 16), legal responsibilities of school personnel fall into the following broad areas, called duties:

1. Anticipation of foreseeable risk to students.
2. Reasonable steps to prevent those risks from occurring.
3. Warning and care addressed toward those risks that cannot be reduced.
4. A duty to aid the injured.
5. A duty not to increase the severity of the injury.

School personnel, through comprehensive safety planning, should be able to anticipate foreseeable risks to students. This includes identifying potential environmental hazards that might result in injury or activities that might potentially result in injury. An example would be activities in physical education classes, such as gymnastics, in which there is great potential for injury.

Education is a key component in taking reasonable steps to prevent accidents or injury from occurring. Students must be informed about safety procedures that need to be employed when involved in certain risky activities. In addition to education, it is important that school personnel do everything they can to eliminate unnecessary risks. Sometimes this includes actually eliminating an environmental hazard.

Education is also a key component to providing warning and care in relation to those risks that cannot be reduced. This includes instruction in correct procedures in such things as waiting for buses, crossing highways, and participating in laboratory or physical education activities.

In most cases, the first three broad duties are addressed to some extent. The last two broad duties are a little more complex and require further discussion and some definitions of legal terms.

Everyone, including school personnel, has a responsibility to provide aid to the injured. The two major legal concepts implied in this duty are what is termed ''responsibility to duty'' and a clarification of the steps that would meet what is termed the ''reasonable man'' test in court. Responsibility to duty simply means that school personnel must provide aid to the injured, and this aid must constitute what is called ''reasonable assistance.'' If reasonable assistance is not used and school personnel do not respond to a responsibility to duty in the case of an accident, then the teacher and school can be held liable for negligence.

If school personnel do respond to a responsibility to duty and provide reasonable assistance, then it is up to legal authorities to decide whether or not the actions taken will meet a ''reasonable man'' test in court. This simply means that the individual acted in a way that is considered reasonable or justified in light of the situation and skill level of the person assisting the injured student.

Organization of School Health Programs

Ultimately the decisions are up to the courts and the legal system in general. There are no simple guidelines that would prevent negligence in these areas. However, if the school personnel are *trained* in emergency care procedures, then certainly the risk of negligence is minimized unless certain other conditions are present. These conditions are discussed in the following paragraphs.

It must be noted that legally, teachers and school personnel work under the concept of *in loco parentis*. This legal term simply means that school personnel are considered "parents" while the students are in their care. As such, they cannot ignore emergency situations when they occur. This fact alone, although the interpretation does vary from state to state, should make it evident that basic emergency care should be a priority of professional training for school personnel.

The last duty of the broad areas constituting the school's legal responsibilities states that the procedures used to treat an injured student must not increase the severity of the injury. This obviously implies that school personnel must employ the correct emergency care procedures when treating an injured student. If a teacher does not feel comfortable in administering emergency care and does not do anything to aid an injured student, then the teacher can be held liable for an act of omission known as *nonfeasance*. In this case, the teacher may be directly contributing to an increase in the severity of the injury.

If the teacher employs the correct emergency procedure but does it wrongly, or employs the incorrect emergency procedure, then the teacher can be found negligent of an act of commission. More specifically, acts of commission in this context involve both *misfeasance* (correct procedure, wrong manner) or *malfeasance* (incorrect procedure). Both of these result in increased severity of the injury.

In some cases, individuals just trying to aid an injured student would not be found negligent because of what is termed the "Good Samaritan" law. However, it must be noted that the guidelines of the Good Samaritan laws and the persons to whom this law applies vary from state to state. It is not a good idea to think that, because of a Good Samaritan law, negligence would not be a factor when trying to aid an injured student.

The purpose of defining some of the legal ramifications is not to dissuade school personnel from helping injured students but rather to have all school personnel view emergency care as a serious responsibility and not one that should be left up to the school nurse or an administrator. Finally, negligence must be proved in a court. Simple accusations made by parents do not constitute negligence. Only evidence that the broad responsibilities were violated is acceptable, and even then it is up to a court to decide if school personnel were negligent in providing or not providing emergency care in a specific situation.

School personnel do have rights when negligence is suspected or accused. Hurt (1976, pp. 202–203) identified five major avenues for defense against negligence. These avenues include showing that the accident was unavoidable;

showing that an act of the defendant's behavior was not the proximate cause; showing contributory or comparative negligence; showing assumption of risk; and claiming immunity. These avenues, if they do indeed represent the situation, can provide a solid defense for the school and school personnel.

THE HEALTH ROOM

Every school should have a full-time school nurse. However, many school districts across the United States do not employ health nurses for each school in the district. In many cases, school nurse responsibilities are performed by public health nurses who are either on call or visit schools once or twice a week.

Regardless of the policies regarding school nursing, every school should have a health room. The health room is a room that contains all materials necessary to meet emergency care problems that arise. The contents of a health room should include a minimum of the following (Commonwealth of Virginia, State Department of Education, State Department of Health, 1980, p. 18):

- Cot or bed
- Blankets (firmly woven, washable)
- Clean sheets
- Splints of several lengths: 1 ft., 2 ft., 3 ft.
- Three 3 ft. × 3 ft. muslin squares for slings and compresses
- 1–in. adhesive tape
- 3 in. × 3 in. sterile gauze (individually wrapped)
- Sterile cotton balls
- Soap
- Clean tweezers
- Snakebite kit (optional)
- Scissors
- Gauze roller bandage, 1 in. and 2 in., sterile
- Band aids
- Medicine droppers
- Safety pins
- Small basin
- Red Cross first aid textbook (may be obtained from local Red Cross chapters)

It should also be noted that facilities should be available in the health room that allow school personnel to wash their hands with antiseptic soap before any open wound is handled or any contact with eyes, mouth, ears, or nose is made. This means that the health room should have hot and cold running water, paper towels, paper cups, and waste basket(s) and that the room should be properly ventilated.

SUMMARY

Basic emergency care is a responsibility of school personnel. However, there are parameters within which school personnel can apply basic emergency care. A philosophy of emergency care, meaningful objectives, and written policies and procedures must be developed in order to have an operational emergency care and safety program in a school setting. Through comprehensive planning, including the involvement of school personnel, the prevention of accidents and the application of quality emergency care can be realized and the benefits of such a program will enhance the overall school health program.

REVIEW QUESTIONS

1. Discuss the importance of written safety policies.
2. Discuss the preparation necessary for handling emergency accidents and illnesses.
3. List some general recommendations to be followed in times of emergency.
4. Define negligence and discuss the major concepts associated with liability.
5. Identify the minimum major items needed for a health room.

REFERENCES

American Red Cross. *Standard First Aid and Personal Safety.* New York: Doubleday, 1981.

Commonwealth of Virginia, State Department of Education, State Department of Health. "Suggestions for Temporary Care of Emergencies in Schools." Richmond: Virginia, 1980.

Florio, A E., W. F. Alles, and G. T. Stafford. *Safety Education.* New York: McGraw-Hill, 1979.

Hurt, T. "Elements of Tort Liability as Applied to Athletic Injuries." *Journal of School Health* XLVI: (April 1976).

———. "Emergency Care—Conceptual Positions." *Emergency Health Care.* Lincoln: U. of Nebraska Extension, 1975.

The Minnesota State School Health Council. "State School Health Council Recommends Medication Policy." *Journal of School Health* **34**: 9 (November 1964).

Mroz, J. H. *Safety in Everyday Living.* Dubuque, Ia.: Wm. C. Brown Publishers, 1978.

Trubitt, H. J. "Legal Responsibilities of School Teachers in Emergency Situations." In Hurt, T., *Emergency Health Care.* Lincoln: U. of Nebraska Extension, 1975.

USDHHS. *Health—United States.* Washington, D.C.: USDHHS, 1982.

Special Medical Problems of School-Age Students

12

There are a variety of student medical problems that school personnel are likely to encounter. However, regardless of the problem, school personnel have a responsibility to understand it, to make every effort to detect potential problems, and to aid students in dealing with specific conditions.

The most common special medical problems seen in schools are discussed in this chapter. It should be remembered that specific criteria for detection of many of these problems were included in Chapter 8.

EPILEPSY ✳

Epilepsy is a neurological disorder. The term *epilepsy* is utilized to describe a wide variety of neurological disorders that result from many different causes. Epilepsy affects about one million Americans. Seventy-five percent of all epileptics are initially diagnosed before the age of 18. Since students generally remain in school until approximately age 17, clearly the schools will be confronted with epileptic students.

The causes of epilepsy and, more specifically, the seizures that are most commonly associated with epilepsy, are numerous. Some of these factors include heredity, high fevers, head trauma, infectious diseases, and poisoning. Obviously, the specific cause will vary from child to child.

Physiologically, epilepsy is a sudden, violent discharge of electrical energy in the brain, which results in what is termed a seizure. There are many different types of seizures that result from this electrical discharge, but the most common are the grand mal, petit mal, and psychomotor.

Grand Mal

Grand mal seizures are considered major motor convulsions and are the most common form of seizure. They are also the most frightening seizure resulting from epilepsy. The preliminary symptoms usually are a headache, tired feeling, or decrease of mental alertness. The seizure is usually initiated by a sudden loss of consciousness. The student may fall, the eyes will often roll upward, respiration momentarily ceases, and the face becomes pale. At this point, uncontrolled muscle spasms occur in the extremities and face. These spasms generally last less than a minute but may persist beyond that time.

During the initial phase, the arms and legs become rigid. Within minutes, the student will seem to relax and begin to moan and move spontaneously. In most instances, the student is drowsy following this type of seizure and falls asleep.

177

If the student has repetitive grand mal seizures without regaining consciousness in the interval, a medical emergency exists. The student must be immediately transported to a hospital for treatment of this rare complication of epilepsy, termed *status epilepticus.* [Haslam, 1985, p. 180]

However, it must be mentioned that in most cases, the student will regain consciousness, and there is no need to summon medical specialists. The student should be kept calm and allowed to rest following the seizure.

Petit Mal

The cause of a petit mal type of seizure is the same as that of the grand mal; however, the actual physical manifestations are drastically different. During a petit mal seizure, the child may appear to be disinterested in things taking place. This is usually revealed in brief episodes of staring or an appearance of daydreaming. Lapses of speech and fluttering of the eyelids are associated with this seizure. In most cases of petit mal, the child does not fall to the floor or have the same convulsions as in the grand mal seizure.

The major problem with petit mal seizures lies in the areas of safety and learning. If a student suffers from petit mal seizures, he or she could possibly become involved in an accident while in a daydreaming state. ''In the case of learning, petit mal seizures may occur so frequently that they interfere with a student's concentration, and thus school performance may decline'' (Haslam, 1985, p. 180). Frequent seizures undoubtedly interfere with memory. Since the onset of petit mal seizures usually occurs between the ages of 5 and 10, many children with this type of epilepsy are not recognized but rather are *criticized* for their lethargy and lack of enthusiasm. Unfortunately, students may experience multiple seizures of this sort, and they are embarrassed to tell the teacher of the problem. Thus, the teacher should be constantly aware of student behavior, including marked changes in academic performance.

Psychomotor Seizures

''The psychomotor type of seizure rarely begins before two years of age and is most commonly seen during the elementary school years'' (Haslam, 1985, p. 180). This type of seizure may begin with visual, auditory, or gustatory hallucinations; abdominal discomfort; headache; or a combination of all three (Haslam, 1985, p. 180). Shortly after these symptoms appear, the student may display unusual movements of the tongue, smacking of the lips, or repetitive motor movements, such as buttoning and unbuttoning an article of clothing (Haslam, 1985, p. 180). ''Most children demonstrate such signs as perspiration, salivation, rapid pulse, pallor of the face, or marked blushing during a psychomotor seizure. For the most part, its duration is a matter of a few minutes, but on occasion a psychomotor seizure may progress to a major motor convulsion'' (Haslam, 1985, p. 180).

Management of the Epileptic

The three areas of utmost concern in the management of the epileptic student include emergency first aid, medical treatment, and the role of the educator (Haslam, 1985, p. 184).

The emergency first aid for psychomotor and petit mal seizures is to keep dangerous objects out of the way of the student. There is literally nothing else that can be done. In the case of grand mal seizures, the following emergency first aid is appropriate:

1. Keep calm. Ease the person to the floor and loosen his [or her] collar. You cannot stop the seizure. Let it run its course and do not try to revive the individual.
2. Remove hard, sharp, or hot objects that may injure the individual, but do not interfere with his [or her] movements.
3. *Do not* force anything between his [or her] teeth.
4. Turn the head to one side for release of saliva. Place something soft under his [or her] head.
5. When the person regains consciousness, let him [or her] rest if he [or she] wishes.
6. If the seizure lasts beyond a few minutes or the person seems to pass from one seizure to another without gaining consciousness, call the doctor for instructions. This rarely happens, but if it does occur it should be treated immediately. [Central Arizona Regional Epilepsy Society, 1980, p. 2]

Most cases of epilepsy cannot be cured in the classical medical sense, but through medication, epilepsy can be controlled and, in most instances, the epileptic can live a normal life and certainly achieve his or her maximum potential in the school setting. Anticonvulsant medications are administered to the student diagnosed with epilepsy. Most forms of medication are not addictive, and they are useful in controlling seizures.

The teacher is in a position to assist the student with epilepsy in living a normal life. The astute teacher can utilize the opportunity of having a child with epilepsy in the class to teach the facts of epilepsy to the entire class so that the social stigma of seizures will be lessened and epileptic students will be allowed to function truly as normal individuals (Haslam, 1985, p. 187).

From a medical standpoint, the teacher can actually provide valuable information to the student's physician. It is difficult for a physician to determine accurately the required dosage of anticonvulsant medication that a student should take. The teacher, during the observation of this student, can answer such questions as, "Is the child sleepy, possibly suggesting too much medication?" or "Has the student had a sudden change in behavior (possibly indicating a reaction to medication)?"

TABLE 12.1

Indicators of Epilepsy

Staring spells (daydreaming)

Lack of response (not paying attention)

Ticlike movements

Rhythmic movements of the head

Dropping things frequently (especially when there is no apparent reason)

Having frequent accidents (again, especially when there is no apparent reason)

Head dropping

Eyes rolling upward

Chewing and swallowing

Sounds and body movements that seem out of place

According to Haslam (1985, p. 187), "Most students with epilepsy who are on medication are well controlled, have normal intelligence, and can be expected to lead normal lives. Cooperation between student, parent, physician, and teacher provides a ready avenue for this goal." For health appraisal purposes, some of the things a teacher can look for when epilepsy is suspected are shown in Table 12.1.

ARTHRITIS

Juvenile rheumatoid arthritis (JRA) is an uncommon childhood disorder. Approximately three new cases per 100,000 population occur each year. The symptoms of JRA will usually occur in children 1 to 10 years of age. A child with JRA might occasionally be encountered by school personnel. Thus it is important to mention in this text that the cause of JRA is unknown. JRA occurs more often in girls than in boys.

The symptoms of JRA vary. The inflammation in the joint causes pain, stiffness, and limited motion. The symptoms may persist for weeks. Anemia and rash are common accompanying symptoms, as well as fever, irritability, and poor appetite. In some cases, involvement of other organs, including the heart, can occur and can make the disease a life-threatening situation.

Since JRA symptoms are very similar to rheumatic fever, the diagnosis of JRA is not simple and at times can take as long as several months. During this time the student is under observation for the appearance of symptoms.

As with the adult form of arthritis, the more severe the condition, the more difficulty the student will have in participating in activities, and even in some cases, in attending classes. Therefore, it is important for the physician, teacher, school nurse, and parents to plan a program of school work and activities that is individually tailored for the students with limitations from JRA.

ALLERGIES

The term *allergy* refers to an excessive response of the body to normally harmless foreign substances called allergens. In most cases, allergies are minor problems because the physical response is slight, causing only minor physical discomfort. Common types of allergic reactions in school-age children are allergic rhinitis, allergic dermatitis, and asthma.

The most common allergens include pollens, molds, house dust, animal danders, feathers, kapok, wool, dyes, food and medicines, and insect stings. When the allergen is absorbed into the bloodstream, it stimulates certain white blood cells, called lymphocytes, to produce special substances known as allergic antibodies. The allergic antibodies react with the allergens and produce allergic inflammation and irritation in particularly sensitive areas of the body, such as the nose, eyes, lungs, and digestive system. The sensitivity may not be present at first contact with the allergen but may develop after repeated exposure.

Allergic reactions may involve any part or system of the body. The most frequent systems or parts of the body involved are the respiratory system and the skin.

Allergic Rhinitis

Allergic rhinitis is the most common allergic disease seen in the school. There are two types of allergic rhinitis: seasonal, also called hay fever, and perennial or nonseasonal. The symptoms include sneezing, nasal congestion, itching, and nasal mucous discharge. The blocked passageways can lead to headache, impaired hearing, and ear infections.

Since there is excessive postnasal drainage, coughing and throat clearing can also be symptoms. In some cases allergic laryngitis may accompany allergic rhinitis.

The ''allergic salute,'' whereby the student pushes up on the bottom of the nose with the base of the hand, is commonly associated with rhinitis. Dark circles under the eyes, puffy eyelids, and chronic breathing through the mouth are also common signs of allergic rhinitis.

Antihistamines are the drugs of choice in treating allergic seasonal or nonseasonal rhinitis. A side effect of antihistamines is drowsiness. Therefore the student might be sleepy and have difficulty in concentrating. If a student is taking antihistamines, it is important that the school personnel be aware of it and observe the length of drowsy periods for the purpose of providing information to the physician so that a correct maintenance dose can be reached.

Allergic Dermatitis

Allergic dermatitis or eczema is a noncontagious, itchy rash that is generally found in the creases of the arms, legs, and neck. However, the rash in some cases can cover the entire body. Substances to which a person is allergic may be important causes of this problem.

Contact Dermatitis

Contact dermatitis is a rash that comes from direct skin contact with many substances, including animals, plants, or chemicals.

Allergic Tension–Fatigue Syndrome

The allergic tension–fatigue syndrome refers to allergic reactions of the body to allergens over a long period of time. The eight most common symptoms of this disorder are:

1. Accompanying respiratory tract allergy.
2. Abdominal discomfort, frequently with nausea.
3. Recurrent headaches.
4. Tenseness and irritability.
5. Facial pallor.
6. Dark circles under the eyes.
7. Tiredness.
8. Musculoskeletal pains. [McGovern, 1976, p. 344]

It is important that this syndrome be identified early since learning may be affected. The syndrome can usually be managed by controlling the allergy. This is done through medication and avoidance of specific allergens that are associated with the condition.

Treatment

The only true treatment for allergies is to remove the allergen from the environment or to desensitize the individual to the allergen. This can be relatively easy if the allergy is to a food or a particular object (e.g., a feather pillow). It is not so easy if the allergens are plant pollens, which are found everywhere in certain environments.

In severe cases, a student may be referred to undergo allergy testing, in which injections of various allergens are administered and the skin is evaluated for a reaction shortly after the injections. This is the only way to positively identify certain allergens. Once the major allergens have been identified, the student can undergo allergy shots over time periods, ranging from several times per week to once a month. The typical allergy shot consists of small amounts of allergens. Usually the amount of allergens is increased with each shot. It is hoped that after a period of time the student's body will become immune (desensitized) to the allergen, and the allergic reaction will not take place when subjected to the allergen. However, it should be noted that allergy shot regimes are expensive and not always successful.

Finally, a number of different drugs can be used to treat the symptoms of allergies. The most popular drugs are antihistamines and bronchodilators. The drugs do not cure the allergy but can be used successfully in reducing the symptoms.

ASTHMA

Approximately 4.5 million school children in the United States suffer from asthma. Of all chronic illnesses, it is the leading cause of school absenteeism (Smith, 1978, p. 311). Asthma is a variable obstruction of the airways. The main symptoms include wheezing; shortness of breath; an irritating, light cough; and tenacious sputum. The symptoms are a result of bronchial tubes in the lungs narrowing, tissues in the bronchial tubes swelling, and the formation of heavy mucus.

The basic cause of asthma is an "increased sensitivity of receptors and chemical mediators in the bronchial system" (Smith, 1978, p. 311). Such things as allergies, cigarette smoke, exercise, emotional upset, and infection can trigger the symptoms. When this happens, the student suffers an "asthma attack."

For many years asthma was thought to be just the byproduct of an emotional upset; there was thought to be little physiological basis to the idea that actual biochemical mechanisms could cause the wheezing and other symptoms associated with it. Emotions do play an important role in triggering attacks, and asthma could certainly be used as a crutch or excuse for certain behaviors. However, there is evidence that many factors cause asthma, not just emotions.

The treatment for asthma, especially if it is related to allergies, is the use of bronchodilators. These drugs dilate the airways and allow the student to breathe without the feeling that he or she is breathing through cotton. Teachers, especially physical education teachers, should be aware of the student's physical limitations so that an asthma attack is not triggered by vigorous exercise. Vigorous exercise, especially if allergens are present in the environment, can aggravate the condition and trigger an asthma attack. However, participation in regular, daily exercise is good for the asthmatic.

Asthma attacks can be a frightening experience for both the student and other students witnessing the attack. Through proper intervention asthma attacks can be effectively dealt with in the school setting. Table 12.2 shows what must be done in dealing with asthma attacks.

Like many diseases, asthma can be acute or chronic. Often students will "grow out" of asthma and, usually after adolescence, may not be troubled again or troubled only occasionally.

Childhood bronchial asthma presents a significant public health problem, with major impact on disruption of the living patterns of the students and their families. It is among the most common of the chronic pediatric diseases, afflicting about 3 percent of all children aged 6 to 16 years. During any school year, it is estimated that asthma causes 28 million disability days for those under 17 years of age (Freudenberg et al., 1980, p. 522).

The influence of asthma on school attendance and performance has not been examined extensively. Several reports have considered various school problems faced by students with asthmatic problems. A Belgian study of asthmatic children followed in a pediatric clinic demonstrated that 80 percent of

TABLE 12.2

First Aid for Breathing Difficulty

In Case of Breathing Difficulty

- Help the child to assume an upright position with shoulders relaxed.
- Talk to the child reassuringly and calmly. His or her anxiety can be lessened if you show you understand and know how to be helpful.
- Encourage the child to drink lots of fluids.
- Encourage the child to take appropriate medication if the child's doctor has prescribed medicine to be used at the time of breathing difficulty. (Check with school nurse for proper school procedure.)
- If the medications do not appear to be working effectively, notify the proper person. According to school regulations, this could be the school nurse, the parent or guardian. Only in rare cases do children with asthma need emergency care.
- If it is possible without embarrassing the child with asthma, turn the episode into a learning experience for the entire class. Explain what asthma is, its effects on breathing, and how classmates can be helpful.

Source: American Lung Association, 1990

the subjects were one to three years behind in their school work (Freudenberg et al., 1980, p. 522). A study based in Brooklyn, New York, revealed that asthmatics who received care in a hospital outpatient clinic missed almost twice as many school days a year as asthmatics treated by private physicians (Freudenberg et al., 1980, p. 522). Parcel and Gilman (1979, p. 878) found that elementary school children suffering from asthma had significantly higher absentee rates than their nonasthmatic schoolmates. This trend diminished as children became older (Freudenberg et al., 1980, p. 522).

✳ DIABETES MELLITUS

Type I, or insulin-dependent diabetes mellitus (IDDM), formerly called juvenile-onset diabetes, is the most common endocrinologic abnormality of childhood (1 to 3.5 per thousand) among school-age children. However, when it does occur, it tends to be more serious in childhood than if diagnosed in later life. Since it is a serious condition and since approximately 5 percent of all people with diabetes display the first symptoms in childhood, it is worth mentioning in this text.

Type I diabetes mellitus is a condition in which the body is unable to metabolize carbohydrates due to an insufficient production of insulin. Insulin is produced by the pancreas and helps in the breakdown of sugar. If not enough insulin is produced, the blood sugar level gets too high and diabetic acidosis, which is an acute life-threatening complication of type I diabetes, can result. If the child does not receive immediate medical attention, coma and death can result. The symptoms of diabetic acidosis include uncharacteristic lethargy, vomiting, and abdominal pain. A student exhibiting these symptoms must receive immediate medical attention.

Members of the school health team will usually be notified if a child or certain children in the school have type I diabetes mellitus. The school nurse should educate those personnel who come into contact with the child or children in order to inform them about the nature of the disease and of the potential seriousness of the condition.

Most students with type I diabetes mellitus will probably already be under the care of a physician when they enter school. The treatment for type I diabetes mellitus includes regular injections of insulin and adhering to a special diet. The diabetic must adhere to the treatment regime in order to avoid a potentially serious medical crisis.

OVERWEIGHT AND OBESITY *

It is estimated that 12 to 30 percent of all children are overweight. The normative values used to define proper weight for height, regardless of age, were developed by the National Center for Health Statistics in 1976. The resulting classifications are as follows:

- *Underweight:* Weight 7 to 12 percent below the median weight for height (10th to 25th percentiles).
- *Lean:* Weigh more than 12 percent below the median for height (below the 10th percentile).
- *Overweight:* Weight 11 to 20 percent above the median weight for height (75th to 90th percentiles).
- *Obese:* Weight greater than 20 percent above the median weight for height (above the 90th percentile).

Naturally, the area of most concern from a health standpoint is that of students who are overweight or obese. Overweight and obese children suffer primarily from a nutritional disorder, although in some cases overweight can be due to glandular problems. The nutritional disorder is simply the consumption of more food energy than one expends, resulting in increased weight. Over a period of time, the small increases in weight add up to a large increase in weight, and in some cases (12 to 30 percent of all school children) to an increase in weight of more than 11 percent of that needed for their height.

Obviously, in such cases there is more than a nutritional disorder involved. Something causes the student to eat more than he or she needs.

It has been shown that obesity is a widespread condition in the United States and other technologically advanced countries. The only really effective treatment is prevention (sound nutrition and regular exercise), especially during childhood.

Comprehensive health education programs that include nutrition education and exercise classes in the schools are feasible in preventing obesity and are important components in overall health care. The causes and disadvantages

TABLE 12.3

Causes and Disadvantages of Obesity

Causes of Obesity

Glandular problem (example: thyroid)

Poor eating habits (overeating, snacking, unbalanced meals)

Lack of proper nutritional knowledge

Lack of exercise

Heredity

Emotional difficulties

Disadvantages of Obesity

Social attitudes toward the ''fat'' student

Psychological traits—more likely to have low self-esteem, feeling of self-consciousness

Movement and agility problems with certain physical activities

Problems concerning clothing, furniture, and so on (example: size of school desks)

Physiological problems (more prone to health risks—high blood pressure, heart and kidney diseases, skeletal or joint problems, i.e., arthritis)

Others: life expectancy reduced, surgery more difficult, and greater incidence of accidents

---

of obesity are shown in Table 12.3. There are both direct and indirect ways of helping the obese student. These ways include the following:

1. Direct ways.
   a. Approach the student directly—talk about the problem, try to influence him or her to talk to parents, see a physician; offer to help in an effort to find the cause.
   b. Have the student talk with the physical education instructor about participating in an exercise program.
   c. Encourage the student to become involved at school and *at home* (example: hobbies or other useful ways of utilizing time).
   d. Inform the student about proper nutrition and eating habits.
   e. Try to help enhance the student's self-image.
2. Indirect methods (assuming that you have tried to talk to the student and received unsatisfactory response).
   a. Present a section in the classroom concerning proper nutrition, eating habits, and exercise.
   b. Try to make the student feel worthwhile, try to help his or her self-image—praise him or her when deserved.
   c. Consult with the school nurse and have the nurse approach the problem.

d. Consult the physical education instructor and see if he or she can help keep the student active.

e. Make up a bulletin board or give out handouts in class regarding nutrition, exercise, and weight control.

DEVELOPMENTAL DISABILITIES

Developmental disabilities refer to a number of different conditions occurring in childhood that are directly related to abnormal brain structure, maturation, or function. The resultant impairment can affect motor skills, adaptive skills, learning skills, and social skills. Too often, an assumption is made that the child with a developmental disability will also have a learning disability; this is not necessarily true.

The most common developmental disabilities found in the school setting are cerebral palsy and mental retardation.

Cerebral Palsy

Cerebral palsy is a general term that is applied to a group of nonprogressive symptoms resulting from damage to the developing brain. This damage occurs before, during, or shortly after birth and results in loss or impairment of control over voluntary muscles. Chief causes of the brain damage are insufficient oxygen reaching the brain, anoxia, complications of labor or delivery, low birth weight, infections, and poisoning.

Of the estimated 750,000 persons who have cerebral palsy, 300,000 of them are children. About 15,000 babies are born with cerebral palsy each year. Even though cerebral palsy may be the general diagnosis, there are six types of cerebral palsy that may result from the brain damage. These six types are as follows:

1. Spastic: abnormally increased muscle tension.
2. Athetoid: recurring slow, involuntary writhing movements of arms and legs.
3. Ataxia: disturbed sense of balance.
4. Tremor: symptoms of fine tremulousness.
5. Rigidity: muscles in a state of semicontraction resulting from slowness in movement.
6. Mixed symptoms: two or more of the preceding types.

There are many learning handicaps associated with cerebral palsy. However, they are not necessarily due to the actual condition of the student suffering from cerebral palsy; rather, they may result from the possible associated dysfunction.

Since the brain is the chief organ affected in cerebral palsy, other types of dysfunction often occur. Some of the dysfunctions include:

1. *Mental retardation,* which occurs in 50 to 60 percent of the cases of cerebral palsy.
2. *Seizures,* which occur in 25 to 35 percent of the cases of cerebral palsy.

3. *Speech problems,* which occur in 70 percent of the cerebral palsy cases.
4. *Visual disturbances,* which occur in 35 percent of the cases.
5. *Hearing problems,* which occur in 20 percent of the cases.

Treatment for cerebral palsy can include medication to control seizures, surgery to lengthen short muscles, physiotherapy, occupational therapy, and counseling (Newton, 1989).

Unfortunately, the stereotype of the individual with cerebral palsy resembles the image of the mentally retarded individual with severe spasticity. This is not an accurate portrait of the cerebral palsy victim. Now that mainstreaming is becoming more common, the child with cerebral palsy stands a good chance of being placed and learning in the regular classroom environment.

Mental Retardation

An estimated 6 million Americans suffer from mental retardation. The incidence of mental retardation is approximately 126,000 new cases per year. A further breakdown of the prevalence of mental retardation by age group is as follows:

*   Birth to 5 years of age: 605,000 cases.
*   Six to 16 years of age: 1,354,000 cases.
*   Sixteen to 21 years of age: 691,000 cases.
*   Over 21 years of age: 3,110,000 cases.

Unfortunately, approximately 80% of the mentally retarded are found in lower socioeconomic areas.

Most mental retardation originates in the prenatal period or in early childhood. However, since the condition is often not diagnosed, many cases are not reported. The chief causes of mental retardation may include:

1. Incomplete development of central nervous system tissue.
2. Lack of brain development before birth.
3. Chromosome abnormalities.
4. Illness affecting the brain.
5. Abnormally long labor.
6. Injury to the brain after birth.

One of the most widespread problems in recognizing mental retardation lies in accurately defining it. Before specific definitions for mental retardation were developed, children and adults were classified as mentally retarded if they were identified as having unusual physical features. Further, the classification of having a low IQ often led to the diagnosis of mental retardation. It was not until 1973, when the American Association on Mental Deficiency altered its definition of mental retardation, that professionals had a more operational definition. According to Grossman (1973, p. 180), the current definition states that ''mental retardation refers to significantly subaverage general intellectual functioning existing concurrently with deficits in adaptive behavior, and manifested during the developmental period.'' Significantly subaverage general intellectual functioning refers to a developmental and intelligence quotient that is below 70 and represents two or more standard deviations from the mean or average of the population tested (Capute, 1985, p. 207). Capute states that:

> of the approximately six million people functioning below an IQ level of 70, 89 percent, or 5.5 million, are mildly retarded . . . [or] educable mentally retarded. The remaining 11 percent, or .5 million, comprise the trainable [mentally retarded and the] severe[ly] and profound[ly] mentally retarded group[s].

Only considerations regarding the educable and trainable mentally retarded will be discussed in this text.

Educable Mentally Retarded (EMR)

The ultimate goal or objective for the individual with an IQ score of 55 to 69 is social and economic independence. Perhaps the most common problem in identifying these groups in the early school years is that they do not deviate that much from the average child and subsequently are not identified until kindergarten or first grade.

Special education programs that are constructed in a multidisciplinary manner have experienced considerable success with EMRs. The more involvement of the EMR student with students with average or above average IQs, the greater chance there is that the EMR will display social and economic independence.

Trainable Mentally Retarded (TMR)

In the words of Capute (1985, p. 209), ''The trainable mentally retarded develops at a rate between one third to one half . . . [the] normal [rate], reaching a mental age of four to eight years by adulthood.'' The TMR child is usually recognized by the parent or pediatrician during infancy or early childhood, primarily because of severe developmental lag (Capute, 1985, p. 210). Educational efforts for the TMR are directed at developing functional reading and writing skills.

LEARNING DISABILITIES

One of the most frequently debated items of special educators and other personnel dealing with school children is answering the question ''What is a learning disability?'' It would be convenient to derive one simple definition that would encompass the entire range of learning disabilities, but since learning disabilities are complex processes, this is nearly impossible.

Kass and Mykleburst (1969, p. 377) published what are termed universal components of learning disabilities. This comprehensive descriptive definition will reflect the complex problem of defining a learning disability. Their definition is as follows:

1. *Learning disability* refers to one or more significant deficits in essential learning processes requiring special education for remediation.

2. Children with a learning disability generally demonstrate a discrepancy between expected and actual achievement in one or more areas, such as spoken or written language, reading, mathematics, and spatial orientation.

3. The learning disability referred to is not primarily the result of sensorimotor, intellectual, or emotional handicap, or of the lack of an opportunity to learn.

- Significant deficits are defined in terms of accepted diagnostic procedures in education and psychology.
- Essential learning processes are those currently referred to in behavioral science as involving perception integration and expression, either verbal or nonverbal.
- Special education techniques for remediation refers to educational planning based on the diagnostic procedures and results.

A conservative estimate of the number of children in the United States school systems with learning disabilities is around 7 percent. Since learning disabilities are particularly hard to define, the exact percentage of students suffering from a learning disability is probably somewhat lower than the actual percentage.

Valett (1969, p. 20), in his book *Programming Learning Disabilities,* listed seven characteristics often observable in learning-disabled children. The seven points include: repeated history of academic failure in educational pursuits; physical and environmental limitations interacting with learning difficulties; motivational abnormalities; vague, free-floating anxiety; erratic, uneven behavior; incomplete evaluation; and inadequate education.

Some of Valett's points, such as repeated history of academic failure or the presence of some physical or environmentally related problem such as vision or hearing loss, are easy to understand. However, some of the points he makes are not as clear. For example, motivational problems, as reflected in repeated failure or rejection by teachers, are more difficult to understand. The anxiety that arises with repeated failure can result in a self-fulfilling prophecy. The student feels that failure is inevitable, so he or she stops trying.

Incomplete evaluations and inadequate education may result in children actually being mislabeled and called slow, retarded, or disturbed. Teachers have been too quick in applying labels to students, and too often these labels have been attached before complete evaluation of the student has occurred. Finally, inadequate education results from classroom activities that are not appropriate for the child. This can create frustration and can often result in an aggravation of any existing problems.

The National Advisory Committee on Handicapped Children formulated the following definition for learning disabilities:

Children with special learning disabilities exhibit a disorder in one or more of the basic psychological processes involved in understanding or using spoken or written language. These may be manifested in disorders of listening, thinking, talking, reading, writing, spelling or arithmetic. They include conditions which have been referred to as perceptual handicaps, brain injury, minimal brain dysfunction, dyslexia, and developmental aphasia. They do not include learning problems which are due primarily to visual, hearing or motor handicaps, to mental retardation, emotional disturbance or to environmental disadvantage. [National Advisory Committee on Handicapped Children, 1968, p. 10]

Cruickshank (1977, p. 31) stated that a learning disability is the direct result of a perceptual processing deficit. Perception and processing are neurologically based, and if the neurological basis for learning disabilities can be identified, a program can be developed to meet the needs of the student. However, most children with learning disabilities will never see a neurologist.

A complete physical evaluation is necessary for a child with a suspected learning disability. In addition to the physical evaluation, an examination of mental status and a physical neurological examination should be performed.

For practical purposes, it is important that school personnel be aware of the following points in identifying a child with a possible learning disability.

1. Atypical spelling errors.
2. Auditory discrimination problems.
3. Letter recognition problems.
4. Initial sound-in-words confusion.
5. Counting and number recognition difficulties.
6. Auditory memory deficits.
7. Visual memory deficits.
8. Gross motor incoordination.
9. Spatial disorientation.
10. Articulation errors.
11. Fine motor problems. [Johnson and Morasky, 1977, p. 33]

INTERDISCIPLINARY TEAMWORK

The child with either a learning disability or developmental disability or both, regardless of the diagnosis, rarely possesses a single problem that would require the service of but one professional. This child needs input from a variety of different specialists who can plan a meaningful educational program, including recommendations for the teacher and parent to aid the child in maximizing his or her learning potential. The ultimate goal in interdisciplinary teamwork is to develop a well-coordinated interdisciplinary rehabilitation program.

MAINSTREAMING AND HANDICAPPED STUDENTS

According to Vlasak (1980, p. 286), ''The legal underpinning of the practice of mainstreaming—the least restrictive environment concept—requires that, whenever possible, handicapped children be educated with children who are not handicapped.'' Although this concept does not absolutely disallow certain handicapped children being educated in separate classrooms or separate facilities, the burden of proof is on school officials to justify removal of any handicapped child from regular classrooms and regular campuses. Access to the regular educational environment must not be restricted because of administrative preference, philosophy, matters of finance, availability of service, or requests by parents (Vlasak, 1980, p. 286).

With the passage of the Rehabilitation Act of 1973 and the Education of All Handicapped Children Act of 1975 (PL 94–142), Congress extended the protection of the least drastic means (least restrictive environment) concept to all handicapped children in the nation. PL 94–142 contains specific language requiring that handicapped children be educated with nonhandicapped children to the maximum extent possible (Vlasak, 1980, p. 285).

More than 90 percent of the handicapped students receive at least some of their education within the mainstream. The courts and legislatures have not excluded the possibility that some handicapped children will require special programs (Vlasak, 1980, p. 286).

ANOREXIA NERVOSA AND BULIMIA NERVOSA

Anorexia nervosa and bulimia nervosa are eating disorders that have emerged as significant health problems in recent years. The onset of anorexia nervosa and bulimia nervosa usually occurs during adolescence and is predominantly a female disorder (Connolly, 1990). The prevalence of anorexia nervosa is from .5 percent to 4.0 percent of the population while bulimia nervosa is from 5 percent to 19 percent of females of high school and college age (Connolly, 1990).

In order to better understand anorexia nervosa and bulimia nervosa it is important to clinically define both conditions. The American Psychiatric Association uses specific diagnostic criteria for defining these eating disorders and are as follows:

Bulimia Nervosa
A.   Recurrent episodes of binge eating (rapid consumption of large amounts of food in a discrete period of time).
B.   A feeling of lack of control over eating behavior during the eating binges.
C.   The person regularly engages in either self-induced vomiting, use of laxatives or diuretics, strict dieting or fasting, or vigorous exercise in order to prevent weight gain.
D.   A minimum average of two binge eating episodes a week for at least three months.
E.   Persistent over-concern with body shape and weight.

Anorexia Nervosa
A.   Refusal to maintain body weight over a minimal normal weight for age and height, e.g., weight loss leading to maintenance of body

weight 15 percent below that expected; or failure to make expected weight gain during period of growth, leading to body weight 15% below that expected.

B. Intense fear of gaining weight or becoming fat, even though underweight.

C. Disturbance in the way in which one's body weight, size, or shape is experienced, e.g., the person claims to "feel fat" even when emaciated, believes that one area of the body is "too fat" even when obviously underweight.

D. In females, absence of at least three consecutive menstrual cycles when otherwise expected to occur (primary or secondary amenorrhea). (A woman is considered to have amenorrhea if her periods occur only following hormone administration, e.g., estrogen).

The cause of anorexia nervosa and bulimia nervosa is not known. What is known is that the conditions are a result of interplay among individual, family, and sociocultural factors (Connolly, 1990). Some of the individual factors include genetic predisposition, substance abuse, depression, low self-esteem, perceived ineffectiveness, helplessness, guilt, anger, and loneliness.

Some of the sociocultural factors related to the development of anorexia nervosa and bulimia nervosa include the increased emphasis on such things as thinness as being desirable for women, the need for women to achieve and be successful, and the sociocultural biases against obesity (Connolly, 1990).

Common family characteristics of women diagnosed with anorexia nervosa or bulimia nervosa include "enmeshment (poor boundary definition or excessive closeness among family members), overprotectiveness, rigidity, and lack of conflict resolution" (Connolly, 1990).

As a result of the interplay between individual, sociocultural, and family factors an adolescent can respond by exhibiting the various characteristics presented in Figure 12.1.

Common physical symptoms of the behaviors displayed in anorexia nervosa and bulimia nervosa include extreme weight loss, hypothermia, insomnia, constipation, skin rash, loss of hair and nail quality, dental caries and periodontal disease, and cessation of the menstrual cycle.

Anorexics may exhibit a loss of 25 percent or more of body weight within several months. Bulimics . . . may exhibit dramatic . . . fluctuations in body weight that affect the body's ability to maintain heat, resulting in a slower metabolic rate. . . . With a slowed metabolic rate, an interruption of sleeping patterns or insomnia may occur. [Bayer and Baker, 1978, p. 3]

Since the function of the intestinal tract often depends on the type and amount of food eaten, constipation is a common physical complaint of people suffering from anorexia nervosa and bulimia nervosa. Also, abuse of laxatives and diuretics can contribute to the problem.

FIGURE 12.1

Behavioral characteristics of anorexia nervosa and bulimia nervosa.

Reprinted with permission from Journal of School Health. Eating Disorders: A Framework for School Nursing Initiatives. Vol. 60, No. 9, October 1990, p. 402. Copyright 1990. American School Health Association, Kent, OH 44240.

Behavioral Characteristics of Anorexia and Bulimia Nervosa

Characteristics	Anorexia Nervosa	Bulimia Nervosa
Drive for thinness	-feels fat when thin	-seeks to avoid obesity
Body image	-distorted-severely -preoccupation with weight	-distorted-varying degrees -preoccupation with weight
Self-concept deficit	-low self-esteem -lack of trust	-low self-esteem -lack of trust
Food-related behaviors	-food rituals -rigid eating patterns -calorically dense foods avoided -sudden increase in cooking, diet books, calories	-chaotic eating patterns -binges (composed of large amounts of food in a short period of time) when feeling bored, angry, depressed, lonely -fad diets-vomits, fasts, exercises after meals -ingests laxatives, diuretics, ipecac to promote weight loss
Individual personality characteristics	-perfectionistic -obsessive	-impulsive -mood swings
Miscellaneous behaviors	-repetitive, frequent exercise -co-addictions possible -wears baggy clothes -social withdrawal -decreased school performance or increased effort to maintain performance	-wears baggy clothes to hide weight loss -repetitive, frequent exercise -co-addictions possible -social withdrawal

Starvation and body purging will often result in deteriorated skin conditions due to body dehydration and associated problems. The protein deficiencies can result in loss of hair and nail quality, and the nutritional deficiencies can also result in dental problems. [Bayer and Baker, 1978, p. 6] Finally, anorexia nervosa and bulimia nervosa can result in a reduction in the female hormone levels. As a result, the absence of menstruation (amenorrhea) can occur.

Both anorexia nervosa and bulimia nervosa sufferers are preoccupied with food. Bulimic binging episodes might be detected easily, whereas self-starvation requires careful monitoring to discover the amount of food that is being consumed. Many young people will exercise vigorously to rid their bodies of calories and fatty tissue (such exercise patterns are compulsive and extreme) and they also will misuse laxatives, diuretics, ipecac, and diet pills.

It is a paradox that many anorexia nervosa and bulimia nervosa sufferers are exceptional students with high aspirations, which are reflected in strong academic performance. However, in the later stages of the disease, these people are characterized by an inability to think clearly, which results in a reduction in academic achievement (Bayer and Baker, 1978, p. 3).

According to Bayer and Baker (p. 3), key factors in identifying those with anorexia nervosa and bulimia nervosa include the following:

1. Weight change over a specific period of time.
2. Menstrual period changes.
3. Eating behavior changes.
4. Personality or behavior changes.

Once diagnosed, the treatment for sufferers of anorexia nervosa and bulimia nervosa usually consists of physical care, counseling including behavior modification, individual therapy, and family and group treatment. The earlier diagnosis is made and treatment begins, the sooner they will recover and live a normal life.

Preventive measures also include more positive interaction with students in attempts to help students feel good about themselves. Other similar factors and specific ways to interact with students are included in Chapter 10. [The national association of Anorexia Nervosa and Associated Disorders (ANAD) can provide anyone with up-to-date, sound information on eating disorders. Information can be obtained by writing to ANAD, Box 271, Highland Park, IL 60035.]

SUMMARY

There are a variety of special medical problems that school personnel are likely to encounter in the school setting. It is important that school personnel understand the wide variety of common problems experienced by large numbers of students in order to make any necessary adjustments in the learning environment to maximize the learning experience for the student with a special medical problem.

This chapter covered many different special medical problems. Because of the nature of this text, only specific information that relates to the school health program was presented. Students needing more information on any of the problems covered are encouraged to do more reading in the area of special education as well as to contact specific health associations whose focus is directed at some of these medical problems.

REVIEW QUESTIONS

1. Discuss the cause and treatment of epilepsy, allergies, and asthma.
2. What are the implications for schools with respect to the special medical problems presented in Chapter 12?
3. What is the difference between a learning disability and a developmental disability?
4. What is meant by anorexia nervosa and bulimia nervosa? What is the cause? Treatment? Implications for the school personnel?

REFERENCES

American Lung Association. *Asthma Alert for Teachers.* New York: American Lung Association, 1990.

Bayer, A., and D. Baker. *Not Just a Skinny Kid.* Highland Park, Ill.: National Association of Anorexia Nervosa and Associated Disorders (ANAD), 1978.

Capute, A. "Mental Retardation." In Haslam, R., and R. Valletutti, *Medical Problems in the Classroom.* Austin: Pro-ed, Inc., 1985.

Central Arizona Regional Epilepsy Society. *Epilepsy Facts.* Phoenix: Cares, 1980.

Connolly, C., and P. Corbett-Dick. "Eating Disorders: A Framework for School Health Initiatives." *Journal of School Health* **60**:8 (October, 1990) 401–405.

Cruickshank, W. *Learning Disabilities in Home, School and Community.* Syracuse, N.Y.: Syracuse University Press, 1977.

Freudenberg, N., et al. "The Impact of Bronchial Asthma on School Attendance and Performance." *Journal of School Health* **50**:9 (November 1980).

Grossman, H. *Manual on Terminology and Classification in Mental Retardation.* Baltimore: Garamont/Pridemark Press, 1973.

Haslam, R., and P. Valletutti. *Medical Problems in the Classroom.* Austin: Pro-ed, Inc., 1985.

Johnson, R., and P. Magrab. *Developmental Disorders: Assessment, Treatment, and Education.* Austin: Pro-ed, Inc., 1978.

Johnson, S., and R. Morasky. *Learning Disabilities.* Boston: Allyn and Bacon, 1977.

Kass, C., and H. Mykleburst. "Learning Disabilities: An Educational Definition." *Journal of Learning Disabilities* **2** (1969).

McGovern, J. "Chronic Respiratory Diseases of School-Age Children." *Journal of School Health* **46**:6 (June 1976).

National Advisory Committee on Handicapped Children. *Special Education for Handicapped Children, First Annual Report.* Washington, D.C.: Department of Health, Education and Welfare, 1968.

Newton, J. *The New School Health Handbook.* Englewood Cliffs: Prentice-Hall, 1989.

Parcel, G., and S. Gilman. "A Comparison of Absentee Rates of Elementary School Children with Asthma and Nonasthmatic Schoolmates." *Pediatrics* **64** (1979).

Rassel, G., J. Tonelson, and C. Appolone. "Epilepsy Workshop for Public School Personnel." *Journal of School Health* **51**:1 (January 1981).

Smith, S. "Some (Not All) Facts About Asthma." *Journal of School Health* **48**:5 (May 1978).

Valett, R. *Programming Learning Disabilities.* Belmont, Ca.: Fearon, 1969.

Vlasak, J. "Mainstreaming Handicapped Children: The Underlying Legal Concept." *Journal of School Health* **50**:5 (May 1980).

Zakus, G. "Treating Adolescent Obesity: A Pilot Project in a School." *Journal of School Health* **51**:10 (December 1980).

Drugs, AIDS, Adolescent Pregnancy, and the Student

13

T hree major health problems, well publicized during the 1980s, were: drug use, misuse, and abuse; AIDS; and adolescent pregnancy. Because each of these serious problems has vast implications for young people, more specifically school-age students, we are devoting a whole chapter in this edition to these topics.

DRUGS AND THE STUDENT

According to the U.S. Department of Education, the United States has the highest rate of teenage drug use of any industrialized nation (USDOE, 1986). This fact is reflected in Table 13.1, which shows frequency of use of selected drugs by age group. It is clear from this table that drug use, particularly alcohol and marijuana use, is high among young people. How young? It is interesting to note that the percentage of students who use drugs by the time they reach the sixth grade has tripled over the last decade (USDOE, 1986). In the early 1960s, marijuana use was virtually nonexistent among 12- to 17-year-olds, but now about one in five from this age group has used marijuana.

In order to combat drug use among school students, it is important for members of the school health team to be knowledgeable in a variety of areas. The United States Department of Education came up with several recommendations for achieving schools without drugs. These recommendations include:

1. Teach standards of right and wrong and demonstrate these standards through personal examples.
2. Help children to resist peer pressure to use drugs by supervising their activities, knowing who their friends are and talking with them about their interests and problems.
3. Be knowledgeable about drugs and signs of drug use. When symptoms are observed respond promptly.
4. Determine the extent and character of drug use and establish a means of monitoring that use regularly.
5. Establish clear and specific rules regarding drug use that includes strong corrective actions.
6. Enforce established policies against drug use fairly and consistently. Implement security measures to eliminate drugs on school premises and at school functions.
7. Implement a comprehensive drug prevention curriculum from kindergarten through grade 12, teaching that drug use is wrong and

TABLE 13.1

Percentage of ''Ever Used'' and Current (Used Within Last Month) Drug Users in Selected Age Ranges

Drug Class (nonmedical use)	Age		
	12–17 Ever Used/Last Month	18–25 Ever Used/Last Month	Over 26 Ever Used/Last Month
Marijuana/Hashish	24/12%	60/22%	27/6%
Hallucinogens	3/1	11/2	6/0
Cocaine	5/2	28/8	10/2
Heroin	0/0	1/0	1/0
Prescribed sedatives	4/1	11/2	5/1
Prescribed tranquilizers	5/1	12/2	7/1
Prescribed stimulants	6/2	17/4	8/1
Alcohol	56/31	93/71	89/61
Cigarettes	45/15	76/37	80/33

Source: Johnson, L. D., *Summary of 1988 Drug Study Report,* Press Release from the Institute for Special Research, University of Michigan, Feb. 28, 1989.

harmful and supporting and strengthening resistance to drugs.

8. Reach out to the community for support and assistance in making the school's antidrug policy and program work.

9. Learn about the effects of drug use, the reasons drugs are harmful, and ways to resist pressures to try drugs.

10. Use an understanding of the danger posed by drugs to help other students avoid them.

11. Communities should help schools fight drugs by providing them with the expertise and financial resources of community groups and agencies.

This section will address the above eleven areas in varying degrees. For the purpose of organization of this section the topics covered will be those about which members of the school health team should have an understanding. These areas include knowledge about: the drugs themselves, indicators of potential drug use, factors identified that increase the likelihood that a student will use drugs, policies schools should adopt so that all members of the school health team can participate in prevention of drug use, what curriculums are available that have proven to be effective in preventing drug use.

Basic Concepts Regarding Drugs

A drug is defined as any chemical that modifies one or more body functions. We are therefore talking about anything from antibiotics to aspirin. The drugs that are popular for recreational use are those that not only modify one or more body functions but also modify mood and behavior. These drugs can be placed into the following major categories: depressants, stimulants, hallucinogens, marijuana, and designer drugs.

Regardless of the category of drug being discussed, there are physiological and psychosocial concepts common to all categories. *Drug use* refers to using a drug for its intended purpose. Inherent in this definition is the assumption that the drug is being taken under a physician's orders or suggestion and is intended to deal with a clinical condition. *Drug misuse* is using a drug for a reason other than for which it was intended. While *drug abuse* is chronically using a drug for a reason other than for which it was intended.

When a person begins taking drugs regularly, the body's response to the chemical can lead to physical dependence to the drug. That is, the body requires the drug in order to function in a normal manner. Along with physical dependence a user is likely to notice that he or she is requiring a larger dose of the drug to achieve the original or intended effect. This is referred to as *tolerance*. Finally, as the drug use continues and becomes a part of the individual's lifestyle, he or she is possibly establishing an emotional attachment to the drug, referred to as *psychological dependence*. In most cases when drug dependence and tolerance have been established, the user may experience withdrawal symptoms if the drug is not taken when there is a physical or psychological need to take the drug. Withdrawal symptoms vary in intensity depending upon the extent of dependence and can range from a simple headache to grand mal seizures (for those with physical dependence) and from anxiety to hallucinations (for those with psychological dependence). When a user is physically dependent and psychologically dependent on a drug, and tolerance has been established, that person is usually considered to be addicted to the drug.

The intensity of effect of any drug is related to the amount of the drug taken—in other words, the greater the dose, the greater the effect. This concept is referred to as *dose-response*.

In addition to dose-response, there are two other major variables that influence how a person responds to a drug. These variables are referred to as *set* and *setting*. Set is the mental expectations a person has with respect to a drug.

If a person's mental expectation is that a drug will relax him or her then the result is relaxation. Setting is the environment that the drug is taken in. The amount of social activity in the environment influences how a person responds to a drug.

Categories of Drugs

As previously mentioned, the major categories of drugs of abuse seen in school environments are those that modify mood and behavior. What follows is a brief overview of those major categories of drugs.

Depressants

Depressants are drugs that decrease functional activity or slow down body processes. In low doses, the effects of depressants are usually experienced in the form of a relaxed state or calmness. Slurred speech, staggering gait, and altered perceptions are symptoms of administration of a higher than normal dose. Finally, a high dose of depressants can lead to respiratory depression, coma, and death. Table 13.2 shows the major types of depressants, the slang terms for the depressant, what it looks like and how it is generally used.

Depressants are highly addictive and traditionally have presented major problems for society. The most abused depressant in the United States as well as in most other countries is alcohol.

Stimulants

Stimulants do the opposite of depressants, they increase functional activity.

In low doses, stimulants increase the level of alertness, which can be interpreted as being "high." In low to moderate doses, the user may experience sweating, headache, blurred vision, dizziness, sleeplessness, and anxiety. Rapid or irregular heartbeat, tremors, loss of coordination and physical collapses are characteristics of abuse of high doses of stimulants.

The more common stimulants can be found in Table 13.3. Stimulants are dangerous and abuse can result in death—e.g., the sports stars and celebrities who have been victims of cocaine-related deaths.

Hallucinogens

Hallucinogens represent a category of drugs that are capable of inducing hallucinations. Hallucinations are a false perception of such things as sights, sounds, physical feelings, and smells. Since hallucinogens are illegal drugs it is difficult to discuss them in terms of dose-response; however, we know that hallucinogens can so disorient the person that they are capable of such things as self-inflicted injuries, injuring others, convulsions, coma, ruptured blood vessels in the brain, and heart and lung failure (USDOE, 1986).

Organization of School Health Programs

TABLE 13.2

Depressants

Type	What Is It Called?	What Does It Look Like?	How Is It Used?
Heroin	Smack Horse Brown Sugar Junk Mud Big H Black Tar	Powder, white to dark brown Tar-like substance	Injected Inhaled through nasal passages Smoked
Methadone	Dolophine Methadose Amidone	Solution	Taken orally Injected
Codeine	Empirin compound with Codeine Tylenol with Codeine Codeine Codeine in cough medicines	Dark liquid varying in thickness Capsules Tablets	Taken orally Injected
Morphine	Pectoral syrup	White crystals Hypodermic tablets Injectable solutions	Injected Taken orally Smoked
Meperidine	Pethidine Demerol Mepergan	White powder Solution Tablets	Taken orally Injected
Opium	Paregoric Dover's Powder Parepectolin	Dark brown chunks Powder	Smoked Eaten

TABLE 13.2 Continued

Depressants

Type	What Is It Called?	What Does It Look Like?	How Is It Used?
Other Narcotics	Percocet Percodan Tussionex Fentanyl Darvon Talwin Lomotil	Tablets Capsules Liquid	Taken orally Injected
Barbiturates	Downers Barbs Blue Devils Red Devils Yellow Jacket Yellows Nembutal Seconal Amytal Tuinals	Red, yellow, blue, or red and blue capsules	Taken orally
Methaqualone	Quaaludes Ludes Sopors	Tablets	Taken orally
Tranquilizers	Valium Librium Equanil Miltown Serax Tranxene	Tablets Capsules	Taken orally

Source: United States Department of Education, 1986

TABLE 13.3

Stimulants

Type	What Is It Called?	What Does It Look Like?	How Is it Used?
Cocaine	Coke Snow Flake White Blow Nose Candy Big C Snowbirds Lady	White crystalline powder, often diluted with other ingredients	Inhaled through nasal passages Injected Smoked
Crack or cocaine	Crack Freebase rocks Rock	Light brown or beige pellets—or crystalline rocks that resemble coagulated soap; often packaged in small vials	Smoked
Amphetamines	Speed Uppers Ups Black Beauties Pep Pills Copilots Bumblebees Hearts Benzedrine Dexedrine Footballs Biphetamine	Capsules Pills Tablets	Taken orally Injected Inhaled through nasal passages

TABLE 13.3 Continued

Stimulants

Type	What Is It Called?	What Does It Look Like?	How Is it Used?
Methamphet-amines	Crank	White powder	Taken orally
	Crystal Meth	Pills	Injected
	Crystal	A rock which resembles a block of paraffin	Inhaled through nasal passages
	Methedrine		
	Speed		
Additional Stimulants	Ritalin	Pills	Taken orally
	Cylert	Capsules	Injected
	Preludin	Tablets	
	Didrex		
	Pre-State		
	Voranil		
	Tenuate		
	Tepanil		
	Pondimin		
	Sandrex		
	Plegine		
	Ionamin		

Source: United States Department of Education, 1986

Table 13.4 shows a variety of common hallucinogens. Drug use surveys show that hallucinogens are used by only a small percentage of school-age students. In spite of this, since they are found in the same marketplace as commonly used drugs, school personnel should be familiar with this category.

Marijuana

Marijuana, a popular recreational drug, was for many years classified under hallucinogens. Although in some textbooks marijuana is still listed under the category of hallucinogenic, it should be pointed out that smoking marijuana does not induce hallucinations in the majority of users. Because of the increasing popularity of marijuana as a recreational drug, most researchers now discuss marijuana as a separate and distinct category of drug.

Marijuana refers to the plant material from a cannabis plant that has been dried and prepared for smoking or ingesting. The plant material from a

TABLE 13.4

Hallucinogens

Type	What Is It Called?	What Does It Look Like?	How Is It Used?
Phencyclidine	PCP Angel Dust Loveboat Lovely Hog Killer Weed	Liquid Capsules White crystalline powder Pills	Taken orally Injected Smoked—can be sprayed on cigarettes, parsley, and marijuana
Lysergic Acid Diethylamide	LSD Acid Green or Red Dragon White Lightning Blue Heaven Sugar Cubes Microdot	Brightly colored tablets Impregnated blotter paper Thin squares of gelatin Clear liquid	Taken orally Licked off paper Gelatin and liquid can be put in the eyes
Mescaline and Peyote	Mesc Buttons Cactus	Hard brown discs Tablets Capsules	Discs—chewed, swallowed, or smoked Tablets and capsules—taken orally
Psilocybin	Magic mushrooms Mushrooms	Fresh or dried mushrooms	Chewed and swallowed

Source: United States Department of Education, 1986

cannabis plant contains an active resin called tetrahydrocannabinol, or THC for short. It is the THC in marijuana that causes the effects most commonly reported—namely euphoria, a sense of well-being.

Concentrations of THC vary with the type of marijuana. For example, marijuana itself has a low concentration while hashish has a much higher concentration. Hash oil has the highest concentration and can produce effects similar to LSD.

TABLE 13.5

Forms of THC

Type	What Is It Called?	What Does It Look Like?	How Is It Used?
Marijuana	Pot Grass Weed Reefer Dope Mary Jane Sinsemilla Acapulco Gold Thai Sticks	Dried parsley mixed with stems that may include seeds	Eaten Smoked
Tetrahydro-cannabinol	THC	Soft gelatin capsules	Taken orally Smoked
Hashish	Hash	Brown or black cakes or balls	Eaten Smoked
Hashish Oil	Hash Oil	Concentrated syrupy liquid varying in color from clear to black	Smoked—mixed with tobacco

Source: United States Department of Education, 1986

Table 13.5 shows important information with respect to marijuana. Although it is unlikely, marijuana can result in some serious psychological problems, namely, paranoia.

Many groups lobby to get marijuana legalized because they argue that it is less dangerous than alcohol, or at best, no more dangerous than alcohol. After all, if alcohol is legal then why not legalize marijuana? This argument does have some major flaws.

First, while the effects of THC, assuming low concentrations such as are found in marijuana, do not produce profound negative effects in most people, marijuana is still a mood modifier with a potential for dependence. Second, the most popular form of using marijuana carries with it a risk of cancer and heart disease with long-term use. Third, some habitual marijuana users develop what has been termed an "amotivational syndrome." In this state, the

Organization of School Health Programs

user has a strong preoccupation with marijuana and life events become centered around marijuana. The result is a person who is so ''laid back'' that he or she literally disengages from a productive role in school or society and is more concerned about marijuana than school or work. While researchers have yet to prove cause and effect between marijuana use and amotivational syndrome the relationship appears to exist. Finally, the greater a student's involvement with marijuana, the more likely it is that the student will begin to use other drugs in conjunction with marijuana (USDOE, 1986).

Despite popularity marijuana does have a compelling negative side. It is not a safe drug. Like cigarettes and alcohol, marijuana is considered a ''gateway drug''—those drugs a person is likely to try because they are simple to take and their effects are not considered to be profound. If a person responds favorably to a gateway drug he or she might be likely to try other drugs, some more powerful.

Designer Drugs

Designer drugs are chemical equivalents to currently available prescription or illicit drugs. All one needs to produce these drugs is a well-stocked chemistry laboratory and a smart chemist. Designer drugs are sold illegally and are marketed as a drug other than what it is. For example, a chemist may produce a designer drug and sell it as heroin or PCP. The users experience a similar effect thinking they have purchased the ''real thing.''

Table 13.6 shows the most common designer drugs. The availability of designer drugs further complicates the nation's drug problems because they provide yet another outlet for drug distribution. In this case it's not drug lords who are the culprits but smart chemists. The bottom line is the chemist gets illegally rich and the user gets illegally high.

Lookalike Drugs

Another popular category of drugs available are called lookalike drugs. These are drugs that contain legal substances, such as over-the-counter substances (e.g., caffeine). The drugs themselves are formed to look like certain prescription drugs or illicit drugs and are sold on the street to naive drug consumers. They purchase what they think is, for instance, amphetamine, because it looks like a popular amphetamine. Although what they have really purchased is perhaps a powdered caffeine, novice users will take the pill, experience the stimulating effect of caffeine and they think it's amphetamine. It is easy to see why some school students are popular consumers of lookalike drugs.

Why Do Students Take Drugs?

There are many reasons why students take drugs. The more common ones include:

- To act grown up.
- To have a good time.
- To fit in with others.

TABLE 13.6

Designer Drugs

Type	What Is It Called?	What Does It Look Like?	How Is It Used?
Analogs of Fentanyl (Narcotic)	Synthetic Heroin China White	White powder resembling heroin	Inhaled through nasal passages Injected
Analogs of Meperidine (Narcotic)	Synthetic Heroin MPTP (New Heroin) MPPP PEPAP	White powder	Inhaled through nasal passages Injected
Analogs of Amphetamines and Methamphetamines (Hallucinogens)	MDMA (Ecstasy, XTC, Adam, Essence) MDM STP PMA 2, 5-DMA TMA DOM DOB	White powder Tablets Capsules	Taken orally Injected Inhaled through nasal passages
Analogs of Phencyclidine (PCP) (Hallucinogens)	PCPy PCE TCP	White powder	Taken orally Injected Smoked

Source: United States Department of Education, 1986

In a study investigating marijuana use and youth, researchers found the most important reason that the subjects offered for taking marijuana was ''to fit in with others.'' The second main reason for children in grades four and five was ''to feel older.'' The third reason for children in grades four and five was ''to have a good time'' (USDOE, 1986).

Other reasons include the influence of family, the media, and peers. Family members are significant role models, particularly during the early school years. If family members use drugs, it is more likely that the child will not respond negatively to the opportunity to use drugs.

Organization of School Health Programs

Television and movies have a great impact on students. The United States Department of Education reports that television and movies had the greatest influence on fourth graders in making drugs and alcohol seem attractive. From the fifth grade on, peers play an increasingly important role while television and movies play a secondary role (USDOE, 1986).

Identification of Potential Drug Abuse

While knowledge about drugs is important for members of the school health team, it is just as important for team members to be able to identify behaviors and signs in students they suspect of using drugs. Table 13.7 shows the most common signs of drug use. Further, Table 13.8 shows the physical and social indicators of drug abuse by category of drug. The information in these two tables provides enough information that would aid or confirm suspicions of drug abuse.

If a student demonstrates the signs shown in Tables 13.7 and 13.8, it is important that the student be referred for a follow-up evaluation. The protocol for referral should be contained in the school policies.

Prevention of Drug Abuse

Use of drugs involves physical, mental, social, and cultural, as well as other, dynamics. As a result of the interaction of these dynamics and factors, students make decisions regarding drug use. Because of the myriad of factors involved in these decisions, it is clear that students must learn concepts, information, and skills besides just drug information. Prevention of drug abuse from an educational standpoint means more than just providing information about drugs.

Sound comprehensive health education programs for grades K-12 can be extremely useful in preventing drug abuse among youth.

The drug education component of a comprehensive health education program must include skill development. The following important drug education curriculum attributes were identified by the Health Promotion Resource Center of Stanford University (Stanford University, 1990) and are appropriately termed *skilled building components:*

- Assertiveness training: Focuses on the development of skills that empower individuals to defend their position in a positive manner.
- Refusal skills: Acquiring the necessary skills to refuse offers of drugs and alcohol.
- Communication skills: Activities that help students to listen and exchange information with their peer group and adults.
- Goal setting: Students learn how to establish meaningful goals both short-term and long-term.
- Coping/Stress reduction: Focuses on helping students to identify stressful situations and how to cope with them in a healthy manner.

TABLE 13.7

Common Signs of Drug Use

Signs of Drugs and Drug Paraphernalia

- Possession of drug-related paraphernalia such as pipes, rolling papers, small decongestant bottles, or small butane torches.
- Possession of drugs or evidence of drugs, peculiar plants, or butts, seeds, or leaves in ashtrays or clothing pockets.
- Odor of drugs, smell of incense or other "cover-up" scents.

Identification with Drug Culture

- Drug-related magazines, slogans on clothing.
- Conversation and jokes that are preoccupied with drugs.
- Hostility in discussing drugs.

Signs of Physical Deterioration

- Memory lapses, short attention span, difficulty in concentration.
- Poor physical coordination, slurred or incoherent speech.
- Unhealthy appearance, indifference to hygiene and grooming.
- Bloodshot eyes, dilated pupils.

Dramatic Changes in School Performance

- Distinct downward turns in student's grades—not just from C's to F's, but from A's to B's and C's. Assignments not completed.
- Increased absenteeism or tardiness.

Changes in Behavior

- Chronic dishonesty (lying, stealing, cheating). Trouble with the police.
- Changes in friends, evasiveness in talking about new ones.
- Possession of large amounts of money.
- Increasing and inappropriate anger, hostility, irritability, secretiveness.
- Reduced motivation, energy, self-discipline, self-esteem.
- Diminished interest in extracurricular activities and hobbies.

Source: United States Department of Education, 1986

- Decision-making skills: Students develop skills to evaluate different behaviors and solutions and alternatives that involve the use of alcohol.
- Self-awareness: Students learn methods of identifying and dealing with personal feelings.
- Consumer awareness: Students learn to critically examine such things as advertising and other efforts to persuade the consumer.
- Drug information: Students learn about the physical, mental, and social effects of drugs.

TABLE 13.8

Physical and Social Indicators of Drug Abuse

Physical and Social Indicators of Drug Abuse

Indicators	*Drugs*
Excessive activity	Stimulants (cocaine, amphetamines, nicotine, caffeine)
Dilated pupils	
Insomnia	
Extreme nervousness or tenseness	
Profuse perspiration	
Tremors of hands	
Lack of interest in activity	Depressants (narcotics, barbiturates, methaqualone)
Drowsiness	
Disorientation	
Staggering or stumbling	
Propensity to fall into a deep sleep	
Distortions of perception (hallucinations)	Hallucinogens (LSD, PCP, marijuana, psilocybin)
Abrupt emotional changes	

The above attributes need to be included in drug education programs at all school levels—elementary, middle, and secondary. Many drug education programs have been developed that contain many of the important attributes discussed above. Figures 13.1, 13.2, and 13.3 show the drug education curricula available at the elementary, middle, and secondary schools as well as the key elements of each curriculum in terms of the information addressed, the skill-building components included, the teaching methods used, and the curriculum philosophy. Descriptions of each curriculum mentioned in Figures 13.1, 13.2, and 13.3 can be found in a book titled *What Works? A Guide to School-Based Alcohol and Drug Abuse Prevention Curricula,* published by the Health Promotion Resource Center of the Stanford Center for Research in Disease Prevention. The address for this center can be found at the end of this chapter.

Community Involvement

The community has a major role in helping prevent and/or deal with drug problems of school-age students. Most communities, regardless of size, have law enforcement agencies, social service and health agencies, parent groups,

ATTRIBUTES OF CURRICULA

ELEMENTARY SCHOOL PROGRAMS

CURRICULUM (alphabetical)	TARGET GRADES	PAGE NUMBER	ALCOHOL	COCAINE	HALLUCINOGENS	INHALANTS	MARIJUANA	STIMULANTS	TOBACCO	SMOKELESS TOBACCO	ASSERTIVENESS TRAINING	REFUSAL SKILLS	COMMUNICATION SKILLS	GOAL SETTING	COPING/STRESS REDUCTION	DECISION MAKING SKILLS	SELF-AWARENESS	RISK FACTOR INFORMATION	CONSUMER AWARENESS	DRUG INFORMATION	AUDIO VISUALS	BEHAVIORAL REHEARSAL/ROLE PLAY	COMMUNITY INVOLVEMENT	GROUP ACTIVITIES	PEER MODELING	FAMILY INVOLVEMENT	OTHER	SUPPORTS LEGAL USE OF ALCOHOL	ADVOCATES LIFELONG ABSTINENCE	PHILOSOPHY NOT CLEARLY STATED
AVALON CARVER PROGRAM	4-6	20									◆	◆		◆	◆	◆		◆	◆	◆	◆		◆				1		◆	
BABES*	P-6	22	◆									◆	◆	◆			◆	◆			◆				2		◆	
ME – ME*	K-6	24							◆	◆		◆	◆		◆	A	◆	◆	◆					◆	
PICADA: 1 – 5*	1-5	26	◆		◆		◆	◆	◆	◆	◆	◆	◆	◆		◆	◆	◆		◆		◆			◆	
POSITIVE ACTION**	K-7	28	◆	◆	◆	◆	◆	◆	◆	◆	◆	◆	◆	◆	◆	◆	◆	◆	◆	◆	◆	◆	◆	◆	◆	◆	3	◆	
PROJECT CHARLIE	K-6	30	◆	◆	◆	◆	◆	◆	◆	◆	◆	◆	◆	◆	◆	◆	◆	◆	◆	◆	◆	◆			◆	
STARTING EARLY	K-6	32	◆						◆	◆		◆	◆	◆	◆	◆	◆	◆	◆	◆		◆		◆	

Table heading groups: DRUG INFORMATION; SKILL BUILDING COMPONENTS (SOCIAL SKILLS, PERSONAL SKILLS, OTHER); TEACHING METHODS; CURRICULUM PHILOSOPHY

* Information based on review of partial curriculum only
** Drug information minimal

A Medicines and Poisons

1 Music
2 Puppets, Storytelling
3 School Support Staff Involvement

FIGURE 13.1

Attributes of elementary drug education curricula. *Health Promotion Resource Center, What Works? A guide to School-Based Alcohol and Drug Abuse Curricula,* Palo Alto, California: Stanford University Press, 1989.

and businesses—each of which can help schools in many ways to prevent drug use among youth. Figure 13.4 shows some of the activities each of the above groups can do to add to the prevention efforts undertaken by the school.

The responsibility of drug education and prevention should not be placed on the school alone. It should be viewed as a total school, community, and family effort.

Drug-Related School Policies

It is important for schools to develop written policies regarding drugs. Written policies reflect that the school is serious about drugs and that drug use, possession, and sale on school grounds and at school functions can have serious repercussions (USDOE, 1989). Also, written policies should not be centered around students only, but should include other school personnel.

The United States Department of Education provides some good guidelines regarding drug policies. According to the USDOE (*Schools without Drugs,* 1986, p. 21) school policies should:

1. Specify what constitutes a drug offense by defining (1) illegal substances and paraphernalia, (2) the area of the school's jurisdiction, for example, the school property, its surroundings, and all school-related events, such as proms and football games, and (3) the types of violations (drug possession, use and sale).

ATTRIBUTES OF CURRICULA

MIDDLE SCHOOL PROGRAMS

CURRICULUM (alphabetical)	TARGET GRADES	PAGE NUMBER	DRUG INFORMATION										SKILL BUILDING COMPONENTS											TEACHING METHODS						CURRICULUM PHILOSOPHY		
													SOCIAL SKILLS	PERSONAL SKILLS							OTHER										
			ALCOHOL	COCAINE	HALLUCINOGENS	INHALANTS	MARIJUANA	STIMULANTS	TOBACCO	SMOKELESS TOBACCO	ASSERTIVENESS TRAINING	REFUSAL SKILLS	COMMUNICATION SKILLS	GOAL SETTING	COPING/STRESS REDUCTION	DECISION MAKING SKILLS	SELF AWARENESS	RISK FACTOR INFORMATION	CONSUMER AWARENESS	DRUG INFORMATION	AUDIO VISUALS	BEHAVIORAL REHEARSAL/ROLE PLAY	COMMUNITY INVOLVEMENT	GROUP ACTIVITIES	PEER MODELING	FAMILY INVOLVEMENT	OTHER	SUPPORTS LEGAL USE OF ALCOHOL	ADVOCATES LIFELONG ABSTINENCE	PHILOSOPHY NOT CLEARLY STATED
AL-CO-HOL	7-8	42	◆			◇		◇			◆	◆	◆	◇	◆	◆	◆	◆	◆	◆	◆		◆	◇	◆			◆		
IT'S YOUR CHOICE	6-8	44	◆			◆			◆	◆	◆	◆	◆			◆	◆			◆		◆		◆				◆		
LIFE SKILLS TRAINING PROGRAM	7-9	46	◆	◆	◆	◇	◆	◆	◆		◆		◆	◆	◆	◆	◆	◆	◆	◆		◇	◆	◆		◇				◆
MN. SMOKING PREVENTION PROG.	6-8	48						◆	◆	◆	◆	◆	◆			◆	◆	◆	◆	◆	◆	◆		◆	◆			◆		
OMBUDSMAN PROGRAM	5-9	50	◆	◆	◆	◆	◆	◆	◆	◆	◆	◆	◆	◆	◆	◆	◆	◆		◆	◆	◆	◆	◆	◆					◆
PICADA: UNDER THE INFLUENCE	6-8	52	◆	◆	◆	◆	◆	◆	◆	◆		◆	◆	◆	◆	◆	◆	◆	◆	◆		◆	◆	◆	◆		◆			
PROJECT ADVANCE	4-9	54	◇	◇	◇	◇	◇	◇	◇	◆	◆	◆	◆		◆	◆	◆	◇		◆	◆	◆	◆	◆					◆
PROJECT SMART	6-9	56	◆			◆			◆	◆	◆	◆	◆	◆	◆	◆	◆	◆	◆	◆		◆	◆	◆						◆
SKILLS FOR ADOLESCENCE (QUEST)	6-8	58	◆	◆	◆	◆	◆	◆	◆		◆	◆	◆	◆	◆	◆	◆	◆	◆	◆		◆	◆	◆	◆					◆
SOUND OFF	6-8	60	◆				◆		◆		◆		◆		◆	◆	◆	◆	◆	◆	◆		◆							◆
WELL AND GOOD	6-7	62	◆			◆		◆		◆	◆	◆	◆	◆	◇	◇	◆	◆	◆	◆		◆	◆	◆		◆				

2. State the consequences for violating school policy; as appropriate, punitive action should be linked with treatment and counseling. Measures that schools have found effective in dealing with first-time offenders include:

- a required meeting of parents and the student with school officials, concluding with a contract signed by the student and parents in which (1) they acknowledge a drug problem, (2) the student agrees not to use drugs, and to participate in drug counseling or a rehabilitation program.
- suspension, assignment to an alternative school, in-school suspension, after-school or Saturday detention with close supervision and demanding academic assignments.
- referral to a drug treatment expert or counselor.
- notification of police.

Penalties for repeat offenders and for sellers may include expulsion, legal action, and referral for treatment.

3. Describe procedures for handling violations, including:

- legal issues associated with disciplinary actions—confidentiality, due process, and search and seizure—and how they apply.

FIGURE 13.2

Attributes of middle school drug education curricula.

Health Promotion Resource Center, What Works? A guide to School-Based Alcohol and Drug Abuse Curricula, Palo Alto, California: Stanford University Press, 1989.

ATTRIBUTES OF CURRICULA

HIGH SCHOOL PROGRAMS

CURRICULUM (alphabetical)	TARGET GRADES	PAGE NUMBER	ALCOHOL	COCAINE	HALLUCINOGENS	INHALANTS	MARIJUANA	STIMULANTS	TOBACCO	SMOKELESS TOBACCO	ASSERTIVENESS TRAINING	REFUSAL SKILLS	COMMUNICATION SKILLS	GOAL SETTING	COPING/STRESS REDUCTION	DECISION MAKING SKILLS	SELF AWARENESS	RISK FACTOR INFORMATION	CONSUMER AWARENESS	DRUG INFORMATION	AUDIO VISUALS	BEHAVIORAL REHEARSAL/ROLE PLAY	COMMUNITY INVOLVEMENT	GROUP ACTIVITIES	PEER MODELING	FAMILY INVOLVEMENT	OTHER	SUPPORTS LEGAL USE OF ALCOHOL	ADVOCATES LIFELONG ABSTINENCE	PHILOSOPHY NOT CLEARLY STATED
ALCOHOL COUNTERMEASURES	10-11	72	◆								◆		◆	◆	◆	◆	◆	◆	◆	◆	◆		◆					◆		
ALPHA INITIATIVE	9-12	74	◆	◆	◆	◆	◆	◆	◆	◆	◆	◆	◆	◆	◆	◆	◆	◆	◆	◆	◆	◆	◆	◆						◆
PICADA: TEENS TEACH TEENS	11-12	76	◆	◆	◆	◆	◆	◆	◆	◆	◆	◆		◆	◆	◆	◆	◆	◆	◆	◆	◆	◆	◆	◆	◆					◆
PREVENTION/INTERVENTION PROG.	7-12	78									◆	◆	◆	◆	◆	◆							◆								◆
SKILLS FOR LIVING (QUEST)	9-12	80									◆	◆		◆	◆							◆	◆	◆	◆	◆	◆				◆

FIGURE 13.3

Attributes of high school drug education curricula.

Health Promotion Resource Center, What Works? A guide to School-Based Alcohol and Drug Abuse Curricula, Palo Alto, California: Stanford University Press, 1989.

FIGURE 13.4

What community groups and agencies can do to help schools fight drug abuse.

Law enforcement agencies and the courts can:

- Provide volunteers to speak in the schools about the legal ramifications of drug use. Officers can encourage students to cooperate with them to stop drug use.
- Meet with school officials to discuss drug use in the school, share information on the drug problem outside of school, and help school officials in their investigations.

Social service and health agencies can:

- Provide volunteers to speak in the school about the effects of drugs.
- Meet with parents to discuss symptoms of drug use and to inform them about counseling resources.
- Provide the schools with health professionals to evaluate students who may be potential drug users.
- Provide referrals to local treatment programs for students who are using drugs.
- Establish and conduct drug counseling and support groups for students.

Businesses can:

- Speak in the schools about the effects of drug use on employment.
- Provide incentives for students who participate in drug prevention programs and lead drug-free lives.
- Help schools obtain curriculum materials for their drug prevention program.
- Sponsor drug-free activities for young people.

Parent groups can:

- Mobilize others through informal discussions, door-to-door canvassing, and school meetings to ensure that students get a consistent no-drug message at home, at school, and in the community.
- Contribute volunteers to chaperone student parties and other activities.

Print and broadcast media can:

- Educate the community about the nature of the drug problem in their schools.
- Publicize school efforts to combat the problem.

- responsibilities and procedures for reporting suspected incidents that identify the proper authorities to be contacted and the circumstances under which incidents should be reported.
- procedures for notifying parents when their child is suspected of or caught with drugs.
- procedures for notifying police.

4. Enlist legal counsel to ensure that the policy is drafted in compliance with applicable federal, state, and local laws.
5. Build community support for the policy. Hold open meetings where views can be aired and differences resolved.

Tobacco

In recent years tobacco smoking has lost its allure among many young people largely due to the efforts of the public and school health programs. However, use of tobacco products still is a problem in schools and deserves mention in this text. Tobacco comes in the form of cigarettes, cigars, and in smokeless tobacco.

The most common form used by students has been, and still is, cigarettes. This is substantiated by the fact that 29 percent of students have tried cigarettes and 19 percent are daily smokers (Inaba, 1991). Cigarettes should be considered a gateway drug (a drug first experimented with before trying other drugs with greater psychoactive effects). According to DuPont "twelve to seventeen-year-olds who are current smokers of cigarettes when compared to youths of the same age who do not smoke are twice as likely to make illegal use of pills such as stimulants and tranquilizers, 10 times as likely to smoke marijuana, and 14 times as likely to use cocaine, heroin, or hallucinogens."

To elaborate on the health hazards of cigarette smoking in this text would be redundant since they have been so well publicized. What does need addressing is what the school policy should be regarding cigarette smoking.

In order to address the issue of school smoking policies some preliminary questions need to be answered. These questions include:

1. What is the legal age for smoking cigarettes in the respective state?
2. Should the school be concerned about a student's smoking behavior if he or she is of age to smoke?
3. Should the school be concerned about the smoking behaviors of faculty and staff?

If the answer to the first question is 18 years of age, then only a select, small percentage of mostly high school seniors are legally smoking. Anyone under 18 smoking cigarettes is doing so illegally. Therefore, the schools should not be condoning illegal behaviors and that should be reflected in policies.

If the answer to the second question is yes, the schools must make a decision as to whether or not they want to accommodate the student who legally smokes. Some schools provide designated smoking areas for students who smoke. Other schools do not accommodate the student who smokes because they do not wish to provide a certain group of students special treatment and they do not want to provide an environment whereby other underage students might be influenced to begin smoking.

The third question has some tricky implications if the answer is yes. If teachers and staff are allowed to smoke within the school premises a special place must be created specifically for them since nonsmokers rights should also be protected.

Overall, one must consider that if the mission of the school is to provide an optimal environment for learning then perhaps smoking should not be allowed in the school at all. It is expected that in the future more and more schools will provide a totally smoke free environment making it near impossible for faculty and staff to find a place to smoke.

The use of smokeless tobacco among young people has increased. The health hazards of smokeless tobacco are not as well publicized as that of cigarette smoking, thus implying, in the minds of students, that it is safe. Smokeless tobacco is anything but safe. Use of smokeless tobacco has been related to cancer of the tongue and mouth at very young ages.

The policy for use of smokeless tobacco should be the same as for cigarette smoking and actually should be included as a part of the same policy.

As can be easily seen in the preceding pages, drugs must be taken seriously and prevention efforts should be viewed as a family, school, and community effort. With good curricula implemented, good community involvement, and strong policies we can expect to see the problem dealt with effectively.

ACQUIRED IMMUNE DEFICIENCY SYNDROME (AIDS)

AIDS (acquired immune deficiency syndrome) is a deadly viral disease that some people have referred to as a modern plague. By the end of 1991 it was determined that approximately 140,000 Americans died of AIDS. Worldwide the numbers are in the millions. It is ironic that AIDS is both a deadly disease yet at the same time a very preventable disease. One of the best ways to begin to prevent the disease is to know something about it.

The actual virus causing AIDS is called the human immunodeficiency virus or HIV for short. The reservoir for this virus is people and the mode of transmission is exchange of body fluids. Transmitting the HIV through exchange is commonly done through sexual contact, particularly contact involving anal intercourse and exchange of blood products.

HIV is transmitted through sexual contact, but it is sexual contact involving anal intercourse that provides the greatest risk for a couple of reasons. First, there is great potential to damage rectal tissue during anal intercourse. Second, AIDS-infected semen has immediate contact with blood if rectal tissue is damaged.

Exchange of blood products can be done through a variety of mechanisms. First, during blood transfusions blood products are exchanged. Second, dirty intravenous needles contain blood. If the blood in the dirty needle contains the HIV and is used by a person then blood products are being exchanged.

Once the HIV enters the body it affects the immune response system by suppressing it. The AIDS victim's immune response system is impaired, eventually rendering the victim powerless to fight off even simple infections.

A person will not get AIDS if they shake hands with a person with AIDS or drink from the same glass. Body fluids must be exchanged. Casual contact with an AIDS victim that does not involve exchange of body fluids does not put one at risk for AIDS. Considering the mode of transmission of AIDS the cases of AIDS are found among some major groups. The percentage of AIDS cases by group include the following:

- Homosexual or bisexual men: 70%
- IV drug users: 20%
- Heterosexual contacts of infected partners: 4%
- Children born to infected mothers: 1%
- Patients with hemophilia: 1%

Stages of AIDS

AIDS is unlike many communicable diseases because of the unique HIV pathogenesis. Once infected with the AIDS virus the victim will progress through three stages.

Stage I AIDS is referred to as the asymptomatic carrier state. This means that the individual has no symptoms but can transmit the virus to others if his or her body fluid is exchanged with a susceptible person. A person in Stage I may never know they have the disease, but they are still capable of transmitting the HIV. At some point, and it may be many years, a person will begin to experience bouts with flulike symptoms. At this point they either have the flu or they are moving into Stage II.

With Stage II AIDS, the individual experiences the typical flulike symptoms—headache, fever, runny nose, and swollen glands—which never really subside or they don't subside for long. Since symptoms are present in Stage II, the victim is said to be suffering from AIDS-related complex or ARC. Once again, the person may stay in Stage II for years experiencing bouts with flulike symptoms. Eventually, the infected person gets weaker and weaker and begins to suffer from what are termed opportunistic infections. At this point, the victim has progressed into the final stage of AIDS, Stage III.

Stage III is referred to as full-blown AIDS. At this point the immune response system of the victim is so weak that they get opportunistic diseases such as rare forms of cancer and pneumonia. As the immune response system becomes more and more depressed the victim has a greater problem with opportunistic infections until eventually the result is death. In terms of incidence it is estimated that by the end of 1991 there were 260,000 Americans with the Stage III AIDS and of that number over 160,000 died. In addition, for every Stage III victim there are 5 to 10 with ARC, or Stage II, and 50 to 100 asymptomatic carriers. When one adds up the total numbers in Stages I, II, and III, it can easily be seen that millions of Americans are AIDS victims. What percentage of Stage I victims will progress to Stage II and what percentage of Stage II will progress to Stage III is unclear.

As of this writing, there is no cure for AIDS. There are some drugs that have shown promise in delaying the onset of Stage III AIDS by blocking the reproductive capability of the virus. This is encouraging and many victims are living longer, but it is still not a cure. Without a cure, prevention becomes even more important.

Education as Prevention

AIDS is pandemic and education is the most effective means available for controlling the pandemic (Black, 1988). Since most AIDS patients are between the ages of 20 and 40 and since the incubation period of AIDS can be long, many AIDS victims were infected as teenagers (Black, 1988).

Young people, particularly teenagers, are at high risk because they engage in health behaviors that increase the risk of exposure to HIV. In addition studies have shown that America's youth have a lack of knowledge regarding sexual issues as well as unmodified sexual behaviors even in light of the AIDS pandemic (Black, 1988).

As with the drug use the educational implications of AIDS education should be directed at both the school and community so that the program is a true school/community effort. AIDS/HIV education is a bit trickier, however, since presentation of material will eventually involve discussing sexual issues. If guidelines are followed it is likely that an AIDS/HIV prevention program will be well received by the schools, communities, and parents. Black (1988) identified six important guidelines for school-based HIV/AIDS education programs. These guidelines are as follows:

1. The score and content of HIV education should be determined locally and should be consistent with parental and community values.
2. School health education about HIV should be developed with broad community participation.
3. HIV information within the curriculum should be taught by professionals who have received special training to deal with the issue.
4. HIV instruction should be provided as one component of a comprehensive, sequential health instruction program.
5. The educational program and materials should be approved by the local school board and other appropriate school personnel prior to use in the classroom.
6. Essential learner outcomes should be established for the instruction and a system implemented to periodically assess the effectiveness of teaching about HIV.

The Coalition of National Health Education Organizations has developed some important recommendations for AIDS education. These recommendations are as follows (CNHEO, 1988):

1. That children and youth be educated about AIDS;
2. Believes that parents have the major responsibility for such education;
3. Resolves that schools include instruction about AIDS as part of a comprehensive health education program K–12;
4. Urges that all school personnel participating in AIDS education receive preparation under the leadership of qualified educators and other health professionals; and
5. That state departments of education and public health assist schools in planning appropriate school–community programs aimed at preventing AIDS.

There are numerous AIDS education programs available. Just because many are published doesn't necessarily mean that they meet the above guidelines. Any prepared curriculum should be evaluated in light of the above guidelines.

AIDS Policies

With the magnitudes of the AIDS epidemic there are obvious policy implications for the school. Figure 13.5 shows a model AIDS policy for local Boards of Education.

Finally, it is likely that schools will have to, at some point, manage a HIV-infected student. How successfully schools deal with HIV-infected students can in part be determined if school students have the right to (Black, 1988):

- Nondiscriminatory school policies;
- Be educated in a school setting by staff who are accurately informed about HIV;
- Have peers who are properly educated about HIV;
- Have a quality support system within the school setting; and
- Privacy and confidentiality of medical records.

The potential is great for discrimination. No one benefits from this. Therefore, school boards must be proactive in stating specific criteria for dealing with HIV-infected students. The above guidelines offer a beginning framework.

Most of us hope and are optimistic that there will be a cure for AIDS soon. Until a cure is found the only feasible way to halt the epidemic is through prevention. With this in mind, the schools must lead the charge.

ADOLESCENT PREGNANCY

Sexual activity of adolescents aged 10 to 19 in the United States is on the rise. A recent study by the Alan Guttmacher Institute has found that there is a 40 percent chance that an American girl will be sexually active by the time she

FIGURE 13.5

A model AIDS policy.
Reprinted with permission from Journal of School Health. *HIV Infection: Educational Programs and Policies for School Personnel. Vol. 58, No. 9, October 1988, p. 319. Copyright, 1988. American School Health Association, Kent, OH 44240.*

Educating Students with Chronic Infectious Diseases: A Model Policy for Local Boards of Education

The _____ Board of Education adopts the following policy for educating students known to have a chronic infectious disease (e.g., AIDS/ARC, CMV, hepatitis B, herpes simplex) and for ensuring a safe and healthy school environment for all students.

1. All children in _____ have a constitutional right to a free, suitable program of educational experiences.

2. As a general rule, a child with a chronic infectious disease will be allowed, with the approval of the child's physician, to attend school in a regular classroom setting and will be considered eligible for all rights, privileges, and services provided by law and existing policy of _____ school district.

3. The school nurse will function as (a) the liaison with the child's physician, (b) the child's advocate in the school (i.e., assist in problem resolution, answer questions) and (c) the coordinator of services provided by other staff.

4. The school will respect the right to privacy of the individual; therefore knowledge that a child has a chronic infectious disease will be confined to those persons with a direct need to know (e.g., principal, school nurse, child's teacher). Those persons will be provided with appropriate information concerning such precautions as may be necessary and should be aware of confidentiality requirements.

5. Based upon individual circumstances special programming may be warranted. Special education will be provided if determined to be necessary by the Planning and Placement Team.

6. Under certain circumstances a child with a chronic infectious disease might pose a risk of transmission to others. If any such circumstances exist the school medical advisor, in consultation with the school nurse and the child's physician, must determine whether a risk of transmission exists. If it is determined that a risk exists, the student shall be removed from the classroom.

7. A child with a chronic infectious disease may be temporarily removed from the classroom for the reasons stated in #6 until an appropriate school program adjustment can be made, an appropriate alternative education program can be established, or the medical advisor determines that the risk has abated and the child can return to the classroom.
   (a) Removal from the classroom will not be construed as the only response to reduce risk of transmission. School personnel should be flexible in developing alternatives and should attempt to use the least restrictive means to accommodate the child's needs.
   (b) In any case of temporary removal of the student from the school setting, state regulations and school policy regarding homebound instruction will apply.

8. Each removal of a child with a chronic infectious disease from normal school attendance will be reviewed by the school medical advisor in consultation with the student's physician at least once every month to determine whether the condition precipitating the removal has changed.

9. A child with a chronic infectious disease may need to be removed from the classroom for his/her own protection when other communicable diseases (e.g., measles or chicken pox) are occurring in the school population. This decision will be made by the child's physician and parent/guardian in consultation with the school nurse and/or the school medical advisor.

10. All staff should use the following routine and standard procedures to clean up after a child has an accident or injury at school. Blood or other body fluids emanating from *any* child, including ones known to have a chronic infectious disease, should be treated cautiously. Gloves should be worn when cleaning up blood spills. These spills should be disinfected with either bleach or another disinfectant, and persons coming in contact with them should wash their hands afterwards. Items soaked with blood or other body fluids should be placed in leak-proof bags for washing or further disposition. Similar procedures are recommended for dealing with vomitus and fecal or urinary incontinence in *any* child. Handwashing after contact with a school child is routinely recommended only if physical contact has been made with the child's blood or body fluids, including saliva.

is 17. In 1982, less than one-third of 17-year-old girls had started having sex. For this group, male and female contraceptive use is, at best, haphazard. As a consequence, in the United States the pregnancy rates of adolescents have reached staggering proportions. Since 1973, about 1.1 million teenagers have become pregnant every year; approximately 11 percent of girls between 15 and 19 years old get pregnant every year; about 500,000 adolescents give birth each year. This places the U.S. teen pregnancy rates at the top of the list among Western nations. In the state of Virginia alone it has been estimated that fifty-three adolescents become pregnant each day. The numbers are riveting. The facts are clear. Adolescent pregnancy in the United States is of epidemic proportions and the human and economic costs of this epidemic are enormous.

Of all those adolescents who give birth each year, approximately 250,000 never complete school. Many of these individuals end up on welfare. In addition, ''girls who have babies at 15 or 16 are likely to have at least one other child before they are 20. Given the stresses on their families, many of these children are at risk of being abused or ending up in foster care'' (*Newsweek,* 1990).

The School's Response

The specific causes of adolescent pregnancy are poorly understood; however, it is realized that a multiplicity of factors each interacting with others contribute to the problem. Exactly what steps need to be taken to stop the spread of this epidemic is a point of debate among many of the nation's experts. Often at the center of this debate are questions about the relative merits of offering family life classes or sex education in the schools. It seems, lately, that the major emphasis of the debate no longer revolves around whether or not family-life or sex education should be offered—93 percent of the U.S. high schools offer some form of sex education (*Newsweek,* 1990)—but whether sex education alone is sufficiently powerful enough to have an effect on the pregnancy rate. Community support for family-life or sex education in the schools is greater today than it has ever been in this country. In 1965, only 65 percent of the public supported school-based sex instruction. Today, however, it is supported by over 85 percent of the public and 86 percent of the nation's teachers.

Many schools, in an attempt to deal with rising adolescent pregnancy rates, have established, with a great deal of controversy, school-based comprehensive health clinics. There are approximately 162 school-based health clinics in 33 states, with the majority being located in or adjacent to high schools. About 14 percent of those clinics are in junior or middle schools. These clinics provide students with comprehensive health services, including family planning. Students are either given prescriptions for contraceptives or are referred to a separate birth control clinic. Studies show that in cities with school-based clinics, teens are more likely to use birth control. At the first such clinic in St. Paul, Minnesota, the adolescent birth rate dropped 50 percent between 1976 and 1984, and has stayed relatively low since then. The clinics appear to be especially effective in poor, urban areas where teen access to health care is limited.

SUMMARY

Drugs, AIDS, and adolescent pregnancy have been well documented as both public and school health problems. It is not likely that these problems will be solved during the 1990s without significant action from members of the school health team. This chapter has provided salient information regarding the nature of the problems as well as how these problems can be addressed. It is hoped that policymakers recognize the importance of a sound school health program in addressing such pertinent problems.

REVIEW QUESTIONS

1. Discuss what is meant by drug use, misuse, and abuse.
2. What are the major categories of drugs of abuse? What are some examples of drugs in these categories?
3. What are some indicators of drug abuse, misuse, or abuse among students?
4. Defend the need for drug education.
5. What are important attributes of drug education curricula?
6. Discuss the pathogenesis of AIDS.
7. Why should the schools be concerned about AIDS?
8. What are some key elements to AIDS policies for the schools?
9. How extensive a problem is adolescent pregnancy?
10. What are some ways in which schools have attempted to confront the issue of adolescent pregnancy?

REFERENCES

American Public Health Association. *Control of Communicable Diseases in Man,* 15th ed. Washington, D.C.: American Public Health Association, 1990.

Black, J. L., and L. H. Jones. "HIV Infection: Educational Programs and Policies for the School Personnel." *Journal of School Health* **58**:8 (October 1988).

Coalition of National Health Education Organizations. "Instruction about AIDS Within the School Curriculum: A Position Paper." *Journal of School Health* **58**:8 (October 1988).

DuPont, R. L. *Getting Tough on Gateway Drugs.* Washington, D.C.: American Psychiatric Press, Inc., 1984.

Futrell, M. H. "AIDS Education through Schools: An Address by Mary H. Futrell." *Journal of School Health* **58**:8 (October 1988).

Johnson, L. D. *Summary of 1988 Drug Study Report.* Press Release from the Institute for Social Research, University of Michigan. Ann Arbor, Mich.: February 28, 1989.

Kantrowitz, Barbara. "Homeroom." *Newsweek* (Summer/Fall, 1990) 50–54.

Lohrmann, D. K. ''AIDS Education at the Local Level: The Pragmatic Issues.'' *Journal of School Health* **58**:8 (October 1988).

Presidential Commission on the Human Immunodeficiency Virus Epidemic. *Journal of School Health* **58**:8 (October 1988).

Rogers, T., B. P. Pitney-Howard, and B. C. Bruce. *What Works?* Palo Alto, CA.: Health Promotion Resource Center, Stanford University, 1990.

United States Department of Education. *Schools without Drugs.* Washington, D.C.: United States Department of Education, 1986.

Child Abuse and Neglect

14

I t is conservatively estimated that at least two million children are abused or neglected in this country every year, of whom as many as 2000 die. Of the two million abused children, as many as 200,000 are physically abused and at least 100,000 are sexually abused. It is generally agreed that child neglect is four to five times more common than child abuse (USDHHS, 1981, p. 8).

The most blatant form of child abuse, physical abuse, is usually the only noticeable form. Unfortunately, many cases of child abuse are never reported, because of unobservable signs (no physical marks) or fear of liability.

Child abuse and *child neglect* are broad terms generically describing three categories: physical abuse, neglect, and sexual abuse, each of which is discussed in this chapter; and much of the information presented is from the results of research done by the Urban and Rural Systems Associates (URSA), a private research corporation that developed child abuse and neglect training materials.

PHYSICAL ABUSE

Physical abuse is any nonaccidental physical injury caused by the child's caretaker. A more operational definition would be "abuse that results in physical injury, including fractures, burns, bruises, welts, cuts, and/or internal injuries" (USDHHS, 1981, p. 6). Physical abuse often occurs in the name of discipline or punishment and ranges from a slap on the hand to the use of such objects as straps, belts, kitchen utensils, and pipes (USDHHS, 1981, p. 6). The types of injuries most frequently found in abused children, in order of frequency, can be seen in Tables 14.1 and 14.2.

> The typical instruments used in physical abuse include the following in no special order: fists, belts, straps, belt buckles, sticks, broomhandles, baseball bats, coat hangers, cords (telephone, ironing, extension, lamp), hairbrushes, lighted cigarettes, matches, cigarette lighters, boiling water and other hot liquids or grease, steaming radiators, open gas flames, hot plates, rulers, shoes and boots, lead or iron pipes, bottles, brick walls, any wall, bicycle chains, knives, scissors, chemicals, pills, alcohol, hot peppers, teeth, guns, any object near at hand. . . .
> [URSA, 1978, as abstracted by ADES, *Forms and Indicators of Child Abuse*, 1980, p. 1]

The indicators of physical abuse are divided into two major categories. These categories include primary and secondary indicators. These are not mutually exclusive categories, but rather a categorized approach for school personnel who suspect child abuse.

TABLE 14.1

Manners of Infliction of Injuries on Abused Children

Manner of Infliction of Abuse	Percentage of Reported Cases
Beatings with instruments	44
Beatings with hands	39
Burning, scalding	9
Kicking	4
Deliberate neglect or exposure	3.8
Locking in or tying	1.7
Strangling, suffocating	1.3
Stabbing, slashing	1.0
Poisoning	.9
Drowning	.2

Source: Gil, D. *Violence Against Children* (Cambridge: Harvard University Press, 1970), p. 121.

TABLE 14.2

Type of Injuries Most Frequently Found in Abused Children

Injury	Occurring in Percentage of Reported Cases of Physical Abuse
Bruises, welts	67
Abrasions, contusions, lacerations	32
Burns, scalding	10
Bone fractures	10
Wounds, cuts, punctures	8
Subdural hemorrhage or hematoma	4.6
Malnutrition (deliberately inflicted)	4.2
Skull fractures	3.9
Internal injuries	3.4
Sprains, dislocations	2
Brain damage	1.5
Poisoning	.9

Source: Gil, D. *Violence Against Children* (Cambridge: Harvard University Press, 1970), p. 119.

Organization of School Health Programs

Primary indicators are those that are easily recognizable through routine physical examination. The three main areas of the body visible to the school personnel are the skin, the face, and the mouth. The primary indicators of abuse can be seen in Table 14.3 (URSA, 1978, as abstracted by ADES, *Forms and Indicators of Child Abuse,* 1980, p. 2).

Secondary indicators are more difficult to identify and usually require a thorough examination and medical history. Naturally, the school personnel are not in a position to notice secondary indicators; however, many of the problems discussed in health appraisals can be signs of physical abuse. The main secondary indicators are listed in Table 14.3.

Once a child is referred for medical treatment or examination, the child may display certain behavior characteristics that are common among physically abused children. These behaviors are usually seen in a hospital or clinic setting and include the following points:

1. Are wary of physical contact by parents or anyone else.
2. Do not look to parents for assurance.
3. Cry hopelessly under examination and treatment. Show no expectation of being comforted. Cry little in general.
4. Seem less afraid than other children when admitted to ward and settle in quickly.
5. Are constantly on the alert for danger.
6. Are apprehensive when other children cry and watch them curiously.
7. Become apprehensive when adults approach some other crying child.
8. Seem to seek safety in sizing up situation rather than in their parents.
9. Are constantly asking in words and actions what will happen next.
10. Are constantly in search of something: food, favors, things.
11. Ask "When am I going home?" or announce "I'm not going home" rather than crying "I want to go home."
12. Neglected/battered children endure life as if they are alone in a dangerous world with no real hope of safety. [URSA, 1978, as abstracted by ADES, *Forms and Indicators of Child Abuse,* 1980, p. 3]

In most cases of child abuse, the parent or guardian is at fault. However, it is difficult always to identify when this is the case.

Several indicators should arouse the suspicions of police and medical personnel pertaining to child abuse. A prime signal is an injury that is inconsistent with an account given by the parent to explain the injury. A typical example of this kind of incongruity would be a report of a child whose hand was "accidentally scalded by hot water." Lacking from the report is any reason why the child did not take the normal action of withdrawing his [or her] hand from the water before it was so severely injured. In this instance it is reasonable to suspect that someone held the child's hand in the water. [URSA, 1978, as abstracted by ADES, *Sample Indicators for Law Enforcement Personnel,* 1980, p. 2]

Primary and Secondary Indicators of Child Abuse

Sign of Abuse	Type of Indicator
Physical Appearance	
1. Skin	Primary
a. Cradle cap, diaper rash, uncleanness.	
b. Cigarette burns, bite marks, grab marks, belt lashes.	
c. Abrasions and lacerations unusual for the child's developmental age.	
d. Injury of external genitalia.	
e. Marks on neck from strangling by hands or rope.	
f. External ears traumatized by pinching, twisting, and pulling.	
g. Unusual skin rashes that defy dermatologic diagnosis.	
h. Burns, particularly of the soles of the feet and buttocks.	
2. Face—nasal bleeding	
3. Mouth	
a. Lacerated lip.	
b. Loosened or missing teeth.	
c. Burns of lips and tongue.	
Medical history	Secondary
1. An unexplained injury in a young child.	
2. An accident history that does not adequately account for the child's injury.	
3. An accident history inconsistent with the developmental age of the child.	

     Organization of School Health Programs

TABLE 14.3 Continued

Primary and Secondary Indicators of Child Abuse

Sign of Abuse	Type of Indicator

Physical examination

1. **Skeletal system**
   a. Tenderness, swelling, and limitation of motion of an extremity.
   b. Deformities of long bones.
2. **Head**
   a. Irregularities of contour resulting from skull fractures.
   b. Signs of intracranial trauma.
3. **Eyes**
   a. Subconjunctival hemorrhages.
   b. Traumatic cataracts.
   c. Retinal hemorrhages.
4. **Ears—ruptured eardrums from blows to the head**
5. **Face**
   a. Displaced nasal cartilages.
   b. Fractures of the mandible.
6. **Chest**
   a. Deformity of chest and limitation of motion due to fractured ribs.
   b. Emphysema.
7. **Abdomen**
   a. Signs of irritation from ruptured organs.
   b. Abdominal masses.
8. **Central nervous system**
   a. Lower motor neuron paralysis from spinal cord injury.
   b. Upper motor neuron paralysis from intracranial injury.
   c. Neurologic signs varying with location and extent of injury.

URSA, 1978, as abstracted by the Arizona Department of Economic Security (ADES). *Forms and Indicators of Child Abuse* (Abstract of URSA Contract to Develop Child Abuse and Neglect Training Materials, 1980). Phoenix: Department of Economic Security, 1980, p. 2.

Certain characteristic injuries provide other signals. These would include cigarette burns, distended fingers and limbs, and nonaccidental bruising patterns. The shape of an instrument imprinted on the skin is a frequent indicator of physical child abuse. For instance, when a lamp cord is looped and used as a whip, it will leave a loop scar on the child's back.

Cases of child torture are publicized widely when they are discovered. These reports have a memorable impact on the public because of the shocking and depraved nature of the crime. Child torture, however, is a relatively rare form of child abuse. More commonly, the abuse takes the form of severe and frequently repeated beatings that go far beyond any normal need for disciplinary punishment. School personnel should suspect child abuse whenever they encounter a child with repeated injuries, injuries in different stages of healing, or complications arising from old injuries that are not adequately explained by the student.

Another indicator that should arouse suspicions is the attitude or conduct of the parent. The parent may be purposely vague or evasive when explaining how the "accident" occurred. The parent may be reluctant to volunteer information. It has . . . been noted that the abusive parent frequently takes the child to many different physicians for treatment. If the battered child is taken to a hospital that is located far from his [or her] home, this could also be an indicator of abuse.

The child's behavior may also arouse suspicions. Statistically, the vast majority of abused children are under three years old. Nearly half of all reported cases involve children under six months old. Abused or neglected children of this age seldom cry. When they do, it is a hopeless, mournful sound that merely accompanies pain and sorrow. The cry is not urgent. It contains no expectation of comfort or relief. Abused children may also be wary of physical contact with adults. Sometimes the child will exhibit extreme fright, reacting to any physical contact with whimpering or attempts to hide. Others show extreme apathy and unresponsiveness. [URSA, 1978, as abstracted by ADES, *Sample Indicators for Law Enforcement Personnel*, 1980, p. 2]

NEGLECT

Neglect refers to "any act of omission, specifically the failure of a parent or other person legally responsible for a child's welfare to provide for the child's basic needs. . . . Most states have neglect and/or dependency statutes; however, not all states require the reporting of neglect" (USDHHS, 1981, p. 6).

Nutritional neglect is defined both as a failure of the caretaker to provide sufficient quantities of food and failure to provide acceptable quality of diet (i.e., appropriate nutrients). An example of nutritional neglect would be a case where a caretaker provides so little food to a child that it suffers malnutrition.

Medical and dental neglect is defined as a failure of the caretaker to recognize medical and dental problems and other appropriate treatment. An example of medical neglect would be a case where a caretaker fails to obtain eyeglasses for a badly cross-eyed child after repeatedly having been informed by school officials that the child had poor eyesight and needs glasses.

Educational neglect is defined as a failure to provide for a child's educational development. An example of educational neglect would be a situation in which a caretaker refuses to permit a child to attend school and makes no other provision for the child's education.

Inappropriate or insufficient clothing is defined as a failure to provide a minimum quantity and quality of clothing to a child. An example of clothing neglect would be a situation in which a child has clothes which are unwashed and torn or clothing inadequate to protect the child from cold and rain.

Shelter neglect is defined as a failure of the caretaker to provide basic minimum standards of adequate shelter (i.e., space, heat, indoor plumbing, electricity, structural adequacy, and sanitation). An example of shelter neglect would be a case where a child's home is inadequately heated, unsanitary, and unsafe due to exposed electrical wires or extreme filth.

Emotional neglect is defined both as a failure of the caretaker to provide appropriately for the developmental needs of the child and as a failure of the caretaker to provide consistency and continuity in the care of the child. An example of emotional neglect is a situation in which a child is fed adequately but is never held or cuddled or provided with the kinds of stimulation and nurturance that children need to develop normally.

Moral neglect is defined as a failure of the caretaker to provide clear expectations for the child regarding ethical and moral issues or where a caretaker exposes the child to immoral influences or exploitation. An example of moral neglect would be a case where a caretaker condones and encourages stealing on the part of the child. [URSA, 1978, as abstracted by ADES, *Forms and Indicators of Neglect,* 1980, p. 1]

The traditional indicators of child neglect include specific detectable evidence in terms of physical neglect, emotional neglect, material neglect, and demoralizing circumstances (unwholesome moral environment). These indicators can be found in Table 14.4.

The indicators presented in Table 14.4 are not intended as definitive diagnostic tools and should not be used as such. They should be useful to school and community health personnel involved in health appraisal and in a diagnostic role, but no indicator should ever be used as a substitute for personal observation, careful interviewing, a sensitivity to the complexity of each case, and an openness to the full and often conflicting range of the available evidence about abuse or neglect. School personnel will often report suspected cases of child neglect to law enforcement personnel.

SEXUAL ABUSE

Sexual abuse is defined as "any contact or interaction between a child and adult in which the child is being used for the sexual stimulation of the perpetrator or of another person. Most states define any sexual involvement of a parent or caretaker with a child as a sexual act and therefore abuse. The most common form of sexual abuse is incest between fathers and daughters" (USDHHS, 1981, p. 7).

Sexual abuse is one of the most difficult forms of child abuse or neglect to identify. In order to attempt to identify children who are being sexually abused, it is important to note the following medical and behavioral indicators (USDHHS, 1981, p. 7).

TABLE 14.4

Indicators of Child Neglect by Category

Indicators	Category
Exploited.	*Physical*
• Excessive responsibilities placed on very young children to care for home and other younger children.	
• Overworked beyond physical endurance.	
• Forced to beg and steal.	
• Forced to sell commodities beyond ability to do so.	
Malnourished and emaciated.	
Failure to receive necessary immunizations.	
Suffers chronic illness and lacks essential medical care.	
Lacks dental care.	
Failure to receive necessary prosthetics, including eyeglasses, hearing aids, and so on.	
Failure to receive proper hygiene.	
• Unbathed.	
• Poor mouth and skin care.	
Failure to attend school regularly because of the parent.	
Without supervision.	
Left alone for hours and days.	
Abandoned.	
• Denied normal experiences that produce feelings of being loved, wanted, secure, and worthy.	*Emotional*
• Rejected through indifference.	
• Rejected overtly—left alone, shouted at, blamed for problems, and so on.	
• Emotional neglect is intangible, but the child's behavior often reveals visible symptoms such as hyperactivity, withdrawal, overeating, fire setting, nervous skin disorders, psychosomatic complaints, autism, suicide attempts, truancy, delinquencies, failure to thrive, aggressiveness, discipline problems, stuttering, hypochondriasis, and overprotection.	

Organization of School Health Programs

TABLE 14.4 Continued

Indicators of Child Neglect by Category

Indicators	Category
• Not kept warm and comfortable at home, at school, and at play.	*Material*
• Not protected from the elements of the weather.	
• Dirty, smelly, with ragged clothes that are generally in terrible disrepair.	
• Wearing of such clothing usually results in ridicule and harassment from the child's peers.	

Filthy living conditions.
- Garbage and dirt strewn about the house and yard.
- Floor and walls smeared with crusted feces.
- Urine smell permeates the house.
- Soiled bedding and chairs.
- Home conditions in total chaos—no evidence of routine housekeeping.

Inadequate shelter.
- Cold.
- Overcrowded.
- Makeshift sleeping arrangements.
- Poor lighting.
- Poor ventilation.
- Fire hazards.
- Poor sanitation as a result of inadequate or unrepaired plumbing.
- Other hazardous conditions existing for children, such as broken porch and stair railings and the like.
- Meals that consistently lack nutritional value.
- Steady diet of potato chips, pop, candy, peanut butter, crackers, etc.

TABLE 14.4 Continued

Indicators of Child Neglect by Category

Indicators	Category
• Continuous friction in the home. • Marital discord. • Immature parents. • Excessive drinking. • Addiction to drugs. • Criminal environment. • Illicit sex relations. • Overly severe control and discipline. • Encouragement of delinquencies. • Harsh and improper language. • Nonsupport. • Values in the home in conflict with society. • Failures to inculcate value system in guidance and care of children (lack of moral training). • Broken home, divorce, and frequent remarriages. • Failure to offer motivation and stimulation toward learning and receiving an education in keeping with child's ability and intelligence. • Failure to provide healthy, wholesome recreation for family and children. • Failure to individualize children and their needs. • Failure to give constructive discipline for the child's proper development of good character, conduct, and habits. • Failure to give good adult example. • Promiscuity and prostitution.	*Demoralizing Circumstances*

URSA, 1978, as abstracted by the Arizona Department of Economic Security (ADES). *Forms and Indicators of Neglect* (Abstract of URSA Contract to Develop Child Abuse and Neglect Training Materials, 1980). Phoenix: Department of Economic Security, 1980, p. 2.

Medical Indicators

1. Bruises in external genitalia, vagina, or anal regions.
2. Bleeding from external genitalia, vagina, or anal regions.
3. Swollen or red cervix, vulva, or perineum.
4. Positive tests for any of the following:
   a. Gonococcus.
   b. Spermatozoa.
   c. Pregnancy.
   d. Venereal disease. [URSA, 1978, as abstracted by ADES, *Sample Indicators of Sexual Abuse,* 1980, p. 1]

Behavioral Indicators

The following list reflects the major behavioral indicators most often shown by children who are sexually abused:

1. Regressive behavior. Molested children (especially young children) may withdraw into fantasy worlds. Sometimes these children give the impression of being retarded when, in fact, they are not.
2. Delinquent or aggressive behavior. Molested children (especially preteen and teen) often act out their anger and hostility on others.
3. Sexual promiscuity. The sexually molested girl or boy may be sexually promiscuous, and their behavior may become very apparent not only to the school, but to the entire neighborhood.
4. Confiding in someone. A molested girl [or boy] may confide in a special friend or teacher. These confidences may not take the form of direct information about being molested, but may involve such statements as ''I'm afraid to go home tonight,'' ''I want to come and live with you,'' ''I want to go and live in a foster home.''
5. Poor peer relationships. Molested children (if molestation had occurred over a long period of time) may not have social skills or may be too emotionally disturbed to form peer relationships. The parent(s) has a vested interest in keeping them emotionally isolated. The child may have such a poor self-image (the ''bad me'' concept) that it overshadows his whole existence.
6. Prostitution. The middle to older molested teenager may turn to prostitution.
7. Extremely protective parent. In incestuous relationships, the parent involved may become exceedingly jealous of the child, often refusing him [or her] any social contact. The parent is afraid that the child will tell but . . . even more afraid of losing the child to others. A father, for example, may pick his teenage daughter up at school every day and become furious if he sees her talking to anyone.

8. Unwillingness to participate in physical or recreational activities. Young children who have been highly sexually stimulated or have been forced to have sexual intercourse with an adult may find it painful to sit in their chairs in school or to play games that require a good deal of movement.

9. Running away. Teenagers who have been molested sometimes resort to escape and run away from the home.

10. Drugs. Teenagers who have been molested may resort to escape through the use of drugs.

11. Confession. The child who has been molested may seek to report the offense. A number of incest cases . . . [in which] a teenager reports may be fictitious, but a thorough investigation should be made to determine the validity of the statement. [URSA, 1978, as abstracted by ADES, *Sample Indicators of Sexual Abuse,* 1980, p. 1]

FAMILY INDICATORS

"Over 90 percent of the perpetrators of child abuse and neglect were the children's own parents" (USDHHS, 1981, p. 8). Child maltreatment is clearly a family problem. The characteristics of the typical family in which child maltreatment occurs would be a family that has a low socioeconomic status and is headed by parents with limited education. As a result, the family is subject to a number of stress factors, including broken family, insufficient income, and inadequate housing. "When families involved in abuse and those involved in neglect are viewed separately, two distinct profiles emerge. The overriding characteristic of neglectful families is that they are headed only by a mother figure, and they tend to have more children than families involved in abuse" (USDHHS, 1981, p. 9).

> The abusive families tend to have both parental figures present and often, consequently, had higher incomes. Stress factors characteristic of these families include lack of tolerance, loss of control during discipline, and a history of abuse as a child. This suggests that problematic family dynamics may play a greater part in families involved in abuse, whereas environmental stress may seem to play a larger part in neglectful families. [USDHHS, 1981, p. 10]

Since abuse and neglect are both critically important, the psychodynamic and family indicators and the early signs of potentially abusive parents will be viewed together. These indicators are presented in Tables 14.5 and 14.6.

LEGAL TRENDS

Prior to 1963, not much had been accomplished legally to help the child who was abused or neglected. It was only in 1962 that the "battered child syndrome" was actually identified by Kempe. This syndrome focused on physical and other signs indicative of internal or external injuries to a child that resulted from acts committed by a parent or caretaker. With the development of this

Organization of School Health Programs

TABLE 14.5

Psychodynamic and Family Indicators of Child Abuse and Neglect

- Many personal and marital problems.
- The parents had poor relationships with their own parents.
- Many parents were themselves abused as children.
- The parents were frequently raised in homes where excessive punishment was the norm.
- They tend to be antagonistic, suspicious, and fearful of people.
- They are isolated, transient, and lack external supports.
- The parents are evasive and contradictory in explaining injuries.
- Frequently, little or no interest is shown for the child's treatment.
- They do not touch the child or involve themselves with the child's care and feeding.
- They fail to appropriately respond to the child's pain.
- Parents may constantly criticize the child and blame him or her for the injury.
- They often neglect their own physical health.
- The parents are afraid of being left alone, especially with the child.
- They have inappropriate expectations of the child.
- The child is seen as someone who is disliked by the parent or who is accusatory and judgmental.

URSA, 1978, as abstracted by the Arizona Department of Economic Security (ADES). *Forms and Indicators of Child Abuse* (Abstract of URSA Contract to Develop Child Abuse and Neglect Training Materials, 1980). Phoenix: Department of Economic Security, 1980, p. 2.

definition, which helped to provide legal criteria for identification of abused and neglected children, states began to pass laws for the reporting of child abuse and neglect.

In 1963, the first child abuse and neglect reporting laws were passed. These laws defined child abuse, identified professionals who had constant access to children, and required that these professionals report suspected cases of child abuse to a statewide agency that could make a complete investigation (USDHHS, 1981, p. 4). By 1967, child abuse and neglect statutes had been passed by all fifty states. However, even though statutes were passed, states varied on their definitions of neglect and the legal ramifications of reporting.

The most significant child abuse-related law was the passing of the Child Abuse Prevention and Treatment Act (PL 93–247). In this act child abuse and neglect were defined as physical or mental injury, sexual abuse or exploitation, negligent treatment, or maltreatment of a child under the age of eighteen by a person who is responsible for the child's welfare (USDHHS, 1981, p. 5).

TABLE 14.6

Characteristics of Potentially Abusive Parents

- Documented history of previous neglect of another child.
- Frequent pregnancies with several children of preschool age.
- Prematurity.
- Out-of-wedlock pregnancy.
- Absent fathers (physically or psychologically).
- Economic stress.
- Retardation of responsible caretakers.
- History of alcohol or drug abuse.
- Social isolation, no supporting network of relatives or friends.
- Unrealistic expectations of child.
- Views the child as "different" from other children.

URSA, 1978, as abstracted by the Arizona Department of Economic Security (ADES). *Forms and Indicators of Child Abuse* (Abstract of URSA Contract to Develop Child Abuse and Neglect Training Materials, 1980). Phoenix: Department of Economic Security, 1980, p. 2.

PL 93–247 was signed by President Nixon in January 1974. The Act was funded for $85 million over a three-year period for the identification, treatment, and prevention of child abuse. As a part of this act, the National Center on Child Abuse and Neglect within the United States Children's Bureau was created. Demonstration projects and programs throughout the country were funded as a result of this act. Grants to states were allocated for the development of child abuse and neglect prevention and treatment programs.

SCHOOL RESPONSIBILITY

Both the individual and the school personnel have responsibilities when abuse or neglect is suspected. School personnel, especially teachers, are in a unique position, because of sustained daily contact, to notice possible abuse or neglect. School personnel must report suspected cases of abuse or neglect immediately. The report can be made to the school nurse, who in turn will report it to law enforcement personnel or to a department of social services. Where no school nurse is present, school personnel are encouraged to report the suspected case to law enforcement personnel or to social services themselves.

The report can be both oral and written. Any report should include the child's name, age, and address. In addition, the parent's name and address, the nature and extent of the injury or suspicions of abuse, and the reporter's name and location should be given.

People making reports of child abuse or neglect are immune from legal prosecution, provided that the report was in good faith. Many states require reporting of suspected child abuse or neglect and state that doctors, social workers, teachers, and law enforcement officials must report suspected cases. There are both criminal and civil penalties for not making the mandated report.

Child abuse and neglect is one of the saddest events that can occur. Not only can these acts result in the death of a child, but they can significantly influence the child throughout his or her entire life. Through an understanding of the various indicators for both abuse and neglect, it is hoped that reporting can be done sooner and help for the child can be obtained.

SUMMARY

Child abuse and neglect in recent years have received much attention from a variety of sources, including the legal system, the health care delivery system, and the media. Child abuse and neglect are very difficult to prove; consequently, any statistics are probably underestimated.

School personnel are in a strategic position to report any suspected cases of child abuse and neglect. Through their efforts, more cases may be identified and more action taken. School personnel have a clear responsibility to become involved, especially when the student's physical, mental, and emotional health are in jeopardy.

REVIEW QUESTIONS

1. Document child abuse and neglect as a national health problem.
2. Discuss the physical, mental, and social indicators of physical child abuse.
3. Discuss the physical, mental, and social indicators of child neglect.
4. Discuss the physical, mental, and social indicators of sexual abuse.
5. Identify characteristics associated with abusive parents.
6. Discuss the role of the school personnel with respect to suspected child abuse or neglect cases.
7. Why do you suppose so many cases of child abuse or neglect go unreported each year?

REFERENCES

American Humane Association. *National Analysis of Official Child Neglect and Abuse Reporting. 1978 Annual Report.* Englewood, Colo.: AHA.

Gil, D. *Violence against Children: Physical Child Abuse in the United States.* Cambridge: Harvard University Press, 1970.

Giovannoni, J. "Parental Mistreatment: Perpetrators and Victims." *Journal of Marriage and the Family* **33** (1971), 649–658.

Helfer, R. E., and C. H. Kempe, eds. *The Battered Child,* 2nd ed. Chicago: University of Chicago Press, 1974.

Jirsa, J. *Child Abuse and Neglect: A Handbook.* Madison, Wis.: Madison Metropolitan School District, 1976.

Kalisch, B. J. *Child Abuse and Neglect: An Annotated Bibliography.* Westport, Conn.: Greenwood Press, 1978.

Kempe, R. S., and C. Henry Kempe. *Child Abuse.* Cambridge, Mass.: Harvard University Press, 1978.

Lynch, A. "Child Abuse and the School-Age Population." *The Journal of School Health* **45** (1975), 141–148.

Martin, H. P., ed. *The Abused Child: A Multidisciplinary Approach to Developmental Issues and Treatment.* Cambridge, Mass.: Ballinger, 1976.

Mussen, P., J. Conger, and J. Kagan. *Child Development and Personality.* New York: Harper and Row, 1979.

Newberger, E. H., and J. H. Daniel. "Knowledge and Epidemiology of Child Abuse: A Critical Review of Concepts." *Pediatric Annals* (March 1976), 110.

Olson, R. "Index of Suspicion: Screening for Child Abusers." *American Journal of Nursing* **76**:1 (January 1976), 108–110.

Polansky, N. A., C. Hally, and N. F. Polansky. *Profile of Neglect: A Survey of the State of Knowledge of Child Neglect.* Washington, D.C.: U.S. Department of Health, Education and Welfare Publication No. (SRS) 76-23037, 1975.

Soeffing, M. "Abused Children Are Exceptional Children," *Exceptional Children* **42** (1975), 126–133.

Urban and Rural Systems Associates (URSA). *Handbook on Child Abuse and Neglect.* San Francisco: URSA, April, 1978.

URSA, 1978, as abstracted by ADES. *Forms and Indicators of Child Abuse* (Abstract of URSA Contract to Develop Child Abuse and Neglect Training Materials). Phoenix: Arizona Department of Economic Security, 1980.

URSA, 1978, as abstracted by ADES. *Forms and Indicators of Child Neglect* (Abstract of URSA Contract to Develop Child Abuse and Neglect Training Materials). Phoenix: Arizona Department of Economic Security, 1980.

URSA, 1978, as abstracted by ADES. *Forms and Indicators of Sexual Abuse* (Abstract of URSA Contract to Develop Child Abuse and Neglect Training Materials). Phoenix: Arizona Department of Economic Security, 1980.

URSA, 1978, as abstracted by ADES. *Sample Indicators for Law Enforcement Personnel* (Abstract of URSA Contract to Develop Child Abuse and Neglect Training Materials). Phoenix: Arizona Department of Economic Security, 1980.

U.S. Department of Health and Human Services. *Child Abuse and Neglect: Curriculum in the Schools.* Washington, D.C.: USDHHS, 1981, PHHS Publication No. 81-30312.

U.S. Department of Health, Education and Welfare. *Child Abuse and Neglect: The Problem and Its Management,* volumes 1, 2, and 3. Washington, D.C.: HEW Publication No. (OHD), 75-30073, 1975.

Walters, D. R. *Physical and Sexual Abuse of Children: Causes and Treatment.* Bloomington, Ind.: Indiana University Press, 1975.

PART IV

Instruction

Health Instruction Patterns

15

reviously in this text, definitions of the major components of the total school health program were provided. The focus of this chapter is on various patterns of providing health instruction, the scope and sequence of health instruction, and the process of developing health instruction units and lesson plans. Clearly, some instructional patterns are more suitable than others for achieving optimal objectives. However, it is important to understand that an impact on health behavior can be attained through means other than direct health teaching.

The term *health instruction* has been selected in this text to distinguish the formal classroom phase of health education from the health education provided by many other people in the school setting. It has been well established that health education is a multifaceted, multidisciplinary concept. There are health-related undertones in nearly everything one does every day.

Health instruction refers to that part of health education that is a sequentially planned and carried out segment of the individual's formal school instruction, regardless of the pattern utilized to deliver that instruction. It may be designed to alter health-damaging behavior or to reinforce behavior that already exerts a positive influence over the total well-being of the individual. The broad concept of school health education was defined in the Report of the 1990 Joint Committee on Health Education Terminology as ''one component of the comprehensive school health program which includes the development, delivery, and evaluation of a planned instructional program and other activities for students preschool through grade 12, for parents and for school staff, and is designed to positively influence the health knowledge, attitudes, and skills of individuals.''[1] Clearly the focus of health instruction is to assist persons, either individually or in groups, to make informed decisions about matters that affect their own health or the health of those around them. The focus of this chapter is on the specific patterns that might be used to organize the health instruction that is presented in school systems. It is important to understand that there is no single ''best'' method of delivering health instruction. The important point is that the instruction is planned and is delivered by qualified personnel if the program is to have the greatest impact.

Some would suggest that the focus of education should be positive behavior change. Perhaps Jesse Ferring Williams stated it best when he stated that health was the ability to do most and serve best. However, it must be

1. Report of the 1990 Joint Committee on Health Education Terminology, *Journal of Health Education* 22, no. 2 (March/April 1991):97–107.

remembered that the decision to engage in either healthful or unhealthful behavior rests with the individual. The role of the health instructor, or anyone in the school system who affects the health of the student, is to provide an opportunity for the student to attain scientifically accurate knowledge upon which to base sound decisions regarding health behavior. Many opportunities arise in the school setting each day that can lead to increased learning about health matters.

Regardless of the methods used in health instruction or the patterns employed to encourage health education, there is general agreement that planning is critical if success is to be realized. If there is to be an impact on students' health knowledge, attitudes, and practices, schools must have a well-organized and sequentially arranged program of health instruction.

If success is to be enhanced, the goals and objectives in terms of outcome variables must be clearly stated. Specific content and the sequential arrangement of that content should be outlined, teaching methods and materials should be suggested, and a plan for the logical and efficient evaluation of all facets of the program should be presented.

If the greatest effect on the health knowledge, attitudes, and practices of both students and teachers is to be attained, it is critical that both formal and informal health education be planned and understood by all school personnel. By planning in this way, school personnel can address the differing health problems of students. This also takes into account the idea that different persons learn in different ways. By using a variety of teaching methods and reintroducing basic content as it relates to the concept being developed, the teacher will probably attain greater success than if one particular concept is presented using but one teaching method.

If a central purpose of education is to develop the individual's rational or intellectual powers and a primary purpose of school health education is to improve health behavior, then critical thinking in terms of curriculum development becomes still more important. Further, the extent to which objectives are met depends a great deal upon the support of administrators, teachers, parents, and other community groups. As such, it is important that these key individuals and groups be involved in the planning process. As has been stated throughout this textbook, teamwork is basic to the success of the total school health program.

Since each school district will have its own pattern for designing and developing curriculums, it is necessary for those responsible for planning the health instruction program to understand some basic organizational patterns that can be utilized in developing that health instruction program. Basic principles of curriculum development, including making decisions relative to approaches, concepts, objectives, goals, content and method selection, and the selection of resource materials are discussed in Chapter 17.

Organization of School Health Programs

ORGANIZATIONAL PATTERNS FOR CURRICULUMS

In general, seven major patterns of curriculum organization have emerged. These patterns include traditional or direct teaching, correlated teaching, integrated or fused teaching, broad fields, core approaches, competency-based or skill-based, and experiential approaches.

Traditional or Direct Instruction

At present in the United States there is a movement called "back to basics," which calls for increased attention to the subjects of writing, reading, and mathematics. President George Bush, who wants to be known as "the Education President," has suggested that there should also be increased emphasis on geography and social studies. The public must be made aware that health is also a "basic." As aptly stated by Oberteuffer, "There is a reciprocal relationship between health and education. An individual in poor health won't derive as much as possible from his [or her] education and it takes an educated individual to make the informed decisions necessary to attain the highest level of health" (1968, p. 72).

In the traditional pattern of instruction, a specific time slot is allocated for each topic or subject in the curriculum. A specified set of objectives has been developed for each subject, and seldom is there much of an attempt to transfer learning from one subject matter to another. Naturally, this transfer will often occur by default, if not by design.

Perhaps the best example of the traditional approach is that used in our postsecondary schools—in colleges and universities. A student selects the courses he or she wants to take, and these courses are offered at specified times. There are no attempts to correlate or integrate subject matter across course lines. Each course is an independent entity.

In the realm of traditional health instruction, instead of specific courses, the various content units within the total health course become the separate courses. This means that there may be several units of health instruction developed, but they are specific elements unto themselves.

For example, the traditional course of health instruction may include units on tobacco, alcohol, other drugs, first aid, consumer health, and disease control. Each unit may be designed for a one-week period; thus, this course will be taught for six weeks. Once the course begins, the teacher discusses the effects of tobacco for one week, then moves to the second unit, which might deal with alcohol use. The third might be on other drugs, and so on, until the final unit has been taught. There is, perhaps, little attention paid to what occurred before or what is to occur after a given unit. Thus, learning is more linear than progressive—progressive teachers might include a common construct such as decision making across the various content units.

The major problem with the traditional approach is the lack of planning and the content overlapping from grade level to grade level. This causes students some consternation. The purpose of a well-developed curriculum is to move the learner from lesser to greater amounts of information and to move the individual from the more concrete to the more abstract. Unless there is planning between grades, the instructor may fail to make this transition.

Ideally, the direct health course will be taught by a specifically trained health instruction specialist (see Chapter 20). This is not generally the case, especially in the elementary schools. Since the children in elementary schools tend to remain in intact classroom groupings throughout most of the school day, the teacher must be a generalist rather than a specialist. Further, when health is taught by the regular classroom teacher, better use can be made of the "teachable moment" for indirect health instruction. If elementary classroom teachers are to teach health, it is important that school administrators plan in-service education programs specifically designed to keep such teachers aware of new developments in the field.

In the junior high school or the senior high school, it is preferable for a professionally trained health instruction specialist to teach health. This person possesses, at minimum, a minor in health instruction and has a desire to teach the health instruction program.

The traditional or direct teaching method has been called the easiest method of teaching health. The advantage of this method is that health instruction retains its own identity as an important part of the school curriculum. It also requires administrative consideration and a recognition of its overall contribution to the total education of the students. If school administrators are not committed to the importance of health instruction, the course will not be well developed and may not be a part of the curriculum.

Correlated Health Instruction

The basic premise of the correlated approach to health instruction is that more than one subject area is used as a vehicle for teaching health. If this organizational method is to be successful, it is important that there be a coordinator working with the teachers. The idea is to attempt to show the relationship between health and the subject matter within which health is being taught. For example, if microorganisms are being studied in a science class, the emphasis might be on studying the basic pathogens of disease and how these pathogens affect health.

If the correlated method of health instruction is to be successful, the specific grade level, the specific health area, and the number of class periods needed to teach the content must be indicated within the total organizational pattern. For those who have questions about where health instruction can be correlated, Sliepcevich and Carroll (1958, pp. 283–292) reported no fewer than 185 correlations in some 17 different subject areas that would work with this type of instructional method.

Integrated or Fused Health Instruction

Integration involves the teaching of health around a central theme or topic. The boundaries of specific topics are ignored, and all aspects of the curriculum are taught as they mutually relate in some genuine association. An example would be the central theme of the Renaissance, wherein an English class might explore the role of literature in advancing health concepts. In art classes, students could develop posters of the period that depict the emergence of medicine, and in history students could write papers about the new discoveries in medicine during the Renaissance.

The integrated approach is particularly appropriate for self-contained classrooms such as are usually found in elementary schools. In fact, many people feel this plan might be the best way to attain maximum learning in elementary school. However, if integration is to be successful, a great deal of time and effort must be taken in planning; far too often, no one is given the sole responsibility for teaching health. In this case, integration can be the quickest way to pay lip service to the existence of the health instruction program, when in fact, it is lost in the effort to teach other subjects. For teachers to integrate health instruction successfully into their subjects, those teachers must have a good command not only of several specific subjects, but also of the content of health instruction. According to Mayshark and Shaw (1967, p. 144), ''Such teachers are few as the rapid increase in subject-matter specialists at the elementary level attests.''

The only way to be sure that either the correlated or integrated health curriculum will work is if someone is given specific responsibility to plan and organize the entire process from start to finish. Naturally, a comprehensive evaluation plan must be a part of this total process.

Broad Fields Health Instruction

Broad fields health instruction is a method of organization that is similar to integration but, although course lines still remain, trunk lines between similar areas of the curriculum exist. Examples of the broad fields pattern would be physical sciences (chemistry and physics) or health and physical education. In the latter case, the same instructor would be responsible for teaching both health instruction and physical education. The success or failure of any type of broad fields instruction rests upon the qualifications and abilities of the teacher. The problem with the broad fields approach is that the instructor may have a major in the primary field and perhaps very little training in the secondary field. Ideally, the teacher would have at least a minor in the secondary field. Unfortunately, the teacher may not have a great deal of interest in teaching the secondary subject; consequently, health instruction may receive little emphasis. If one agrees with the idea that attitudes are better caught than taught, what type of attitude would be shown by a teacher who does not want to teach health in the first place?

The school lunchroom can provide opportunities for informal health education.
Photo courtesy, Michigan Department of Health

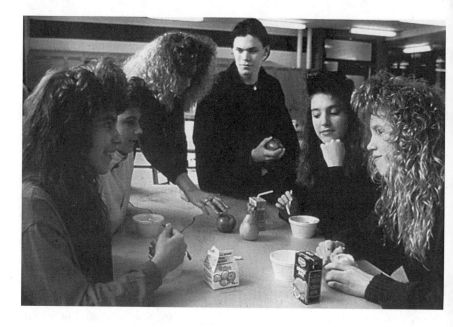

Core Health Instruction

The core approach is similar to the integrated or fused approach in that a group of subjects becomes the focal point for learning. Loose course lines are retained, and it is this concept that differentiates the core approach from the integrated approach. Many of the positive aspects of the integrated approach are retained, yet the core approach overcomes several of the shortcomings of the integrated approach. Ample time for health instruction can be provided as long as those responsible for planning hold health instruction as a priority. Many elementary schools employ a modified form of the core approach, and it seems particularly appropriate for them. The core approach is also employed in some secondary schools, but in general, direct instruction would be more appropriate for both the junior high school (grades 7, 8, and 9) and the senior high school (grades 10, 11, and 12).

Competency/Skill-Based Health Instruction

Competency-based or skill-based instruction became popular during the 1970s when several national reports suggested that American students were not as competent in several selected areas of education as were their foreign counterparts. As a result, many school districts tried to quickly develop competency statements in selected areas of the curriculum, most notably science and mathematics. In competency- or skill-based health instruction, specific competency statements are written as the specific outcomes expected to be achieved as a result of the health instruction program.

Organization of School Health Programs

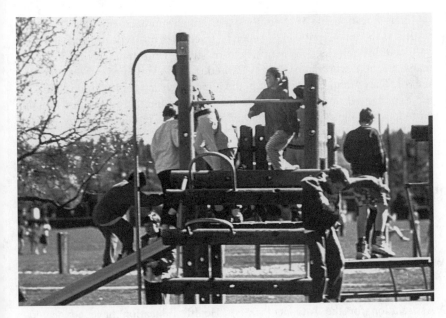

Learning basics of stretching and exercise at a young age will help in instilling positive attitudes toward the physical dimension of health.
Photo courtesy, Health and Welfare, Canada

Unfortunately, competency statements generally are written in the present. This means that the competencies, if attained by students, may well be quite applicable to present conditions, but may not be appropriate or as appropriate, in the long-range plan. For example, a basic, though controversial competency in the area of human sexuality might be that the individual practices birth control when engaging in sexual activities. However, now that the major health problem of AIDS has emerged, this competency might be quite risky and certainly, if still advocated, written in much different terminology.

A second problem associated with the competency/skill-based approach is the fact that it is predicated on "best" behavior. Who is to determine that behavior? Further, since in many cases the health education curriculum is not developed by health education specialists, there is a major chance that the competencies that might be developed may not be appropriate for select grade levels. It is also important that the learning activities and content be directly related to the competencies, which severely limits the teacher in his or her creativity since it is the competency that is evaluated, not the ability of the student to apply knowledge in a variety of situations.

Experiential Approach to Health Instruction

In the experiential approach to health instruction there are no core themes, nor are there any course lines. The curriculum is totally individualized, and students are allowed to study what they wish—as in the Summerhill approach to learning (Neil, 1977).

It is questionable if a purely experiential approach produces the same results as the other approaches, since instructors in this type of approach teach only within their specific major field of study. Unfortunately, there are not many teachers who majored in health education available in the elementary school. They are more prevalent in the junior high and senior high school. For the experiential approach to work, the school administration must be committed to the idea of health instruction and must employ persons who are qualified in health instruction.

COMPREHENSIVE HEALTH INSTRUCTION

More and more health professionals are calling for comprehensive health education for all schools at all grade levels. Unfortunately, about the only point of agreement as to what constitutes "comprehensive" is the idea that a comprehensive school health program consists, at a minimum, of three parts: health instruction, health services, and a healthful school environment. More recently, such organizations as the American School Health Association and the Association for the Advancement of Health Education have advocated a broader approach to comprehensive school health programs. In addition to the three traditional areas of instruction, services, and environment, they also include school food services, guidance and counseling, physical education, school-site wellness programs, and integrated school/community programs to define the comprehensive school health program. Regardless of the definition used, all definitions include the concept that the instructional program should be orderly and progress through a succession of health topics sequentially arranged from grade to grade. This sequential arrangement of topics will help in avoiding the crisis orientation, or "band-aid" approach, to health instruction.

Recently the 1990 Report of the Joint Committee on Health Education Terminology was released. This committee consisted of representatives from eight organizations committed to school health. The organizations were: the American School Health Association; the Association for the Advancement of Health Education; the Society for Public Health Education; the American Academy of Pediatrics; the American Public Health Association (both the School Health Education and Services Section and the Public Health Education and Health Promotion Section); the Association of State and Territorial Directors of Public Health Education; the Society of State Directors of Health, Physical Education and Recreation; and the American College Health Association. This group defined the comprehensive school health program as "an organized set of policies, procedures, and activities designed to protect and promote the health and well-being of students and staff which has traditionally included health services, healthful school environment, and health education. It should also include, but not be limited to guidance and counseling, physical education, food service, social work, psychological services, and employee health promotion." Within the context of that definition, the committee

Organization of School Health Programs

indicated that comprehensive school health instruction refers to the development, delivery, and evaluation of a planned curriculum for grades preschool through 12, with goals, objectives, content sequence, and specific classroom lessons which include, but are not limited to, the following major content areas:

- Community health.
- Consumer health.
- Environmental health.
- Family life.
- Mental and emotional health.
- Injury prevention and safety.
- Nutrition.
- Personal health.
- Prevention and control of disease.
- Substance use and abuse.

Previously the Committee to Establish Guidelines for Comprehensive School Health Education (1984, p. 5) developed nine criteria for the comprehensive school health program. These criteria included (but were not limited to):

1. Instruction intended to motivate health maintenance and promote wellness and not merely to prevent disease or disability.
2. Activities designed to develop decision-making competencies related to health and health behavior.
3. A planned, sequential pre-K to 12 curriculum based upon students' needs and current and emerging health concepts and societal issues.
4. Opportunities for all students to develop and demonstrate health-related knowledge, attitudes, and practices.
5. Integration of the physical, mental, emotional, and social dimensions of health as the basis for study of the following topic areas: causes, control, and prevention of disease and disorders; community health; consumer health; environmental health; family life; growth and development; nutritional health; personal health; safety and accident prevention; substance use and abuse.[2]
6. Specific program goals and objectives.
7. Formative and summative evaluation procedures.
8. An effective management system.
9. Sufficient resources: budgeted instructional materials, time, management staff, and teachers.

These nine points are discussed further in the chapters that follow.

Previously in this chapter, seven organizational patterns for health instruction were discussed. We will now turn to a discussion of patterns for health instruction that could be employed regardless of the type of curriculum

2. Mental health is omitted as a separate topic area, since it is embodied in all the content areas included under this definition.

FIGURE 15.1

Vertical organization for
the health curriculum.
*Adapted from: Fodor, J.,
and G. Dalis,* Health
Instruction, *4th ed.
(Philadelphia: Lea and
Febiger, 1989), p. 106.*

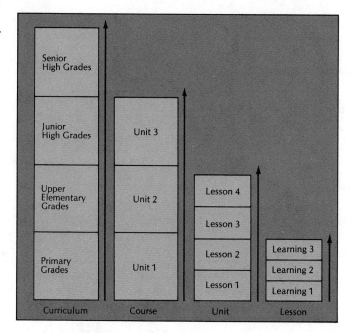

organization used in the school. Before embarking on that discussion, it is
important to understand both the vertical and horizontal perspectives of curriculum planning.

Vertical Planning

Vertical organization, simply stated, is the ordering of content and learning
so that new learning builds on what was learned in a previous grade level.
This type of planning should pervade the total school curriculum and should
not be confined to only one aspect of it.

Learning that occurs at the primary level should produce a movement
toward more abstract learning at intermediate and secondary levels. For example, before a student can spell words, he or she must know the alphabet.
Similarly, the student must know words and how they fit together before sentences can be constructed. The student then learns that groups of sentences
form paragraphs, that groups of paragraphs form themes, and that groups of
themes can produce an unlimited number of books, plays, and other literary
works.

This type of vertical learning occurs at all levels of the curriculum,
through the course, unit, and even the individual lesson. Fodor and Dalis
(1989, p. 106) developed a diagram of the concept of vertical organization that
illustrates this concept (see Figure 15.1).

Figure 15.1 shows the relationship between lower-level learning and how
that leads to more abstract learning at the upper levels. Bloom and his associates (1956, pp. 201–207) set forth a taxonomy of educational objectives in
the cognitive domain that also represents this vertical organization. These

objectives progress from lower levels (knowledge) through four stages and ultimately culminate in the student being able to evaluate various situations he or she faces. The six stages of the taxonomy are knowledge, comprehension, application, analysis, synthesis, and evaluation. This cognitive taxonomy was followed by one developed by David Krathwohl and his associates (1964, pp. 50–54) for the affective or attitudinal domain. The five phases of the affective taxonomy include receiving, responding, valuing, organizing, and characterizing.

Obviously, when considering vertical organization, one must question how many topics should be covered in each grade level. Since health education covers a broad range of topical areas, it is not practical to think that all areas can be covered in any given grade level. Thus, it becomes obvious that if health instruction is to be meaningful, several things must be considered. Foremost among these criteria should be the following:

- The maturity level of the students.
- The needs of the students.
- The needs of the community.
- The type of material being taught in other subject matter in the same grade.
- The legal requirements.
- The availability of materials to teach the course.
- The priority of each topical area within the total curriculum pattern.

Naturally, these seven points are not all-inclusive. Each local school district should use these criteria plus any local ones that may aid in the selection of grade placement for selected topic areas. The important thing to remember is that there is no universally agreed-upon topic that should be placed at any given grade level. Thus, local districts have the responsibility to convene a group of persons interested in the health of the school-age child for the purpose of developing a rationale for grade placement of health topics.

Horizontal Planning

This concept refers to within-grade organization, regardless of the topical area, so that the learning from topic to topic occurs in an interrelated fashion. An example of this is to use a health text for a reading assignment; then, using the data from the reading assignment, selected mathematics concepts could be developed. This also serves as a motivational element for the individual, since the interrelated nature of learning is exemplified in this arrangement. The key element here is to be sure the various learning components complement each other and lend support to constructs developed in other areas.

The purpose of considering horizontal organization when developing a curriculum is that it leads to a smooth transition from subject matter to subject matter. By turning Figure 15.1 90 degrees, one can see the relationship of horizontal to vertical organization (see Figure 15.2).

Figure 15.2 shows that concepts developed in science carry through physical education to health instruction and vice versa. In like manner, concepts

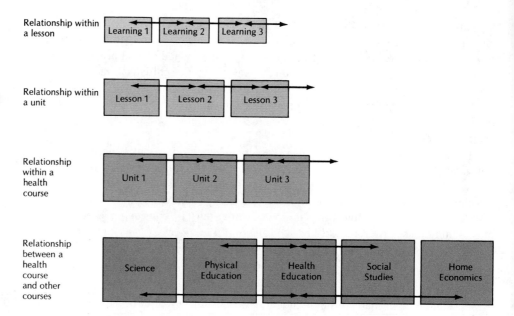

Relationship within a lesson

Learning 1 — Learning 2 — Learning 3

Relationship within a unit

Lesson 1 — Lesson 2 — Lesson 3

Relationship within a health course

Unit 1 — Unit 2 — Unit 3

Relationship between a health course and other courses

Science — Physical Education — Health Education — Social Studies — Home Economics

FIGURE 15.2

Horizontal organization for the health curriculum.

Adapted from: J. Fodor and G. Dalis, Health Instruction, *4th ed. (Philadelphia: Lea and Febiger, 1989), p. 108.*

developed in health instruction impact on both physical education and social studies and carry over into home economics. Each unit flows into the next unit, each lesson flows into the next lesson, and each learning builds a foundation for the learnings to follow.

EMERGING PATTERNS OF HEALTH CURRICULUM

Early attempts at health instruction were based primarily upon the selection of a textbook, often without specific regard to the needs and interests of the students. The teachers were generally not well versed in the subject matter, so the course became rather tedious at best. Textbooks, in general, are written to cover a wide range of topical areas, since they are designed to be "comprehensive." As such, the same basic content is covered in each textbook for each grade level. This is further complicated by the fact that teachers using a textbook rely on that text to provide basic content information. In these cases, the teacher often tends to concentrate instructional efforts on those topics with which he or she is most familiar. Because of this, students feel that they get the same material in health, year after year.

The Cycle Plan

According to Rash and Pigg (1979, p. 8), the cycle plan of instruction first appeared in 1933 in the state of Indiana. However, the first widespread use of the cycle plan was in the state of Oregon in 1945–46. The basics of that program, entitled "Oregon's Four-Cycle Health Curriculum," are still in evidence today.

The four-cycle plan was specifically developed to promote cumulative health learning. A series of studies and surveys was completed to identify the needs and interests of students, teachers, parents, and the community at large. Once the needs were identified, the scope of the curriculum was framed.

The four cycles were based upon the grade level equivalents of 1–3, 4–6, 7–9, and 10–12. The "cycle" was a refresher element that was built into the curriculum. The question was when, or in what order, various topics should be taught, and what topics should be taught at each grade level.

Analysis of the survey data provided a great deal of insight for the persons given the responsibility of developing the plan. Children had voiced an on-going complaint that there was a great deal of repetition in their existing health instruction course and that some topics were totally ignored. Thus, the health instruction subcommittee of the Oregon State Joint Committee for Health and Physical Fitness faced the problem of vertical and horizontal curriculum organization.

At that time, Oregon state law on health and physical education specified that health curricula in all elementary and secondary schools in the state must include instruction in (1) personal hygiene, (2) community health and sanitation, (3) communicable diseases, (4) nutrition, (5) mental health, (6) safety education, (7) first aid, (8) choice and use of health services and health products, (9) physiology of exercise, (10) structure and functions of the human body, and (11) effects of alcoholic drinks, stimulants, and narcotics.

Using the results of input from experts in medicine, dentistry, education, and public health, as well as input from students, parents, and specific research data relative to the various health problems of children at different developmental levels, the health instruction subcommittee developed specific objectives designed to help students deal more effectively with personal, family, and community health problems.

The four-cycle plan was designed to promote cumulative health learning. A cycle was defined as a three-year period of time; thus, in twelve years of school, four cycles were to be realized. This initial plan for the state of Oregon is presented in Table 15.1.

One disadvantage of Oregon's four-cycle plan was that each health area was placed in only one grade level in each three-year cycle. This initial placement then dictated where the topic would be placed in subsequent cycles, since the philosophy of the program was that each topic should be repeated in each cycle. For example, personal hygiene was initially placed in grade 1 of the first cycle. Thus, it was placed in the first grade level of the ensuing cycles (grades 4, 7, and 10). There was not a lot of reasoning behind where the topic was initially placed, but the plan was reorganized in 1948, since it became readily apparent that some topics should be repeated more often than once every three years. This repetition of topics became the refresher element of the curriculum. This means that some basic content may be repeated using a different teaching method in subsequent years. This serves as a review or refresher for the student. When doing this, it is critical that the refresher

TABLE 15.1

Four-Cycle Plan of Health Instruction in Oregon Schools

Areas	Cycle 1; Grades			Cycle 2; Grades			Cycle 3; Grades			Cycle 4; Grades		
	1	2	3	4	5	6	7	8	9	10	11	12
I Structure and functions of the human body	X			X			X			X		
II Personal hygiene*	X			X			X			X		
III Physiology of exercise		X			X			X			X	
IV Nutrition		X			X			X			X	
V First aid and safety education		X			X			X			X	
VI Choice and use of health services and health products			X			X			X			X
VII Communicable diseases†			X			X			X			X
VIII Community health and sanitation			X			X			X			X
IX Mental health‡	X			X				X				X

*This unit also includes instruction in the area "Effects of alcoholic drinks, stimulants, and narcotics."

†This unit also includes instruction on the noncommunicable diseases.

‡On the three lower levels, appropriate instruction on mental health is included in the units on personal hygiene. The unit on mental health, recommended for grade 12, also includes instruction on family-life education.

element be just that. It should not dominate the health instruction course; rather, it should serve as a stepping-stone to the development of new or more abstract knowledge.

For the most part, the four-cycle plan was a traditional or unit plan for health instruction. Although the nine major topics were rotated on a cyclic plan, specific units of instruction for each of the grades specified within the plan were developed. Each unit was taught for a predetermined period of time. By doing this, the minimum time for health instruction specified in the law would be met.

In general, teachers feel quite comfortable with the unit approach. If they complete the unit, there is a certain amount of reassurance that all the material that should be covered is, in fact, covered. The problem with this approach is

Organization of School Health Programs

the fact that student needs may be neglected in the effort to ''get through each unit.'' The specifics of how to develop units are presented in Chapter 17.

Conceptual Approaches to Health Instruction

There have been two major conceptual approaches developed for health instruction. The first was developed in the early 1960s by the Health Education Curriculum Commission (HECC) of the American Association for Health, Physical Education, and Recreation. The second was through the effort of a group of educators initially supported by the Samuel Bronfman Foundation and subsequently supported by the 3M Company. The curriculum developed by this latter group of educators is known as the School Health Education Study (SHES).

Health Education Curriculum Commission (HECC)[3]

In 1959, the vice president of the health education division of the American Association for Health, Physical Education, and Recreation appointed a commission on curriculum development. This committee was given the responsibility of developing a plan to improve health education in the public schools. From the time of the initial appointment of the committee until its first formal meeting in 1962, committee members met informally at the various professional conferences that they attended.

Over the course of several years of discussion, the commission decided to explore a conceptual approach to health education. In order to do this, they felt that there were three major tasks to complete:

1. Identify crucial health problems of the 1960s and 1970s.
2. Consider these problems as they relate to health education instruction areas.
3. Identify health concepts related to the problem areas by well-known research and program specialists.

After completion of these three tasks, schools would be given any materials that might result.

Fourteen different crucial health problems were identified by the commission. These 14 included accident prevention, aging, alcohol, disaster preparedness, disease and disease control, economics of health care, environmental conditions, ionizing radiation, evaluation of health information, family health, international health, mental health, nutrition, and smoking. Each of these problem areas was sent to a research expert and a program expert in the problem field. These experts were asked to tell the commission the basic knowledge a health-educated individual should possess about the problem area. In other words, these experts were asked to develop some basic concepts about a particular program area. Once this task had been completed, the concepts had to be put into a usable format. In order to accomplish this, the

3. For a detailed discussion of the HECC, see American Association for Health, Physical Education, and Recreation (AAHPER) (1967).

commission developed a justification for the inclusion of each of the 14 problems with particular reference to the significance of the topical area to children and youth.

An example of the stated concepts from one area of the commission's work is presented here. These concepts pertain to the problem area of alcohol (AAHPER, 1967, pp. 10–12):

Beverage alcohol (ethyl alcohol) is the product of the fermentation of grains and fruits.

Alcohol is a depressant, or anesthetic, not a stimulant.

The mature individual will make his [or her] own decisions regarding drinking.

The intoxicating effects of alcohol are in direct relationship to the concentration of the alcohol in the blood.

In societies where social drinking is acceptable, the use of alcohol should be in relation to the responsibilities of the user.

Intoxication and alcoholism are not synonymous.

Alcoholism and intoxication must be considered community problems, the solution of which requires an informed and conscientious citizenry.

Alcoholism is now recognized as an illness that can be successfully treated.

State laws regarding the use of alcohol (when driving, by minors, etc.) have their foundations in the experiences of society and are worthy of being respected.

Following the development of each of the concepts, a content outline was prepared. By way of example, for the concept ''Alcoholism is now recognized as an illness that can be successfully treated,'' a content outline for that concept included:

- About one in 13 drinkers becomes an alcoholic.
- The recovered alcoholic has no tolerance for alcohol; he [or she] can live successfully as long as he [or she] does not try to drink.

It is obvious that this content is rather sparse at best, but it was an attempt to provide teachers with some guidance for the development of a health education curriculum.

The total document, containing all 14 topic areas, justifications, and 96 supporting concepts and content outlines, was published in 1967. It did provide a good reference work for curriculum planners, administrators, and teachers. However, no attempt was made by the commission to prioritize the concepts or to develop any type of sequential arrangement of them. Further, they did not attempt to define any goals or behavioral objectives, nor did they suggest any learning activities, resource materials, or evaluation methods. Their focus was on the content of health instruction, and everything else was left to individual teachers.

It is suggested that, because of all the omissions in the HECC document, its use was not as widespread as had been hoped or anticipated. This may also have been because of the emergence of a more sophisticated approach, the School Health Education Study.

The School Health Education Study (SHES)

In 1960 the Samuel Bronfman Foundation asked Dr. Granville Larimore, then First Deputy Commissioner of the New York State Department of Health and a member of the NEA–AMA Joint Committee on Health Problems in Education, to suggest to the Bronfman board several projects in health or education that should receive funding consideration. Dr. Larimore suggested the following: (1) graduate medical education, (2) a study of the effectiveness of the mass media, and (3) school health education. After hearing presentations on these three programs, the foundation decided to provide $200,000 to study the status of health education in the nation's schools.

A total of 135 school systems were involved in the School Health Education Study. Covering 38 states and involving some 1101 individual elementary schools and 359 secondary schools, this survey remains the broadest of its type ever completed in the United States. Test instruments were administered to students in grades 6, 9, and 12. Of 17,634 usable answer sheets returned to the researchers, a weighted sample of 2000 scores for each of the three grade levels representative of the makeup of the school sample was selected for analysis. Additionally, administrators in each of the sample districts were sent a questionnaire that dealt with administrative practices and instructional patterns.

Analysis of the responses to the inventories showed that the state of health education in this country was "appalling." It was concluded that cooperative action between schools and various community resources to bring about improvement in health instruction was definitely needed.

The major problems that emerged as a result of this survey (Sliepcevich, 1964, pp. 11, 12) were:

1. Failure of the home to encourage practice of health habits learned in school.
2. Ineffectiveness of instruction methods.
3. Parental and community resistance to certain health topics.
4. Lack of coordination of the health education program throughout the school grades.
5. Insufficient time in the school day for health instruction.
6. Inadequate professional preparation of staff.
7. Disinterest on the part of some teachers assigned to health teaching.
8. Failure of parents to follow up on needed and recommended health services for children.
9. Indifference toward and hence lack of support for health education on the part of some teachers, parents, administrators, health officers, and other members of the community.

10. Neglect of the health education course when combined with physical education.
11. Inadequate facilities and instructional materials.
12. Student indifference to health education.
13. Lack of specialized supervisory and consultative services.

From these findings, it was obvious a great deal of work and innovation in curriculum design for health instruction was needed.

As a result of the findings of the nationwide school health survey, the advisory committee for the survey approved a proposal that focused directly upon the development of experimental curriculum materials for the schools. It was proposed that a team of experts be convened and be given the specific charge to develop experimental materials. Experimental school districts that had professionally prepared teachers and administrators who were supportive of the idea of health instruction and who would be competent to conduct the experimentation of classroom curriculum materials were to be selected.

The writing team that was selected included the following persons (positions indicated are those held by the person at the time they were appointed):

- Elena M. Sliepcevich, director of the study
- William H. Creswell, Jr., professor of health education, University of Illinois
- Gus T. Dalis, consultant in health education, office of the Los Angeles County Superintendent of Schools
- Edward B. Johns, professor of school health education, University of California, Los Angeles
- Marion B. Pollock, assistant professor of health education, California State College, Long Beach
- Richard K. Means, professor of health education, Auburn University
- Ann E. Nolte, associate director of the study
- Robert D. Russell, associate professor of health education, Southern Illinois University

A great deal of care went into the selection of the writing team. It is obvious that those who were selected were accomplished in writing skills and were creative health educators who possessed a wide range of experience in the theory and practice of health education. All of them had actual teaching experience, and were experienced in supervision and in teacher preparation and education.

This team was immediately confronted with several problems—such as identifying health instruction content areas that should be high priority; developing some sort of curricular framework that included a rationally based scope and sequence for the health topics; and preparing experimental classroom materials, following the framework, that could be used in the tryout school districts.

Organization of School Health Programs

Since several of the members of the writing team had also been involved with the AAHPER Health Education Curriculum Commission, they realized that the approach used by the commission had met with less than optimal success. They felt that a more universal framework, one that could be accepted and used in a wide variety of school districts, had to be developed. They were not trying to develop a national curriculum, but rather were trying to develop a conceptual organization or structure that would allow local school districts a great deal of flexibility yet also provide a stability not present in the HECC work.

The writing team decided that since health was the central topic toward which all the material would be directed, it was critical that a definition of health be central to the entire effort. It was also decided that eight major sources of data should form the foundation for this new curriculum. These eight sources of data included:

1. Growth and development characteristics of learners.
2. The needs and interests of students as suggested by published research.
3. The role of education in a changing society.
4. Current studies in other areas of the curriculum and new trends in curriculum development.
5. The needs of communities as evidenced by investigations and expository writings.
6. The increase and acceleration of knowledge.
7. The theories about learning and behavioral change.
8. The extent and frequency of current health problems among school-age children as revealed in morbidity and mortality data. [SHES, 1967, p. 14]

Responsibility for making recommendations for the tryout centers rested with William H. Creswell, Jr., a member of the advisory committee as well as part of the writing team. At that time, Dr. Creswell was also the secretary for the NEA–AMA Joint Committee on Health Problems in Education. He visited numerous public school systems to determine if they met the criteria for inclusion as a tryout center and if they wanted to participate as a tryout center. Four school districts that met the criteria wanted to participate. These districts were Alhambra, California public schools; Evanston, Illinois public schools; Garden City and Great Neck, Long Island, New York public schools; and Tacoma, Washington public schools.

The writing team first met in January 1964 to become familiar with the task of identifying the health concepts an educated person should know and understand by the time that person completed a high school education. Since this was the same basic charge given the Health Education Curriculum Commission, members of the SHES writing team felt that the concepts being developed by the HECC might be appropriate for their own use. Although the HECC agreed that their work could be used, it soon became obvious that the concepts they were developing would not be ready in time to meet the time line set by the SHES writing team. Because of this, the SHES personnel had to develop a new point of view and develop some broad concepts of school health education.

Robert Russell proposed an initial point of view that health was a unified concept of well-being that had physical, mental, and social dimensions. It is the interaction of these three dimensions that constitutes the well-being of the individual, thereby empowering the person to lead a more personally satisfying and socially useful life. These dimensions of health are described thus:

> Health is a quality of life involving dynamic interaction and interdependence among the individual's physical well-being, his [or her] mental and emotional reactions, and the social complex in which he [or she] exists. Any one dimension may play a greater or lesser role than the other two, at a given time, but the interdependence and interaction of the three dimensions still hold true. As an example, an individual's way of life may require a greater emphasis upon one particular dimension of health . . . different individuals may be deemed ''healthy'' without necessarily exhibiting identical proportions of the three dimensions of well-being. At certain times and under particular circumstances, one dimension may be more in need of attention than another in order to maintain and promote a state of optimal health. . . . [SHES, 1967, pp. 10–11]

The writing team met on the campus of UCLA in the summer of 1964 along with representatives from each of the tryout centers. After a five-week period, a conceptual framework for the development of an experimental health instruction program emerged. What evolved was a refinement of the initial point of view developed by Dr. Russell, a description of three key concepts (growth and development, interaction, and decision making) that became the unifying elements of the curriculum; ten major concepts that represented the eight foundational elements; numerous concepts developed from the standpoint of the physical, mental, and social dimensions; and a draft of a teaching–learning guide for two of the ten major concepts.

The three key concepts were felt to be representative of a life-cycle process common to all humankind; thus, they would be fundamental to the overall concept of health. The ten major concepts, which represented the scope of health instruction, were:

> Growth and development influences and is influenced by the structure and functioning of the individual.

> Growing and developing follows a predictable sequence, yet is unique for each individual.

> Protection and promotion of health is an individual, community, and international responsibility.

> The potential for hazards and accidents exists, whatever the environment.

There are reciprocal relationships involving man [humanity], disease, and environment.

The family serves to perpetuate man [humanity] and to fulfill certain health needs.

Personal health practices are affected by a complexity of forces, often conflicting.

Utilization of health information, products, and services is guided by values and perceptions.

Use of substances that modify mood and behavior arises from a variety of motivations.

Food selection and eating patterns are determined by physical, social, mental, economic, and cultural factors. [SHES, 1967, p. 20]

Subconcepts were developed in the physical, mental, and social dimensions for each of the ten concepts. These subconcepts were designed to provide a clue to behavioral outcomes. They represent some 31 different health topics. From the subconcepts, long-range goals that depicted overall learnings as a result of participating in the total curriculum, and behavioral objectives written at four progression levels (grades K–3, 4–6, 7–9, and 10–12) representative of a hierarchy of learning (vertical and horizontal organization) were developed. The specific behavioral objectives were written for each concept in the cognitive (knowledge), affective (attitudinal), and practice (behavioral) domains. These objectives reflect specific outcomes for each concept within each of the various grade level progressions. This model is represented in Figure 15.3.

It is important to point out several major differences between the approach taken by the Health Education Curriculum Commission and the SHES writing team. Both groups of writers began with the same basic idea, to identify critical or useful content areas around which health instruction methods and materials might be developed. However, to a large extent, this is where the similarities end. Whereas the HECC identified areas for the curriculum and then identified research and content specialists to develop the concepts about the problems they had identified, the SHES group began with a central concept, that of health, and let everything grow from that central concept. The SHES group also developed experimental materials in the form of teaching–learning guides. The SHES writing team also developed behavioral objectives based upon a concept of four progression levels and the idea that each level of progression should contain greater levels of abstraction for the students to "meld" into a knowledge base.

Competency-Based Instruction

A new trend in health instruction as a result of the "back-to-basics" movement is for states to define various curricular areas in terms of minimum skills necessary to function in today's fast-paced society. Those who attempt to

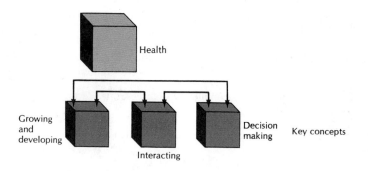

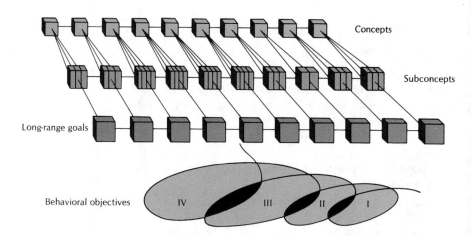

FIGURE 15.3

The school health
education study
curriculum design.
*Source: School Health
Education Study (SHES),*
Health Education: A
Conceptual Approach to
Curriculum Design *(St.
Paul: 3M Education Press,
1967), p. 27.*

identify these minimum competencies must have an eye to the future and what
skills will be needed to function in a future society. This idea was stressed by
the NEA–AMA Joint Committee on Health Problems in Education (Joint
Committee, 1972, p. 3). This committee stated that we should focus our concerns rather than merely continue to react to "crisis" situations.

Another factor that has led several states to define minimum competencies
for curricular areas is that of accountability, which means that the schools
should document the fact that students are learning skills that will enable them
to function in society.

Competency-based health instruction necessitates three factors. These
three factors are:

1. Program goal—stated in terms of student long-range outcomes.
2. Competency—possession of select skills and knowledges to the
   degree that they can be demonstrated.
3. Performance indicator(s)—a specific description of a specific skill
   or behavior in a prescribed setting.

One of the more recent attempts to define minimum competencies or skills
for elementary school children has taken place in the state of Arizona. The
Arizona State Legislature enacted legislation that mandated the development

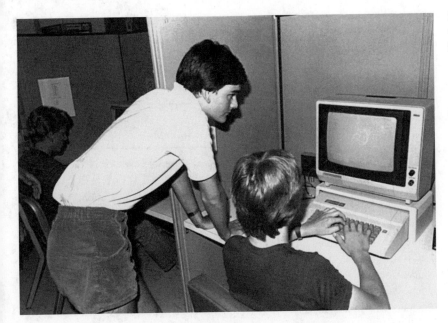

Use of computers is one way to individualize instruction.

of competency or skill charts for all curricular areas in public schools. Since health instruction is mandated in the common schools (elementary school grades 1–8), minimum competencies in health instruction had to be developed.

The initial minimal skill statements were drafted in the summer of 1983. In February, 1989 a second group of educators, laypersons, physicians, parents, nurses, and representatives of community agencies began work on revising these minimum skills. The statements that were developed were termed "essential skills." For each "essential skill," key indicators and suggested evaluation for that indicator were produced. The committee stated that the ultimate goal of the comprehensive school health promotion program was to help young people achieve their fullest potential in and out of school by attaining their highest level of health and wellness as students and as adults. Students should learn to accept responsibility for personal health decisions and practices, work with others to maintain a healthy environment, and become informed consumers of health information, health services, and health products.

The committee further defined "comprehensive health essential skills" as a process that instructs, motivates, and assists students and school personnel to adopt and maintain healthy practices and life-styles, and advocates community and environmental programs to facilitate this goal. The essential skills were developed for four progression levels, K–3, 4–6, 7–8, and 9–12. Selected examples of these minimum skills and key indicators for each of the progression levels are presented in Table 15.2.

Although the competencies may not be as all-inclusive as might be hoped, they do represent a concerted effort on the part of educators and laypersons to develop a scope and sequence of health instruction that provide a great deal

TABLE 15.2

State of Arizona
Health Education
Course of Study/Skill Requirement

Grades K–3

Essential Skill	*Key Indicator*
Students will understand stress and the importance of managing it.	Recognize that everyone experiences stress.
Students will understand the causes, controls, and effect of indoor and outdoor pollution on human health.	Define the word "pollution."
Students will understand types of injuries.	Describe the difference between intentional and unintentional injury.
Students will understand the uses of drugs and medicine.	State the difference between prescription and nonprescription medication.
Students will understand safe food handling.	State the importance of safe food storage and cleanliness in handling food.
Students will understand that they grow differently to become unique individuals.	Demonstrate awareness that sequential growth and development are unique to each child.
Students will understand responsibilities to self and others, associated with sexuality.	Recognize that there are body areas which deserve privacy.
Students will understand the difference between advertisements and educational messages.	Recognize that the major purpose of advertising is to sell a product.
Students will understand the basic causes of illness and disease.	List causes of illness and disease, e.g. heredity, environment, life-style, and germs.
Students will understand techniques in dental hygiene and care.	Demonstrate proper brushing and flossing.
Students will understand their own roles, contributions, and responsibilities as family members and how those may change.	Describe how individual family member attitudes affect family life.
Students will develop and maintain an adequate level of physical fitness.	Participate in activities to improve (i) cardiovascular endurance, (ii) flexibility.

TABLE 15.2 Continued

Grades 4–6
Essential Skill   *Key Indicator*

Students will understand the importance of positive self-concept to health and well-being.	Identify personal strengths.
Students will understand the relationships between community health problems and environmental pollution.	Describe pollution problems specific to the community.
Students will understand types of injuries and their causes.	Analyze the leading types and causes of injury by age group.
Students will know the basic nutrients and their functions.	List the three nutrients in food that provide the human body with energy (CHO, protein, fat).
Students will know the major factors which influence growth and development.	Demonstrate knowledge that genetic makeup influences individual characteristics.
Students will understand the human reproductive process.	Recognize how conception takes place.
Students will understand the roles of advertising and other influences on the selection of health products and services.	Identify the effects of advertising and peer pressure on health product choices.
Students will understand the differences between communicable and noncommunicable diseases.	List diseases that are not contagious, e.g., heart disease and asthma.
Students will understand factors important to healthy vision and hearing.	Identify the parts of the ear and eye.
Students will understand changing family roles throughout the life cycle.	Recognize that their levels of dependence upon the family change as they mature.
Students will develop and maintain an adequate level of physical fitness.	Participate in activities to improve (i) cardiovascular endurance, (ii) flexibility, (iii) muscular strength and endurance, and (iv) body composition.

TABLE 15.2 Continued

Grades 7–8
Essential Skill   *Key Indicator*

Essential Skill	Key Indicator
Students will understand the importance of being aware of feelings of self and others.	Use self-assessment and goal setting as a means to improve feelings about self.
Students will recognize the causes and prevention of emotional, physical, and sexual abuse.	Define emotional, physical, and sexual abuse.
Students will understand basic eating disorders.	Examine the harmful effects of eating disorders.
Students will understand that life begins and progresses through various stages from conception to death.	Describe the physical changes that take place in the body during puberty and the need to promote respect for self and others.
Students will understand factors involved in developing positive relationships.	Describe the importance of self-discipline in making decisions regarding self and others.
Students will understand that there are reliable and unreliable sources of health information and health-related products.	Demonstrate knowledge of where to go for reliable information regarding health services and products.
Students will understand common community health problems that agencies need to address.	List community health agencies and their responsibilities.
Students will understand the characteristics and classifications of various diseases.	Define and provide examples of acute, chronic, communicable, noncommunicable, degenerative, metabolic, hereditary, and congenital diseases.
Students will understand basic dental safety and first aid.	Identify activities requiring teeth protectors.
Students will understand the different types of family units and the major factors that affect them.	Describe ways in which social factors impact family units, e.g., marital status and local, state, and federal government.
Students will apply learned skills and strategies in a variety of sport activities.	Participate in team sports, e.g., basketball, field/floor hockey, flag/touch football, soccer, softball, team handball, and volleyball.

TABLE 15.2 Continued

Grades 9–12 *Essential Skill*	*Key Indicator*
Students will analyze and understand the importance of effective life management skills to psychological and physical health and well-being.	Identify and describe life management skills which contribute to psychological and physical well-being.
Students will understand major environmental health concerns and the functions of local, state, federal, and international resources which address these concerns.	Summarize major environmental health concerns.
Students will understand advanced first aid procedures.	Explain symptoms of, and basic first aid procedures for, unconsciousness, shock, and fractures.
Students will know the issues and impact of drug abuse in our society.	Analyze the economic impact of substance abuse on national health care costs.
Students will understand that nutrient needs vary according to age, development, activity level, and body type.	Evaluate and compare RDAs for different age groups, gender, activity levels, and growth.
Students will know the major factors which influence growth and development.	Analyze the influence of genetics on individual characteristics.
Students will understand factors involved in developing positive relationships.	Discuss double standards and conclude that boys and girls have equal responsibility in regard to sexuality.
Students will understand distinctions among health professions.	Demonstrate knowledge of licensing and certification standards for health professions.
Students will know how local, state, federal, and international organizations provide community health services.	Evaluate local, state, federal, and international efforts to contain community health problems, e.g., smallpox, infant mortality, and HIV.

TABLE 15.2 Continued

Grades 9–12

Essential Skill	Key Indicator
Students will understand risk reduction and disease prevention methods.	Review community resources that assist in reducing risk behavior and disease.
Students will understand self-care concepts and practices.	Identify the components of personal health and wellness.
Students will understand that personal development is necessary to successfully assume multiple adult roles and responsibilities.	Analyze qualities and skills which may lend themselves to specific life choices.
Students will demonstrate proficiency in a variety of rhythmic activities.	Perform fundamental movements of aerobic dance and participate in a variety of routines.

Source: Arizona Department of Education. *Arizona Comprehensive Health; Essential Skills.* Phoenix: The Department of Education, August, 1990.

of latitude for local school districts to develop their own course of study. This also ensures both vertical and horizontal organization.

In 1976, Pigg published a study (pp. 15–16) he had done among more than 175 colleges that offered degree programs in health education. This study was designed to determine the perception of health educators relative to competency-based health instruction. Among his findings were the following:

1. There was no consensus among health educators about what constitutes competency-based instruction.
2. In those states where mandatory competency-based education had been mandated, the teacher training institutes had more elaborate competency-based training programs than in states where this had not been mandated.
3. Health educators make little use of competency-based education materials available from the American Association of Colleges for Teacher Education.
4. The value of competency-based education is viewed many different ways by professional health educators.

Thus, if competency-based health instruction is to be used, several questions must be considered (Rash and Pigg, 1979, p. 35):

1. Is competency-based education of value in this setting?
2. Who will specify what the minimum competencies should be and how will they go about determining these competencies?
3. What competencies should be demonstrated by those given the responsibility to define minimum competencies in health instruction?

4. If minimum competencies are specified, does this detract from individualized instruction and the individuality of students exposed to it?

5. What competencies should be required of teachers who teach competency-based health instruction?

6. How does competency-based health instruction interface with other curricular areas?

7. What are the implications of competency-based instruction for in-service education of teaching and nonteaching staff?

8. How and by whom will students be evaluated to determine if they possess the minimum competencies specified?

If school district curriculum planning committees consider all eight of these questions, any competency-based instruction programs they develop are likely to be more effective.

SUMMARY

In this chapter, seven patterns of curriculum organization and four types of organizational patterns for the health instruction course have been offered. It should be rather obvious from the discussion of each type that there is no "right way." Each approach has positive and negative features. In reality, one would probably not find any of these approaches in a "pure" form anywhere in this country. Rather, one would probably notice that a combination of the approaches would not only be utilized, but also would be best suited for most local situations. The key element here is that the local district must analyze its current curriculum pattern and determine how health instruction can best interface with that total curricular picture.

Since several basic elements are included in all of the approaches presented in this chapter, suggestions for these elements are offered in Chapter 16.

REVIEW QUESTIONS

1. What do you think Jesse Ferring Williams meant when he stated that health was the ability to do most and serve best? Do you feel Dr. Williams was realistic in his orientation?

2. What are seven major patterns used to organize the school curriculum? Briefly discuss the major components of each of these patterns.

3. If you were to organize a course of health instruction for a school, what curricular pattern would you select? Discuss the advantages and disadvantages as well as administrative considerations for the pattern you have selected.

4. How would you define comprehensive health instruction? What makes your definition superior to other definitions that have been suggested?

5. Distinguish between vertical and horizontal organization of the curriculum. Why is it important for an educator to understand these two concepts?

6. Some people have said that the textbook that has been ordered for a school formulates the curriculum. How do you feel about this concept? What are the implications of this idea for a course of health instruction?

7. The authors discuss four types of approaches to the development of the health instruction course: textbook, cycle, conceptual, and competency-based. If you were to have the responsibility to select one approach for use in your school, what approach would you select? Why would you select that particular approach?

8. Distinguish between a concept, a long-range goal, and a behavioral objective.

9. The School Health Education Study writing team consisted of eight experts in the field of health instruction and curriculum development. Where is each of these eight individuals currently working? What additional contributions to the field of health instruction has each of these persons made?

10. Why do you think that the School Health Education Study writing team defined health as a quality of life?

11. Why do the authors state that it is probably unrealistic to think that any of the approaches to curriculum development will be found in a pure form in any school today?

REFERENCES

American Association for Health, Physical Education, and Recreation. *Health Concepts: Guides for Health Instruction.* Washington, D.C.: AAHPER, 1967.

Arizona Department of Education. *Arizona Comprehensive Health; Essential Skills.* Phoenix: The Department, August 1990.

Bloom, B. (ed). *Taxonomy of Educational Objectives, Handbook I, Cognitive Domain.* New York: David McKay, 1956.

Boyer, E. *High School: A Report on Secondary Education in America.* New York: The Carnegie Foundation for the Advancement of Teaching, 1983.

Committee to Establish Guidelines for Comprehensive School Health Education. "Comprehensive School Health Education as Defined by the National Professional School Health Education Organizations." *Health Education* 15:6 (Oct/Nov, 1984).

Fodor, J. T., and G. T. Dalis. *Health Instruction: Theory and Application,* 4th ed. Philadelphia: Lea and Febiger, 1989.

Joint Committee on Health Problems in Education of the NEA and AMA. "School Health—1985." *School Health Review* 3:3 (May–June, 1972).

Kime, R. E., R. G. Schlaadt, and L. E. Tritsch. *Health Instruction, An Action Approach.* Englewood Cliffs, N.J.: Prentice-Hall, 1977.

Krathwohl, D. et al. *Taxonomy of Educational Objectives, Handbook II, Affective Domain.* New York: David McKay, 1964.

Lohrmann, D., and D. DeJoy. "Utilizing the Competency-Based Curriculum Framework for Curriculum Revision: A Case Study." *Health Education* 18(6):36 (Dec 1987/Jan 1988).

Mayshark, C., and D. Shaw, *Administration of School Health Programs.* St. Louis: C. V. Mosby, 1967.

Menhke, P., P. Garton, and R. Barnes. "Experience with Competency-Based Curriculum Design: A School and Community Health Model." *Health Education* 14(3):14 (Mar/Apr, 1984).

Neil, A. S. *Summerhill: A Radical Approach to Child Rearing.* New York: Wallaby, 1977.

Oberteuffer, D. "Health and Education—An Appraisal II." *The Journal of School Health* 38:2 (1968).

Pigg, R. M. "A National Study of Competency-Based Health Education." *Health Education* 7:4 (July–August 1976).

Pollock, M. *Planning and Implementing Health Education in Schools,* Mountain View, Cal.: Mayfield Publishing Company, 1987.

Rash, J. K., and R. M. Pigg. *The Health Education Curriculum.* New York: John Wiley & Sons, 1979.

"Report of the 1990 Joint Committee on Health Education Terminology." *Journal of Health Education* 22(2):97–108 (March/April, 1991).

School Health Education Study (SHES). *Health Education: A Conceptual Approach to Curriculum Design.* St. Paul: 3M Educational Press, 1967.

Schumacher, M. *The National Association of State Boards of Education HIV/AIDS Education Survey: Profiles of State Policy Actions.* Alexandria, Virginia: National Association of State Boards of Education, 1989.

Sliepcevich, E. M. *School Health Education Study, A Summary Report.* Washington, D.C.: The School Health Education Study, 1964.

———, and C. B. Carroll. "Correlation of Health with Other Areas of the High School Curriculum." *The Journal of School Health* 28:9 (September 1958).

16

Considerations When Developing a Curriculum

The primary purpose of health instruction is to provide learning opportunities that help students develop habits, skills, and attitudes that will contribute to their optimal well-being. The degree to which this purpose is reached is directly proportional to the amount of support given the program by administrators, teachers, parents, students, and the community. In this chapter, basic issues that must be addressed when developing a health instruction curriculum are presented. Before discussing these issues, it is important that the individual have a basic knowledge of the need for health instruction and the current status of the field.

THE NEED FOR HEALTH INSTRUCTION

We are a product of our life-styles, and our life-styles tend to be ones of excess. If one examines the major causes of death in this country, it becomes abundantly clear that chronic, not acute, conditions are almost omnipresent.

As medical science controls acute health problems, the individual survives longer, often only to be devastated by chronic health problems. Unfortunately, not a great deal is known about the multiplicity of factors that interact to result in the development of one or more chronic conditions. There is no vaccine at present that will prevent cancer, but we do know that over 80 percent of certain types of lung cancer could be prevented if people would not smoke cigarettes. This is not a medical problem; it is one of education and life-style.

The need for some type of health care far precedes the colonization of America. It is certainly beyond the scope of the present text to relate all the history of health instruction, for Dr. Richard Means (1975) has done that quite well. However, it is important to understand the basic foundation upon which current health instruction is built.

A HISTORICAL LOOK AT HEALTH INSTRUCTION[1]

Although one could develop a lengthy treatise about health in ancient civilizations, suffice it to say that there are records of health-related activities dating from the Code of Hammurabi, developed in 2000 B.C. Records of Hebrew,

1. Adapted from R. L. Means, *Historical Perspectives on School Health* (Thorofare, N.J.: Slack, 1975), pp. 1–17.

Egyptian, Greek, and Roman civilizations all testify to the fact that health and fitness were important to those people. The concept of a sound mind and a sound body seemed to pervade these societies.

When the fall of the Roman Empire plunged the world into the Dark Ages, religion was a major contributor to a seeming decline in hygienic practice. In religious doctrine of the times, it was considered "sinful" to observe one's own body; obviously, numerous health problems arose. However, during the massive disease outbreaks of this period, some types of health practices must have occurred; otherwise, it is quite likely that the totality of civilization would have perished.

Although problems abounded during the Dark Ages, when feudalism arose, the concept of a sound mind and a sound body became more than an ideal, it became a practicality in terms of readiness for combat. Peasants stayed fit so they could protect their feudal lords, thus preserving their livelihood.

Just as religion helped bring on the Dark Ages, it was also instrumental in bringing about the Renaissance. Since religious leaders wanted people to follow their teaching, it was important that people be able to read and understand what was being said. Thus, the same leaders who had stated that to view one's body was sinful began to urge people to learn to read and to keep themselves clean.

Many of the leaders of the Renaissance produced books and other documents that dealt with health topics. Some of these leaders included Sir Thomas Elyot, Martin Luther, Richard Mulcaster, François Rabelais, John Milton, and John Locke. These persons might be considered true proponents of health instruction. Perhaps the most far-reaching document of the time relative to health education was written by John Locke. He wrote extensively on the value of good nutrition, adequate sleep, proper clothing, and vigorous exercise. In fact, much of what he said is totally applicable in today's society.

When the colonists arrived in America from England, they brought ideas relative to health and education. Although they endured great losses and became quite isolated from each other, these pioneers were convinced that education was an inherent good and that all children should have reading and writing skills. Massachusetts was the first of the colonies to pass a mandatory education law.

Because of the rigors of pioneer life, these people became physically strong; however, many of their health practices were based upon misconceptions. These misconceptions were particularly prevalent when persons afflicted with such health problems as mental illness and epilepsy were often prosecuted for being witches, or they would consume potions thought to have the power to drive out evil spirits in the mistaken idea that this would cause the individual to be "cleansed." It has been said that in pioneer days, a person who became ill only had a 50 percent chance of getting a correct diagnosis of his or her illness and then only a 50 percent chance that the prescribed treatment would be effective. The problems were compounded by the fact that teachers were more concerned about ensuring literacy than about prevalent health practices.

Numerous essays about health were written in the mid-1800s. In 1832, Horace Mann advocated the training of teachers in health topics so that they could pass this information on to their students. He felt that by this practice students would stay healthier; thus, they would be able to learn more.

Closely following Mann's work was the publication of a document entitled *A Report of the Sanitary Commission of the State of Massachusetts*. This document has often been referred to as the initiation of the field of public health in America. Written by a self-educated man named Lemuel Shattuck, the report called for such things as sanitation programs; studies on the health of school-age children, on the control of communicable disease, and on the effects of alcohol; the preaching of health in church; and numerous other reforms, many of which are applicable today. As stated by Shattuck (1850, pp. 178–179):

It has recently been recommended that the science of physiology be taught in the public schools; and the recommendation should be universally approved and carried into effect as soon as persons can be found capable of teaching it. . . .

Every child should be taught early in life that to preserve his [or her] own health and the lives and health of others, is one of the most important and constantly abiding duties. . . . By knowing and avoiding the causes of disease, disease itself will be avoided, and he [or she] may enjoy health and live; by ignorance of these causes and exposure to them, he [or she] may contract disease, ruin his [or her] health and die. Everything connected with wealth, happiness and long life depends upon health; and even the great duties of morals and religion are performed more acceptably in a healthy than a sickly condition. . . .

The Shattuck report had many far-reaching consequences. It began a whole reform movement in the field of public health and resulted in a refocusing of efforts to safeguard the health of all people. In fact, the state of Massachusetts began requiring hygiene as a compulsory school subject in 1850 (Irwin and Mayshark, 1967, p. 20).

In 1842, the French legislature began requiring school districts to employ a physician whose duties included periodic inspection of buildings and grounds. This began a more concerted health effort in Europe; by the end of the nineteenth century, the majority of school districts there utilized the services of a physician as a regular school staff member.

In 1870, the American Public Health Association was founded. Although the Association took a strong position on school health instruction and services, the School Health Education Section (now called the School Health Education and Services Section) was not constituted until some 80 years later.

The first appearance of what might be considered health instruction in this country was in the form of states' requirements for the teaching of the harmful effects of drugs, alcohol, and narcotics. Carrie Nation and her group, the Women's Christian Temperance Union, founded in 1874, gave a great deal of visibility to the evils of "John Barleycorn" and other mood-altering substances. Studies examining today's school codes reported in 1982 that the education codes in 43 states required instruction on the effects of drugs and alcohol on health (Noak, 1982, p. 8). However, a more recent study conducted by Lovato, Allensworth, and Chan (1989) showed that although 43 states had a legal basis for health education that had been established through educational codes or other state legislation, only 29 states required drug and alcohol abuse prevention and only 20 states required tobacco-use prevention. One may wonder what occurred relative to the status of health education over the seven-year time span.

When Theodore Roosevelt became President of the United States, he brought to the office an increased sense of responsibility for the health of the nation's citizens, but particularly for the school-age child. In 1909, he convened the first White House Conference on Children and Youth. From this initial conference came the statement, ''Every needy child should . . . be instructed in health and hygiene.''[2] Also considered were health services and the environmental aspects of the school in order to promote optimal learning. Although the focus of the first White House Conference on Children and Youth was on the care of dependent children, the impetus for school health was clearly evident. In fact, it was from an initiative developed at this conference that the United States Children's Bureau was created. The Children's Bureau began to assume a major role in the conduct of subsequent White House Conferences. Although all the conferences have been important, the 1930 Conference on Child Health and Protection was truly significant in promoting the total school health program because detailed recommendations for school health services, teacher responsibilities for health, and maintaining a safe and sanitary school environment were made.

It was two years after the first White House Conference on Children and Youth that the American Medical Association and the National Education Association got together to form their Joint Committee on Health Problems in Education. This committee was formed so that the American Medical Association could learn more about education and the National Education Association could learn more about medicine as it affected the school-age child. By combining both areas of expertise, the cause of the school health program could be advanced. This committee is now disbanded, but it left a legacy that included classic texts in the areas of health instruction, school health services, and healthful school living.[3]

Simultaneously with the development of the Joint Committee, the Department of Superintendence of the National Education Association was working at reforming the total school curriculum. In 1918, they issued a report

2. Proceedings of the Conference on the Care of Dependent Children: U.S. Department of the Interior, Office of Education, Document No. 721. Washington, D.C.: Government Printing Office, 1909, p. 8.

3. For a more complete discussion of the contributions of the Joint Committee, see R. L. Means, *Historical Perspectives on School Health*, pp. 113–115.

entitled *Report on the Seven Cardinal Principles of Education for Secondary Schools*. This document provided a great deal of emphasis on achieving goals in education. It also gave a boost to health education, in that health was the first of the seven principles listed. The seven cardinal principles as offered by the Department of Superintendence (U.S. Department of the Interior, 1918, p. 3) are as follows:

1. Health.
2. Command of fundamental processes.
3. Vocational training.
4. Citizenship.
5. Worthy home membership.
6. Worthy use of leisure.
7. Ethical character.

In 1926, the Department of Superintendence issued its fourth yearbook, entitled *The Nation at Work on the Public School Curriculum*. Dr. Thomas Wood (1926, pp. 221–238) was given the task of authoring an entire chapter devoted to health and physical education in that publication. This reaffirmed the commitment of the department to the idea of health instruction as an integral part of the total school curriculum.

In 1937, the department adopted a new charter and became the American Association of Secondary School Administrators. At about the same time, the Educational Policies Commission of the National Education Association revised the seven cardinal principles of secondary education into a classic document entitled *The Purposes of Education in American Democracy* (1938). The new document regrouped the seven cardinal principles into four major groups of educational objectives, each with health as a fundamental dimension. These four groups were:

1. Self-realization.
2. Human relationships.
3. Economic efficiency.
4. Civic responsibility.

As an example of the importance of health, when the commission discussed the first objective—self-realization—they stated that the health-educated individual will possess three major attributes:

1. The educated person understands the basic facts concerning health and disease. Health conditions our success in everything; thus, schools should place great emphasis on health as an outcome of education. The schools would save more than their own total cost if they could see to it that the oncoming generation of adults used its resources for health more wisely.

2. The educated person protects his [or her] own health and that of his [or her] dependents. If the person knows basic facts about health and disease, he [or she] applies these facts to maintain health in both the physical and mental dimension. He [or she] seeks competent medical care for himself [or herself] and his [or her] family and is alert for early symptoms of disease but lives a life of preventive maintenance. The emphasis should be positive, dealing with the healthful functioning not the breakdown of the organism with disease, and should promote both mental as well as physical health.

3. The educated person works to improve the health of the community. The health-educated person has a global view of his [or her] role in society. The value of good health is clear for the individual and his [or her] family and the individual should work to extend this benefit to the community; if all neighbors are healthy, the entire community benefits. Healthy people should show an active concern for all conditions which threaten the safety or injure the health of others. This concern can be shown through promoting the health work of schools and other social agencies and encouraging study and action concerning the economic, physical, and social conditions which cause disease and imperil the health of the mind and body. [NEA, 1938, p. 63]

Individuals who are currently being given the responsibility of planning the curricula for schools would be well advised to secure a copy of the Educational Policies Commission document and read it quite carefully. The recommendations contained and the philosophy espoused in that 1938 document are as applicable today as when they were originally written.

Perhaps the landmark health-related publication prepared by the American Association of Secondary School Administrators was their 1942 publication entitled *Health in Schools*. This was the twentieth yearbook of the Association and contained an elaborate discussion on a wide range of school health topics. Such topics as philosophy, organization and administration of school health, a healthful school environment, professional preparation of personnel, coordination of health-related emergencies, legal components, mental hygiene, communicable disease, and first aid were included. This document was so popular that it was revised and reissued in 1951, using the same title.

In 1950, the Department of Elementary School Principals of the National Education Association published a book entitled *Health in the Elementary School*. This ten-chapter book, written by several authorities, dealt with the total scope of the school health program, including foundations, healthful school living, school health services (including handicapped services), health instruction, and the role of various personnel within the school health program.

Although different from the White House Conferences on Children and Youth, the 1955 White House Conference on Education, attended by representatives of both education and medicine, tried to determine what schools should accomplish. A total of 14 goals were developed, each of which included health as a desired outcome. These 14 goals present as realistic a picture today as they did when they were developed about 40 years ago. The 14 recommended outcomes include:

1. The fundamental skills of communication—reading, writing, spelling, as well as other elements of effective oral and written expression; the arithmetical and mathematical skills, including problem solving.
2. Appreciation for our democratic heritage.
3. Understanding of civic rights and responsibilities and knowledge of American institutions.
4. Respect and appreciation for human values and for the beliefs of others.
5. Ability to think and evaluate constructively and creatively.
6. Effective work habits and self-discipline.
7. Social competence as a contributing member of the family and community.
8. Ethical behavior based on a sense of moral and spiritual values.
9. Intellectual curiosity and eagerness for lifelong learning.
10. Esthetic appreciation and self-expression in the arts.
11. Physical and mental health.
12. Wise use of time, including constructive leisure pursuits.
13. Understanding of the physical world and man's relation to it as represented through basic knowledge of the sciences.
14. An awareness of our relationships with the world community. [Committee for the White House Conference on Education, 1956]

In 1959, the Educational Policies Commission stated:

> The elementary curriculum, among other things, teaches the essentials of safety and personal health and promotes physical coordination and skill. The programs of all secondary-school students should include English, social studies, science, mathematics, and fine arts, as well as physical and health education. [NEA, 1959, p. 8]

Although the previously cited documents, reports, and publications reflect the importance of the existence of a total school health program, it was not until 1963, with the publication of the National Education Association's Project on Instruction, *Schools for the Sixties*, that a firm statement specifically dealing with health instruction had been developed. This statement reads in part:

> . . . the content of health instruction belongs in the school curriculum because such knowledge is necessary, is most efficiently learned in school, and no other public agency provides such instruction. [NEA, 1959, p. 31]

It should be obvious by this time that preparing people to live personally satisfying and socially useful lives, free of illness, disease, and disability, is a central theme in American education. If this goal is to be accomplished, it is critical to include health instruction as a part of the basic education of all school-age children and youth. In the same manner that language arts teachers teach communication skills; that mathematics teachers teach computational abilities; that science teachers teach organizational principles and how individuals fit into the total ecological mosaic; that teachers of the humanities help students develop creativity and aesthetic expression; the skills of daily living to promote health and well-being should be taught in well-developed and planned health instruction programs. Health instruction helps students synthesize other parts of the curriculum and apply them to problems of everyday living (AMA, 1982, p. 1).

All of the foregoing gave rise to what has been called the single most significant enterprise in school health education since 1960, the School Health Education Study, which was completed in early 1972. A total of ten conceptual areas covering over 30 health topics were developed by the SHES writing team. These concepts were then placed into a framework that could be utilized by school districts to organize their own school health instruction program. (For a detailed description of the School Health Education Study (SHES), see Chapter 15). At present, at least 50 different organizations and agencies have specific policy statements that support school health instruction.

Several important evaluation efforts have occurred since the publication of the School Health Education Study. Most notable are the School Health Education Evaluation (*Journal of School Health,* October, 1985), and the National Adolescent Student Health Survey (American School Health Association, Association for the Advancement of Health Education, and the Society for Public Health Education, Inc., 1989). These studies are discussed in Chapter 18.

Most recently, the United Nations held a World Summit for Children and produced a World Declaration on the survival, protection, and development of children. The declaration was released September 30, 1990, just after the release of *Healthy People 2000,* listing the health promotion and disease prevention objectives for the nation (USDHHS, 1991).

The purpose of the World Summit for Children was to undertake a joint commitment and make an urgent universal appeal in the attempt to improve the future for children. For example, over 100 million children in the world are without schooling, and two-thirds of these children are girls. One-half million mothers die each year from causes related to childbirth. The challenge to all is clear. In fact, virtually all nations at the World Conference on Education for All, conducted in Jontien, Thailand in 1989, agreed to increase significantly educational opportunities for both children and illiterate adults. Health education should be a part of that education.

Within *Healthy People 2000,* the health goals for the nation are presented and discussed. Of the nearly 300 specific objectives that are presented within that document, nearly 200 of them could be impacted by quality health education within the schools. In fact, Goal 8.4 states:

> Increase to at least 75 percent the proportion of the Nation's elementary and secondary schools that provide planned and sequential kindergarten through 12th grade quality school health education. (p. 255)

HEALTH INSTRUCTION DEFINED

The definition of health instruction has evolved over the decades from 1918,[4] when the term *health education* was first proposed by Sally Lucas Jean (1951, p. 963), considered by many to be the "mother of health education." Prior to this time, the term *hygiene* was used to designate health teaching.

As an indication of the futuristic thinking of health educators of the time, Lucy Oppen proposed the idea that the goal of health education was action, not just the acquisition of factual knowledge. She also stated that both direct and indirect means should be used in teaching health, that it could be integrated across the total curriculum, but that it should be given its own time allotment (Means, 1975, p. 38).

It should be noted that the majority of attempts to define hygiene or health education were not definitions, but rather were indications of the goal of health education. However, in 1934, the Health Education Section of the American Physical Education Association stated that health education "is that organization of learning experiences directed toward the development of favorable health knowledges, attitudes and practices" (Means, 1975, pp. 15–16).

At this same time, the NEA–AMA Joint Committee on Health Problems in Education proposed that "health education is the sum of all experiences which favorably influence habits, attitudes and knowledges relating to individual, community and racial health" (Anderson and Creswell, 1980, p. 242). Some 14 years later, they revised their definition slightly to state that "health education is a process of providing learning experiences for the purpose of influencing knowledge, attitudes or conduct relating to individual, community and world health" (Anderson and Creswell, p. 242).

Following their definition of health set forth in their constitution in 1945 (health is a state of complete physical, mental, and social well-being, not merely the absence of disease or infirmity), the World Health Organization (1954, p. 4) focused on health education. Their 1954 definition has a broader scope than most, encompassing a global view:

> The aim of health education is to help people achieve health by their own actions and efforts. Health education begins, therefore, with the interests of people in improving their condition of living, . . . in developing a sense of responsibility for their own health betterment and for . . . the health of their families and environments.

4. The New York City Health Department established a division of health education about 1915, so there is some controversy over the specific origin of the term *health education.*

Embodied in this definition is the concept of individual responsibility for one's own health and well-being. This responsibility then extends to the family and ultimately to the community. By staying healthy, individuals will benefit others as well as themselves.

In 1961, the NEA–AMA Joint Committee (p. 7) redefined health education as "the process of providing learning experiences which favorably influence understandings, attitudes, and conduct in regard to individual and community health." This definition omits the concept of world health, perhaps because the committee felt that the individual does little on a global basis. At any rate, the definition emphasizes the process aspect of health instruction, while recognizing that health status may be influenced by all the experiences of the individual. The definition intimates that if health instruction is to be meaningful, it must be carefully planned and organized; it cannot rely on incidental instruction.

In 1966, the National Committee on School Health Policies of the NEA and AMA (1966, p. 1) stated:

> Health education programs are a vital force in closing the gap between scientific health discoveries and their application. Health education is an applied science concerned with man's [the individual's] understanding of himself [or herself] in relation to health matters in a changing society. It is not the hygiene of yesteryear. It is not physiology, anatomy, biology, physical education, or physical fitness. It is an academic field and subject. [1966, p. 1]

The Health Education Curriculum Commission (HECC) of the American Association for Health, Physical Education, and Recreation (AAHPER) (1967, p. 49) embraced this definition when they developed their pamphlet "Health Concepts: Guides for Health Instruction." This guide was designed to provide teachers and administrators with basic guidelines for the development of health education curricula using a conceptual approach (see Chapter 15).

The writing team for the School Health Education Study (1967, pp. 9–11) envisioned health education as a tri-dimensional concept. They saw health as a unity of physical, mental, and social well-being; health behavior as knowledge, attitudes, and practices; the focus of health education as individual, family, and community. "Health is a quality of life involving dynamic interaction and interdependence among the individual's physical well-being, his [or her] mental and emotional reactions, and the social complex in which he [or she] exists" (p. 11). Following this, they defined health education as:

> An important entity among the subject areas of the curriculum which, through organization of health knowledge, is primarily concerned with the well-being of individuals and groups. The goal of health education is not directed at a high level of health simply for health's sake, but rather to help each individual view health as a way of life that will help to attain individual goals and utilize one's highest potential for the betterment of self, family, and community. . . . Health

education is an applied field of learning that relies largely upon the knowledge of the physical, biological, and medical sciences and related fields for its subject matter and upon the application of behavioral science.

Beginning as early as 1951, AAHPER's Committee on Terminology in School Health Education (1951, p. 14) defined health education as "the process of providing learning experiences for the purpose of influencing knowledges, attitudes, and conduct relating to individual and group health." This statement was revised in 1974 (AAHPER, 1974, pp. 33–37) as follows:

> A process with intellectual, psychological, and social dimensions relating to activities which increase the abilities of people to make informed decisions affecting their personal, family, and community well-being. This process, based on the scientific principles, facilitates learning and behavioral change in both personnel and consumers including children and youth.

As with the prior definition, process is emphasized; however, the definition is sufficiently broad to recognize life-related experiences, in addition to planned learning activities, as impacting upon the health status of the individual.

In 1970, President Richard Nixon appointed a national committee to examine the status of school and community health education in the nation. After listening to thousands of hours of testimony at hearings across the nation, in 1973 the committee (AAHPER, 1974, p. 17) made the following statement:

> Health education is a process that bridges the gap between health information and health practices. Health education motivates the person to take information and do something with it—to keep himself [or herself] healthier by avoiding actions that are harmful and by forming habits that are beneficial.

In like fashion, the Office of Health Information, Health Promotion, and Physical Fitness and Sports Medicine (OHIP) of the United States Department of Health and Human Services (1980, p. 1) defined health education as "any combination of learning opportunities designed to facilitate voluntary adaptations of behavior (in individuals, groups, or communities) conducive to health."

More recently, another statement defining health education was released by the Joint Committee on Health Education Terminology. This committee was comprised of representatives from eight different health-related organizations: American Public Health Association (School Health Education and Services Section and the Public Health Education and Health Promotion Section); American Academy of Pediatrics; Society of State Directors of Health, Physical Education, and Recreation; Association for the Advancement of Health Education; American College Health Association (Health Education Section); Society for Public Health Education; Association of State and Territorial Directors of Public Health Education; and the American School Health

Association). This group reviewed all of the previous definitions of health education, updated the various terms that had been defined, and added relevant new definitions. The definitions developed by the Joint Committee are as follows:

> *Health Education Process:* that continuum of learning which enables people, as individuals and as members of social structures, to voluntarily make decisions, modify behaviors, and change social conditions in ways which are health enhancing.

> *Health Education Program:* a planned combination of activities developed with the involvement of specific populations and based on a needs assessment, sound principles of education, and periodic evaluation using a clear set of goals and objectives.

> *Comprehensive School Health Program:* an organized set of policies, procedures, and activities designed to protect and promote the health and well-being of students and staff which has traditionally included health services, healthful school environment, and health education. It should also include, but not be limited to, guidance and counseling, physical education, food service, social work, psychological services, and employee health promotion.

> *School Health Education:* one component of the comprehensive school health program which includes the development, delivery, and evaluation of a planned instructional program, and other activities for students preschool through grade 12, for parents and for school staff, and is designed to positively influence the health knowledge, attitudes, and skills of individuals. [Joint Committee, 1990, pp. 105–106]

Health Instruction in the Curriculum

In the previous section many definitions of health were discussed and, though worded differently, the goal of each is the same. Perhaps the most definitive statement from the standpoint of official sanction for school health instruction appeared in the 1979 *Surgeon General's Report on Health Promotion and Disease Prevention* (p. 143). In discussing opportunities for action, the Surgeon General says:

> More than 40 million children and youth spend most of their day in school. No group is more able than school teachers to provide information and instruction that can help young people make decisions that promote good health.

> Comprehensive school health education activities can: enhance a child's skills and personal decision making; promote understanding of the concepts of health and the causes of disease; and foster knowledge about the ways in which one's health is affected by personal decisions related to smoking, alcohol and drug use, diet, exercise, and sexual activity.

In 1981, the Education Commission of the States made specific recommendations to state education agencies regarding school health education. The commission recommended the following:

1. Encourage local school boards and administrators to include health education in the curriculum in elementary and secondary schools.
2. Promote health education as a responsibility shared by the family, school, and community.
3. Promote the development of comprehensive school health education programs.
4. Support the development and improvement of school health education programs using all means available to them in their official capacities.
5. Provide technical assistance to local school districts who are planning and implementing school health education programs.
6. Encourage the undertaking of participatory planning for school health programs.
7. Ensure the presence of trained and qualified teachers in school health education programs.
8. Assist in developing an information exchange system about health education.
9. Encourage and assist local districts to evaluate their school health programs.
10. Encourage federal agencies to channel categorical funds to enhance comprehensive school health education program development. [Education Commission of the States, 1981, pp. 5–14]

Despite the fact that nearly all state legislatures and boards of education have developed positions or policy statements about school health, it is estimated that only several hundred programs of formal health instruction may be operating in the more than 15,000 school districts in the United States.

CURRICULUM DEFINED

In a traditional sense, the term *curriculum* has been used to connote the totality of courses of study offered in any given school. More recently it has also been taken to mean the totality of courses in a given subject matter. Thus curriculum is a plan that includes the content to be taught to individuals expected to learn. One must remember, however, that the student will learn from unplanned learning experiences too; thus, this broad concept of curriculum must encompass all learning experiences, both planned and unplanned.

The use of television monitors for showing close-ups of demonstrations in classrooms has the advantage of getting each student close to the demonstration.

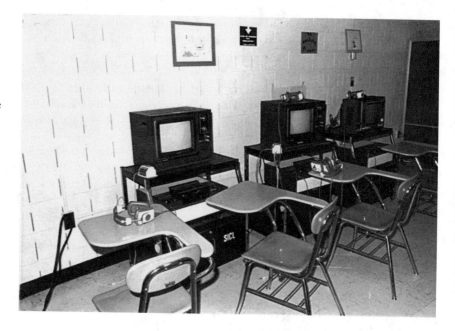

In 1942, Mortimer Adler posed an interesting question. He stated that there were two basic categories into which all human efforts could be placed: the operative and the cooperative. Operative efforts are those activities wherein the individual acts upon nature to attain an effect nature alone cannot attain. Examples are producing lumber and eventually a house, or extracting iron ore from the earth and fashioning it into an automobile. Cooperative efforts, on the other hand, are those efforts in which individuals cooperate with nature, thereby facilitating what should occur. Medicine would be an example. A physician does not ''create'' health; the physician generally assists the organism regain its natural balance with nature. This same idea could be put forth for a gardener. The gardener assists nature, but it is not the gardener who causes the seeds to germinate and develop into a plant. Thus Adler's (1942, p. 211) question: ''If, in one instance nature is waiting for human intelligence to act upon it and in the other, nature is already operational but striving to go further, what is education—operative, or cooperative?''

Obviously, this question could be and is debated whenever educators gather. The question is not whether one or the other is correct, but rather, have both viewpoints been considered? If one reexamines the definitions of health education elaborated earlier in this chapter, one must ask, ''Does our plan or curriculum in health education facilitate learning from both an operative and cooperative viewpoint?''

Reexamining the diagram of the total school health program from Chapter 1, it becomes clear that the curriculum, or plan or schedule of classes, flows out of philosophy. Willgoose (1982, p. 62) has stated, ''Curriculum commands

Organization of School Health Programs

a central position in a body of experiences." He purports that life philosophy, educational philosophy, and aims and objectives for the curricular area precede the actual curriculum. The curriculum itself then encompasses content, methods, materials, and evaluation.

One must examine the classical definition of curriculum as all the courses of study in a school, while retaining the more modern definition of curriculum as the courses for a specific subject matter. A curriculum should contain an orderly arrangement of elements, in order to show the nature of the relationships between these elements, as influenced by the educational system from which they are derived. The structure of the curriculum must coincide with the philosophy, goals, and objectives of the educational system wherein the curriculum is located (SHES, 1967, p. 3).

Learning Theory

Central to any discussion of curriculum and planning for development of curriculum is *learning theory*. Numerous texts have been published that deal with learning theory and the scope of this text precludes a detailed explanation of all the theories that have been set forth. According to Hilgard and Bower (1981), learning is the process by which an activity originates or is changed through reaction to an encountered situation provided that the characteristics of the change in activity cannot be explained on the basis of native response, tendencies, maturation, or temporary states of the organism (e.g., fatigue, drugs, etc).

Although many may ascribe to the learning theory definition, it is unclear exactly how learning occurs. As a result, numerous theories about learning have been expressed and published in the printed literature. According to Hill (1963) two major schools of thought relative to learning theory have emerged—the connectionist and the cognitive theories. Connectionist theory has its roots in the work of Thorndike and was first published in *Animal Intelligence* (1898). This theory holds that learning is a process of making connections between a stimulus and a response (the S–R theory, sometimes called operant conditioning). As such, all actions are responses to stimuli. The response is learned through trial and error in such a fashion that the individual "learns" the "best" response by responding randomly until a particular response continues to produce some sort of "reward" for the respondent. An individual who "learns" produces the same responses over and over until they become habits. Pavlov's famous experiments with salivating dogs is an example of connectionist theory in action.

Individuals who subscribe to the connectionist theory of learning tend to write behavioral objectives in terms of linkages. These linkages are explicit and detailed and the objectives are specified in measurable, behavioral outcomes. The method of writing behavioral objectives that was espoused by Mager (1962) is an example of connectionist theory objectives. This concept is discussed more fully in Chapter 17.

On the other hand, cognitive theorists concentrate on the individual's perception of the environment and how that knowledge affects behavior. Similar to Gestalt theory, cognitive or field theory is exemplified by the work of Abraham Maslow, John Dewey, Carl Rogers, and Jean Piaget. This theory contends that an individual can solve problems without having to go through the rather laborious task of trying several erroneous responses prior to discovering a correct response. This theory takes into consideration the social or environmental context in which the problem must be solved. The central theme of cognitive theorists is that the individual perceives his or her surroundings and, based upon these perceptions, solves a problem—the individual looks at the total picture, not just a single element within the picture. For example, when a thirsty individual is given a choice of food or water, the water will most likely be selected prior to the food. When a cliff diver is standing on the edge of the cliff just prior to the dive, he or she will survey the entire scene including the flow of the water and the wind currents, as well as visualizing the dive that must be completed.

Individuals who subscribe to the cognitive theory of learning write behavioral objectives in terms of interactions. These interactions serve as motivational devices and the learnings that occur transfer from one situation to another. The concept of interaction is stressed not only in objectives that are written, but also predominates in the classroom activities that are enacted. Concentration is on defining and modifying perceptions, thus producing behavior change.

WHO PLANS THE CURRICULUM?

The United States is experiencing an awareness of health and fitness probably never before realized in this country. There is increased emphasis on total well-being. As a result, many people feel that they are "instant experts" in the area of health. One need merely look at the burgeoning of health spas, natural food stores, and pseudo weight-loss clinics, or read the various health-related schemes in the newspaper, to realize that everyone is trying to "get in on the act."

It is good to have an increased interest and awareness of health and fitness, but it is a completely different matter to plan, implement, and evaluate a total school health program. It is obvious that a myriad of organizations including voluntary health agencies, official health agencies, and many commercial companies, each with a slightly different vested interest, exists in every community. Each one of these organizations would like to have input into the school curriculum. Many of them have provided a great deal of well-developed material as resource aids for the teacher. Many of the agencies are willing to conduct special in-service workshops for teachers who wish to use the material they have developed. However, unless the curriculum is coordinated, it could well become a "disease-of-the-month" approach that has little impact on the well-being of students.

Organization of School Health Programs

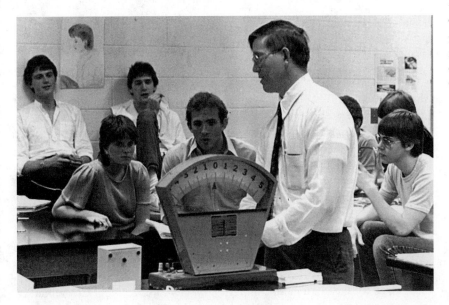

The teacher is a critical factor in promoting the mental health environment of the classroom.

A Shared Responsibility

Health education should be a shared responsibility between the home, the school, and the community. In Chapter 1, a conceptual model for the total school health program was presented (see Figure 1.1). In that model, this shared responsibility was clearly represented. Thus, cooperative planning is certainly a necessity. Earlier in this chapter it was suggested that people learn from all their experiences, not just academic ones. Through cooperative planning for the school health program, concepts and constructs developed in formal school programs can be reinforced by the community health organizations and in the teachings of the home.

The Home

The home provides the individual with primary values and beliefs. It is the cornerstone for future learnings. It is in the home that continual reinforcement of school learnings can occur. It is important that there be two-way communication between the school and home, not just for the sake of health instruction, but also for follow-up to the school health services program. Specific needs of children can and should be communicated to the school by parents or guardians.

Since parents have primary responsibility for the health of their children, they should be encouraged to work closely with the school toward this end. Naturally, this assumes an open-door policy on the part of the school. Parents should be encouraged to participate in the school health program, perhaps by joining parental groups or even by contributing their particular expertise as a resource person in the classroom. Educators should do all they can to increase the cooperation between the home and the school when developing curriculums.

The School

This is the most obvious place where learning occurs. It is important that school administrators keep an open mind and be aware of the changing nature of society. This "ear-to-the-ground" approach should also apply to the changing needs and interests of students within the school. School administrators have primary responsibility to assure that the student is exposed to experiences that promote optimal learning. They also have a responsibility to keep the community and the home informed of school policies and actions, as well as other occurrences that may impact on the student. This responsibility cannot be abdicated or assigned to any other person or group. Schools should also have a curriculum development committee for health instruction. It is preferred that this committee be chaired by someone who is professionally qualified in health instruction, preferably someone who has been nationally recognized by the National Commission on Health Education Credentialing, Inc. as a Certified Health Education Specialist (CHES). (This is discussed more fully in Chapter 20.) Contact with the community is an essential part of the job of administration if the school is to assume a responsible place in society. This is why all policies from the school should be written and available to the community.

The Community

Any student is a part of the community. Community organizations can support the school health program by making various resources—material, personnel, and monetary—available. Giving students the opportunity to use the community as a "living laboratory" also contributes greatly to overall learning.

Professional Societies and Private
Medical and Dental Practice

The professional societies in the fields of medicine, nursing, education, and dentistry certainly have a stake in the health status of the school-age child. Members of these societies can be influential in aiding the passage of bond issues to promote school health programs and can contribute a great deal in terms of their knowledge of the growth and development patterns of children. This will considerably improve the functioning of any committee planning a health instruction curriculum.

Persons representing these societies should be invited to serve on both school and community health councils. They may also have their own school health subcommittee within their professional society. In these cases, the representative to the school and/or community health council could be from that subcommittee. By having these persons involved, cooperation between the members of the profession and the school can be encouraged and enhanced.

This expert advice could also extend to the development of standards for the health of school personnel. An excellent example of community support for school programs is the way the New York Medical Society cooperated with the New York City Board of Education to institute a special health education curriculum into the elementary schools in the city. The Medical Society assisted in raising funds to implement *Growing Healthy* (see Chapter 18) and that particular curriculum has now been disseminated, along with the necessary materials, to nearly all elementary schools within New York City.

Other resources available from private practitioners and professional societies include small grants for the purchase of health-related materials, the donation of medical and dental models or instruments to the schools, and the provision of guest speakers.

Official and Voluntary Health Agencies

In any attempt at developing a comprehensive school health program, it is important to maintain a balance among the various segments of the community. Most official and voluntary health agencies have developed helpful resource material. Having representatives from these agencies help in the curriculum planning process will aid greatly in drawing the school and community health programs into close harmony. Examples of curriculum developed by voluntary health agencies are presented in Chapter 18.

Service Clubs

Many service clubs have a direct involvement in school health programs. Rotary, Kiwanis, and Optimist Clubs are examples of service clubs that have done a great deal in promoting the health of the school-age child. Other service clubs that help promote health education programs include the Lions Club (hearing, diabetes, glaucoma, and vision screening programs) and the Elks (muscular dystrophy). Another example of service club activities in health include the Polio Plus program of Rotary International. This program was specifically designed to assist global efforts to eradicate poliomyelitis, worldwide, by the year 2000. In like manner, Kiwanis International has a program entitled Young Children: Priority One, a special preschool through age 5 program. All of these programs could be incorporated into a comprehensive school health program. By using the varied resources of these organizations, the school is again participating in outreach. These clubs will often assist the school in obtaining resources by conducting fund-raising activities or by providing direct funding for specified projects.

Private Industry

This is one group often overlooked in the curriculum development process. However, logic dictates that persons who are employed in local industry are often products of the local school system. Illness is a major expense to industry each year. Increased costs as a result of health insurance claims, loss of productivity, workman's compensation claims, and loss of top executives as a result of premature death and/or disability are all of major concern to industry. By supporting a comprehensive school health program, industry is investing in the future health of its own work force.

Youth Groups

It is obvious that those who belong to youth groups will usually be those who are also in school. Young people are both participants in and benefactors of the school health program. Further, when determining the interests of youth, whom better to ask than youth? There is a tripartite responsibility ascribed to youth in this regard—that they willingly participate in both planned and unplanned learning experiences, willingly work toward improving their health, and voice their interests and concerns about the health program. Students are active, not passive, participants in the learning process.

According to Rash and Pigg (1979, p. 45):

> Success in the school health program hinges as much if not more on the cooperative efforts of the students as on any other members of the school. The students may very well be the final authority in the success of the school health program. It is they who consider, choose, or discard, and practice or not practice in the health conservation measures that are being encouraged.

Parent–Teacher Association

As was stressed in the section dealing with parents, continual contact between the school and parents is a necessary component within the curriculum development process. Too often the argument used to reduce or eliminate health education in the schools is that material taught in schools may well contradict what is taught in the home. Through close contact with the local Parent–Teacher Associations (sometimes called Parent–Teacher–Student Associations), many of these problems can be anticipated and alleviated.

It should also be realized that PTA or PTSA groups generally have a health chairperson. Further, the National Congress of Parents and Teachers, in cooperation with the Center for Health Promotion and Health Education (formerly the Bureau of Health Education) of the Centers for Disease Control, U.S. Department of Health and Human Services completed a series of demonstration projects designed to increase community understanding and support for school health education programs. It is clear that the PTA is committed to the concept of health education.

BASIC PRINCIPLES FOR CURRICULUM DEVELOPMENT IN HEALTH INSTRUCTION

Too often, educators think of planning a curriculum in one specific content area without giving consideration to the total educational responsibility of the school. Vested interests often surface throughout the curriculum. When these problems are compounded by public accountability of education and the

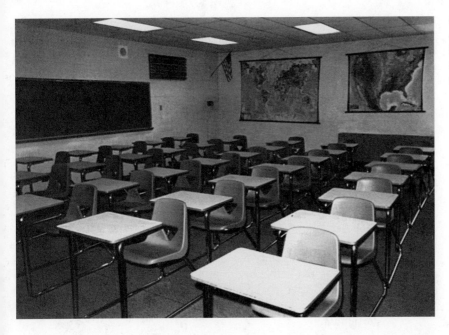

Consideration of classroom flexibility is important when developing the curriculum.

"back-to-basics" movement, it becomes clear that there is no single way to plan a curriculum that is "best." A curriculum planning process that produces an acceptable and effective curriculum in one school district may not produce the same results in another. It is important that those responsible for developing curricula be aware of some basic curricular principles, then temper those principles to meet the local situation.

Basic Assumptions

When discussing basic principles of curriculum development, one must make the assumption that quality has priority in a school district's educational goals. This does not mean that breadth of the total curriculum must be sacrificed for depth. What it does mean is that planning is an integral part of the total process, and this planning cannot be piecemeal.

A second assumption is that the curriculum must be dynamic. Flexibility and responsiveness must be integral parts of the planning process. Knowledge is expanding at an alarming rate, and those planning the curriculum must take this into consideration.

A third assumption is that curriculum planning must be continuous. If the second assumption is correct, then the third is obvious. We must be ready to revise the curriculum as aspects of it become outmoded or as new knowledge develops. Communities are dynamic entities, as are students. Their needs and interests, as well as the demands of society, will change. Educators must be ready to alter the curriculum to stay abreast of those changing needs, interests, and demands.

As noted on p. 291, health education curriculum planning is a shared responsibility. The home, the school, and the community all play vital roles to ensure that the curriculum meets the needs of the students.

Finally although no master plan will serve all needs, general guidelines can be developed that help ensure that students receive comparable education regardless of the system, school, or classroom. Unfortunately, this may be more a goal toward which to move than a reality in practice.

The Health Instruction Curriculum

Johns (1972–73), in citing Hilda Taba and others, has developed a guide for developing health education curricula. This guide contains 14 major steps:

1. Orientation of the persons engaged in the planning.
2. Appraising the existing health education curriculum.
3. Developing a philosophy.
4. Identifying community health needs.
5. Identifying individual health needs.
6. Planning to meet legal requirements.
7. Considering authoritative opinion about school health education curriculum.
8. Formulating objectives of school health education.
9. Developing scope.
10. Developing sequence.
11. Organizing learning experiences.
12. Selecting an organizational plan.
13. Implementing the curriculum.
14. Evaluating.

Orientation of Persons Engaged in the Planning

Earlier in the chapter the importance of having wide representation on the planning committee was discussed. It is important that all persons know exactly what is to be accomplished in the planning process. All persons on the committee must agree with the task definition and have input into the development of the process. Once these procedures have been developed and adopted, each member of the committee must know and accept his or her individual responsibility within the total process—then each member must perform.

Appraising the Existing Health Education Curriculum

The decision to develop or revise a health education curriculum may arise from one of two factors: the belief that health education is a part of the basic education of a child, or the realization that the current curriculum does not meet the needs and interests of the students, the community, or society at large. Obviously, this second assumption connotes that some evaluation of the strengths and weaknesses of the current program has taken place.

Organization of School Health Programs

Developing a Philosophy

For any educational endeavor to succeed, it must be built on a firm foundation of fact and philosophy. If sound philosophy pervades the selection of content, methods, learning experiences, and resource materials, it is questionable if the curriculum will stray far from excellence.

The philosophy for the health education program should arise from three major sources: an analysis of society and culture, studies of learners and learning theories, and a description of what constitutes health education. Concerning the first source, those responsible for developing curricula must have a finger on the "pulse of the community." They must also have a feel for how the school fits into the overall community scheme.

As for the second source, if we do not understand how people learn, how can we develop good curricula? We must know what conditions must be in place for optimal learning to occur. Regardless of the learning theory or theories to which a school district ascribes, the philosophy of the district should reflect that theory and it should be reflected in the curriculum. The key word is "relevance." The curriculum must meet the needs of today's youth while remaining futuristic for tomorrow's adults.

The third source involves knowing how health education is defined by those responsible for developing the curriculum. It is also important to know how it is perceived in relation to the total education of the individual. By knowing this, planners will be able to identify many of the problems they must face when selecting an organization plan for the curriculum.

Identifying Community Health Needs

At this stage, the multidisciplinary nature of the planning process becomes obvious. Local health officials should have data on community health needs readily available. If they do not, the committee may need to undertake a community needs assessment. This might require the services of an outside consultant to be sure that the results of the survey are an accurate picture of the needs of the community. Often local colleges or universities will be able to assist in planning, conducting, and analyzing a community needs assessment.

Identifying Individual Health Needs

Since the curriculum is to be planned for a specific group of students, it is important that their health problems be examined. The maturity and the receptivity of the learners must also be considered in much the same manner as it is considered in learning theory. This information can be gained through direct observation and research about the learners, by getting input from a variety of sources that deal with children and youth, and by speaking directly with students. Another good source of information is the health records of the children. The school nurse should have these records readily available. Formal needs assessments may also be conducted.

Planning to Meet Legal Requirements

On the surface, this category may appear obvious. However, the curriculum committee must consider such things as mandated topics to include topics that are precluded from inclusion (such as sex education) and any time specifications that must be met. As noted by Lovato et al. (1989), the legal mandates for health education vary widely by state. For example, several states do not have legal mandates for the teaching of drug and alcohol abuse prevention, tobacco use prevention, or HIV/AIDS education. Further, when select topics are required, the context in which the education is to occur varies widely as well. If no legal mandates exist, the committee should search the board of education records to determine specific policies. If none are found, it becomes important for the committee to recommend policies to the board and perhaps eventually to the state legislature.

Considering Authoritative Opinion

As the saying goes, "There is no sense in reinventing the wheel." Committees are well advised to secure and examine curricula developed in other school districts to see if parts of these programs might be adapted for their use. It is suggested that sources such as those found in Chapter 18 be consulted. Contact with the state facilitator for the National Diffusion Network is also suggested.

Formulating Objectives

Although this area will be discussed in greater depth in Chapter 17, the sources for objectives should be mentioned at this point. Objectives for the health instruction curriculum arise from two major sources: the purpose of education, and the desired student outcome measures (knowledge, attitudes, and behaviors). These objectives help in formulating the basis for the formal evaluation of the instructional program used in steps two and fourteen.

Developing Scope

There should be provisions for a sequential program that includes the movement from lesser to more advanced knowledges from grades K through 12. The program is based upon the studies of learner characteristics, with particular reference to readiness for learning and the maturity level of the students.

Developing Sequence

As discussed in Chapter 15, sequence involves both horizontal and vertical planning. One must be sure that the course of study builds on prior knowledge, both within and between grade levels. As with scope, maturity and readiness for learning must be considered when planning the sequence of a curriculum.

Organizing Learning Experiences

One must be sure that students possess basic skills necessary to complete various classroom assignments. This principle also refers to horizontal and vertical organization of the curriculum. Learning experiences should build upon each other, and the concept of transfer of learning should pervade this process.

Selecting an Organizational Plan

Several curriculum plans were presented in Chapter 15. These included the traditional or direct approach, the cycle approach, the conceptual approach, and the competency-based approach. Each of these approaches could be incorporated into the various administrative patterns discussed in Chapter 15. The planning committee must be aware of the overall administrative plan used in the school curriculum and take care that the health instruction curriculum follows that pattern, regardless of the specific curriculum plan used for the health instruction course. The key here is to assure, regardless of the type of organization used, that adaptability and flexibility are built into the plan so that as new medical knowledge emerges, as new materials evolve, or as society changes, the curriculum can be adapted accordingly.

Implementing the Curriculum

This is the point where the program moves off paper and into action; it may be the most difficult of all the 14 steps in this process. If the reader subscribes to the idea that the true curriculum is what happens to the learners when they enter the classroom door, this problem becomes even more formidable.

It is hoped that, if all the procedures developed in the first step have been followed, the committee has garnered "good press" and will not meet with community or administrative resistance to the implementation of the curriculum. If the community has been kept appraised of what the committee has been doing, the program will become operational more smoothly and efficiently. Since there are several sensitive topic areas within the scope of health instruction, it would be best to have discussed these topics with school administrators, community leaders, and parents prior to the implementation stage of the process. Unfortunately, this is not always the case; thus, many well-developed plans have remained just that—plans.

Evaluation

Evaluation will be discussed more extensively in Chapter 19. However, a brief introduction at this point seems warranted.

Evaluation is an assessment process that is used to assess progress toward predetermined goals. This assessment also helps determine the degree to which the program matches current recommended practice. The critical variable is how to use the evaluation. If a lot of data are collected and never used, should the effort have been expended to collect the data in the first place?

Evaluation should be used as a basis to determine both strengths and weaknesses of an educational program. Once these two facets have been identified, the processes of revision, reinforcement, or both, should occur.

SUMMARY

In this chapter, the need for health instruction was developed from a historic perspective. This same perspective was used when defining health instruction and curriculum.

Specific considerations for curriculum development, including learning theory, the groups who should be involved in the planning process, basic assumptions about curriculum development in general, and principles for health instruction curriculum development were presented.

Factors to consider when selecting an organizational approach for the curriculum and when developing concepts, long-range goals, behavioral objectives, content, methods, learning opportunities, and resources are discussed in the next chapter. Additionally, schemes for developing units and lesson plans are presented.

REVIEW QUESTIONS

1. How did the authors define the primary purpose of health instruction? Do you agree or disagree with their statement of purpose? Why?
2. Many people have stated that health instruction belongs in the home and not in the school. How would you react to that statement? How would you go about justifying the inclusion of a health instruction program in the school curriculum?
3. What is the importance of the seven cardinal principles of education for secondary schools from both a historical and practical standpoint?
4. How can health instruction further the four purposes of education in America?
5. Why is it important to have a basic understanding of the roots of health instruction?
6. The term *hygiene* is seldom used to describe health instruction today. Why do you think that the professionals in the field have moved away from the use of this term?
7. The true curriculum of a school is what happens to the child as he or she enters the classroom. What is meant by this statement? Do you agree or disagree with this concept? Why?
8. Distinguish between operative and cooperative human effort.
9. You have been given the responsibility to plan a curriculum for a school district. How would you accomplish this task? Whom would you involve and why would you involve them?
10. Do you agree with the authors' basic assumptions about curriculum development? Why or why not? What additional assumptions do you feel should be set forth?
11. Briefly describe the two major theories of learning that seem to be present in education today. In addition to the theorists mentioned by the authors of the text, are there others who typify the two theories that are explained? Who are some of these additional theorists, and what is the nature of their theory of learning?
12. Why do you think it has been so difficult to determine how people learn?

13. Do you agree with the definition of learning that is presented in this chapter? Why or why not?

14. Why is Lemuel Shattuck considered a man who was ahead of his time by many persons in health?

REFERENCES

Adler, M. J. "In Defense of the Philosophy of Education." In N. B. Henry (ed.), forty-first yearbook of the National Society for the Study of Education, Part I, *Philosophies of Education.* Chicago: The Society, 1942.

American Association of Secondary School Administrators. *Health in Schools,* twentieth yearbook of the association. Washington, D.C.: National Education Association, 1942.

American Association of Secondary School Administrators. *Health in Schools,* revised twentieth yearbook of the association. Washington, D.C.: National Education Association, 1951.

American Medical Association, Medicine/Education Committee on School and College Health. *Why Health Education in Your School?* Monroe, Wis.: The American Medical Association, 1982.

American Physical Education Association, Health Education Section. "Definition of Terms in Health Education." *Journal of Health and Physical Education* **5** (December 1934).

Anderson, C. L., and W. H. Creswell, Jr. *School Health Practice.* St. Louis: C. V. Mosby, 1980.

Committee on Terminology in School Health Education. "Report of the Committee on Terminology in School Health." *The Journal of Health, Physical Education, and Recreation* 22:7 (July 1951), p. 14.

The Committee for the White House Conference on Education. *A Report to the President.* Washington, D.C.: Government Printing Office, 1956.

Cornacchia, H. J., L. K. Olsen, and C. J. Nickerson. *Health in Elementary Schools,* 8th ed. St. Louis: Times Mirror/Mosby College Publishing, 1992.

Education Commission of the States. *Recommendation for School Health Education: A Handbook for Policymakers,* Report No. 130. Denver: Education Commission of the States, 1981.

Expert Committee on Health Education of the Public. *First Report.* World Health Organization Technical Report Series, No. 89, Geneva, Switzerland: The World Health Organization, 1954.

Health Education Curriculum Commission (HECC) of the American Association for Health, Physical Education, and Recreation. *Health Concepts: Guides for Health Instruction.* Washington, D.C.: AAHPER, 1967.

Healthy People 2000: National Health Promotion and Disease Prevention Objectives. Washington, D.C.: U.S. Government Printing Office, Publication No. (PHS) 91–50212, 1991.

Hilgard, E. and G. Bower. *Theories of Learning,* 5th ed. Englewood Cliffs, NJ: Prentice-Hall, Inc., 1981.

Hill, W. F. *Learning: A Survey of Psychological Interpretations.* Scranton, Pa.: Chandler Publishing Company, 1963.

Irwin, L. W., and C. Mayshark, *Health Education in Secondary Schools.* St. Louis: C. V. Mosby, 1967.

Jean, S. L. "Stars to Steer By." *American Journal of Public Health* **44** (August 1951).

Johns, E. B. "School Health Program Development and Evaluation," unpublished course syllabus for Public Health 230, School Health Curriculum Development. Los Angeles: University of California, 1972–73.

Joint Committee on Health Education Terminology. "New Definitions: Report of the 1972–73 Joint Committee on Health Education Terminology." *The Journal of School Health* **44** (1974).

Lovato, D., D. Allensworth, and F. Chan. *School Health in America: An Assessment of State Policies to Protect and Improve the Health of Students,* 5th ed. Kent, Ohio: American School Health Association, 1989.

Mager, R. F. *Preparing Instructional Objectives.* Palo Alto, Cal.: Feron, 1962.

Means, R. L. *Historical Perspectives on School Health.* Thorofare, N.J.: Charles B. Slack, 1975.

National Adolescent Student Health Survey: A Report of the Health of America's Youth. Oakland, California: Third Party Publishing Company, 1989.

National Committee on School Health Polices. *Suggested School Health Policies.* Washington, D.C.: The National Education Association, 1966.

National Education Association (NEA). *Schools for the Sixties.* New York: McGraw-Hill, 1963.

National Education Association, and American Association of Secondary School Administrators, Educational Policies Commission. *An Essay on Quality in Public Education.* Washington, D.C.: The Association, 1959.

National Education Association, and American Association of Secondary School Administrators, Educational Policies Commission. *The Purposes of Education in American Democracy.* Washington, D.C.: The Commission of Administrators, 1938.

National Education Association and American Medical Association (NEA–AMA) Joint Committee on Health Problems in Education. *Health Education.* Washington, D.C.: National Education Association, 1961.

National Education Association Center for the Study of Instruction (CSI). *Schools for the 70's and Beyond: A Call to Action.* Washington, D.C.: the Association, 1971.

National Education Association, Department of Elementary School Principals. *Health in the Elementary School,* twenty-ninth yearbook of the Department of Elementary School Principals. Washington, D.C.: The National Education Association, 1950.

Noak, M. *State Policy Support for School Health Education: A Review and Analysis.* Report 182–1. Denver: Education Commission of the States, 1982.

Office of Health Information, Health Promotion, and Physical Fitness and Sports Medicine. "Definitions from OHIP." *Focal Points.* Atlanta: Bureau of Health Education, U.S. Government Printing Office (June 1, 1980).

President's Committee on Health Education. *The Report of the President's Committee on Health Education.* New York: Department of Health, Education, and Welfare, Health Services and Mental Health Administration, 1980.

Proceedings of the Conference on Care of Dependent Children. Washington, D.C.: U.S. Department of the Interior, Office of Education, Document No. 721, U.S. Government Printing Office, 1909.

Rash, J. K., and R. M. Pigg, *The Health Education Curriculum.* New York: John Wiley & Sons, 1979.

"Report of the 1990 Joint Committee on Health Education Terminology." *Journal of Health Education* 22(2):97–108 (March/April, 1991).

School Health Education Evaluation. *Journal of School Health,* Special Issue, 55(8) (October 1985).

School Health Education Study (SHES). *Health Education: A Conceptual Approach to Curriculum Design.* St. Paul: 3M Educational Press, 1967.

Shattuck, L. *Report of the Sanitary Commission of the State of Massachusetts.* Boston: Dutton and Wentworth (facsimile edition), 1850. Reprinted in 1948 by Harvard University Press.

Surgeon General's Report on Health Promotion and Disease Prevention. *Healthy People.* Washington, D.C.: U.S. Department of Health and Human Services, Government Printing Office, 1979.

United Nations: World Declaration on the Survival, Protection and Development of Children and Plan of Action for Implementing the World Declaration on the Survival, Protection and Development of Children in the 1990s. New York: United Nations, Sept. 30, 1990.

U.S. Department of the Interior, Bureau of Education. *Cardinal Principles of Secondary Education.* Bulletin 1918, No. 35. Washington, D.C.: Government Printing Office, 1918.

Willgoose, C. E. *Health Teaching in Secondary Schools,* 3rd ed. Philadelphia: CBS College Publishing, 1982.

Wood, T. D. "Health and Physical Education." In *The Nation at Work on the Public School Curriculum,* fourth yearbook, Department of Superintendence, National Education Association. Washington, D.C.: The Department, 1926.

World Health Organization. *The First Ten Years of the World Health Organization.* Geneva, Switzerland: The World Health Organization, 1954.

Yager, R., P. Kabarec, and B. Atwood: "Assessing and Designing Statewide Comprehensive School Health Education Programs. *Health Education* 15(4):19 (June/July, 1985).

Planning the Curriculum

17

I n order to develop an effective health instruction curriculum, the three major components of curriculum—knowledge of society, knowledge of the learner, and knowledge of the content of the discipline—must be successfully integrated into the total pattern. One might liken the curriculum development committee to a weaver given three colors of thread. Singularly, the three colors do not signify much, but when skillfully joined together, an intricate pattern can emerge.

SELECTING AN ORGANIZATION PLAN

In Chapter 16, five basic assumptions about curriculum development were set forth. These five were:

1. Quality has priority in a school district's educational goals.
2. The curriculum must be dynamic.
3. Curriculum planning must be continuous.
4. Curriculum development is a shared responsibility.
5. No master plan will serve all districts or schools.

Additionally, 14 major steps in planning the curriculum were set forth and described.

In Chapter 15, seven major patterns of curriculum organization (traditional, correlated, experiential, integrated or fused, competency-based, broad fields, and core), two perspectives for curriculum planning (vertical and horizontal planning), and four methods of developing the health instruction program (textbook cycle, textbook, conceptual, and competency-based) were presented and discussed. The discussion of all these elements provided a foundation upon which to base the decision as to what approach to use in planning.

If one reexamines the model presented in Chapter 1, it becomes clear that the philosophy of the role of education in society becomes the major building block for the development of the curriculum. The specific organizational pattern that is ultimately selected is less important than the specificity of planning and the quality, objectivity, and practicality of what is ultimately presented.

Naturally, the health instruction curriculum must conform to the overall curricular pattern used in the school. If it is different, it is quite likely that the health instruction program will not become a part of the total school curriculum.

It must be remembered that the specifics of subject matter areas can be developed in many ways. Obviously, if an integrated approach to learning is used, health instruction will assume a different look than if a broad field

Individualization of instruction necessitates a thorough knowledge of one's students.

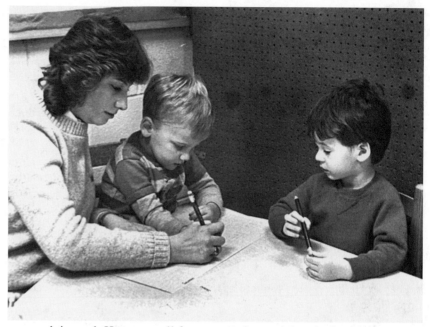

approach is used. However, all four ways of organizing the health instruction course can be successfully implemented in any of the organizational plans used in a school. It must also be recognized that seldom will any of these approaches be found in a school system in a pure form. Rather, what is found is a combination of approaches developed in a manner comfortable for the individual teacher, but one that meets the needs and interests of the learner, while satisfying society that learning is actually taking place.

Fodor and Dalis (1989) have suggested five steps that will aid in systematically organizing health knowledge for the purpose of planning and conducting health instruction:

1. Collecting data or information relative to the health needs of the individual and society.
2. Grouping similar health data or information under broad health topics/themes, problem areas, or generalizations.
3. Identifying generalizations to be stressed within each health information grouping.
4. Developing instructional goals and objectives for each generalization to be stressed.
5. Periodically repeating Steps 1 through 4 to identify, group and make ''room'' for new knowledge (p. 31).

What is omitted from these five steps is the development of philosophy; however, it is intimated in Step 1. When collecting data prior to developing the health instruction curriculum, it is important that a variety of data sources be utilized. Two of the three major components of the curriculum, the learner and society, are paramount in this process.

Organization of School Health Programs

In order to determine the needs and interests of the learner, surveys must be done. Several such surveys have been completed over the years, the most notable of which are those conducted by Lantagne in the early 1950s (Lantagne, 1952, pp. 300–346), by the Denver Public Schools in 1953 (Denver Board of Education, 1954), by the School Health Education Study in the early 1960s (Sliepcevich, 1964), and by Byler, Lewis, and Trotman in 1969. In 1983, Pigg (pp. 29–35) reported six major studies involving over 25,000 students, teachers, administrators, and parents in five separate states and one study involving a national sample. More recently, Trucano (1984) surveyed the health interests and concerns of over 5,000 kindergarten through 12th grade students in the state of Washington. In addition, several major, national evaluation studies have been conducted—the School Health Education Evaluation (Connell, Turner, and Mason, 1985), the National Adolescent Student Health Survey (1989), and two in the area of fitness, National Children and Youth Fitness Study (1985), and National Children and Youth Fitness Study II (1987). Although these studies were evaluative in nature, they all pointed to specific needs of children and youth.

All of the studies pointed to the same general conclusion: Students are interested in their overall health and well-being; students have basic health needs that can be addressed in school settings; students lack general knowledge in health and health-related topics; and the basic interests of children in selected health topics have not varied a great deal over nearly three decades. In fact, if some of the historic studies of the needs of children were examined, it is questionable whether the basic needs and interests of children have changed a great deal over the past 50 years.

Following the guidelines developed in these major studies, local curriculum planners should be able to devise a survey that will gather current information about the health needs and interests of their students. Fodor and Dalis suggest that during the first week of class, teachers might have students list those things they would like to learn in a health course or have them write or discuss the topic "What Health Means to Me" (1989, p. 18).

Several societal data sources exist. The local or state health department will be able to provide specific data concerning health problems that have been identified. Each state has data relative to mortality and morbidity within the communities of the state. In addition, *Healthy People 2000* (the national health goals for the nation) includes a tremendous amount of information that can be used to plan curricula. In that document, nearly 300 health goals for the nation for the year 2000 are specified. An analysis of those objectives shows that nearly 100 of them can be impacted by comprehensive school health programs. One must not overlook the legal mandates for health instruction. As noted previously, health instruction is mentioned in the education codes of more than 40 states (Lovato, Allensworth, and Chan, 1989). There are also numerous health education textbooks that contain content felt to be important for children to learn at various grade levels. Often these textbooks have been reviewed for content and appropriateness by various state agencies or committees empowered to prepare a state textbook adoption list.

By doing a sample survey among parents, the curriculum development team can gain insight into the perceptions of those with school-age offspring relative to the health needs of the community. By discussing the intent to develop a school health instruction program within the meetings of the community health council, community needs become known and considered in the curriculum development process. In those cases where a community health council does not exist, a more tedious procedure of surveying or talking with various community resources will be needed. Once the data have been collected, the analysis phase is initiated. By grouping the responses of students with the responses of parents and community members, broad content areas should begin to emerge.

Examining specific responses will identify the topics that are of most concern with each content area. These topics of concern become the basis for emphasis within the curricular framework and may form the basis for the generation of concepts. It is questionable that the respondent population will demonstrate a thorough knowledge of fact; therefore, someone well versed in the content of health instruction (the third major component of curriculum development) will have to be involved in these analyses. It is preferred that this individual is a certified health education specialist (C.H.E.S.) as determined by the National Commission on Health Education Credentialing, Inc. This person can develop generalizations about the content; the generalizations begin to give shape and direction to the curriculum.

The remainder of this chapter focuses on the specifics of writing concepts, long-range goals, and behavioral objectives. Suggestions for the development of units and lesson plans as well as for the selection of content, methods, learning opportunities, and resources are presented.

DEVELOPING CONCEPTS

It should be apparent by this time that a conceptual approach to learning is likely to produce results superior to other approaches. Traditional teaching focuses upon memorization and recall of facts. Students are regarded as "sponges," and the classroom is representative of knowledge. As time progresses, the sponges absorb knowledge and, at the right moment, they can be squeezed and the knowledge they gained can come rushing out. Unfortunately, knowledge gained in this fashion can appear quite unorganized. It often emerges in helter-skelter fashion; the various segments do not seem to be related.

A conceptual approach, on the other hand, provides a means of organizing thoughts or knowledges. Concepts themselves provide a framework for thinking; they provide a way to interrelate knowledge; thus, they provide a relatively stable and permanent system for storing knowledge. Taba (1962, pp. 119–120) feels that once basic ideas are identified, a curriculum can be developed that provides for a continual reexamination and use of the ideas on an increasingly deeper and more formal level. This concept is manifested both in the cycle plan and the conceptual plans, presented in Chapter 15.

Perhaps the best or most complete definition of the term *concept* was formulated by Woodruff in 1964:

> A concept is a relatively complete and meaningful idea in the mind of a person. It is an understanding of something. It is his own subjective product of his way of making meaning of things he has seen or otherwise perceived in his experience. At its most concrete level, it is likely to be a mental image of some actual object or event. [p. 82]

From the preceding it can be seen that a concept is a personal understanding that arises out of one's perception of experiences. Thus, a concept, per se, cannot be taught. However, teaching can be directed toward a concept. Learning opportunities should be provided in sufficient number and with sufficient focus that the student begins to develop much the same concepts that have been written by the curriculum planners.

Concepts are the result of understanding. As more concepts are developed, it is hoped that understanding is increased. The more understanding the person has, the more likely that person is to make informal choices. Thus, it stands to reason that if a student develops many health concepts, this is indicative of understanding which, in turn, should lead to more healthful decisions.

The question then arises: "What is a good concept?" It would be utopian to think that everyone would agree upon the specific criteria for identifying a well-written concept. Drawing upon the work of Brookbeck (1965, pp. 44–93), Gage (1965, pp. 884–887), and Phenix (1964, p. 306), Sorochan and Bender (1979, pp. 170–171) suggested 13 criteria for a good concept. These criteria are:

1. A generalized or summary statement about pieces of content or information.
2. An abstract idea of what the detailed and specific content is all about.
3. Representing meanings of an object or an event.
4. Representing a class, a process, or a property expressed by a symbol.
5. Reflecting or supporting a basic theory or law (that explains behavior, cause, and effect).
6. Defined in terms of observable individuals.
7. Specifying what is the same in different individuals.
8. Generalizing about time.
9. Valid if it yields successful predictions or outcomes.
10. Implicating desirable behavior, ability, or skill.
11. Reworded or organized at various levels of complexity.
12. Always symbolized and easily evolved from pictorial material.
13. Moving from specific to general, from simple to complex, and from concrete to abstract.

The implications to be drawn from the preceding list are that concepts continually evolve, that they change with one's age, moving from simple to abstract and from an "I" or "me" orientation to a more social orientation.

Although complex concepts may be too advanced for young children, it is suggested that, when using the conceptual approach to a health instruction curriculum, the organizing concepts for that curriculum be representative of higher levels of complexity. They should represent ideas commonly held by high school graduates. The reasoning here is that concepts are not taught; they are taught *toward*. It is the learning opportunities, specific behavioral objectives, and content that need to be developed at the maturity level of the learner. A concept may be abstract, but the ways the teacher moves toward that concept must be specific. The ten concepts developed by the School Health Education Study writing team (Chapter 15) are good examples of a higher level of concept being used as a curricular organizing element.

SELECTING CONTENT

The question ''Do concepts dictate content or does content dictate concepts?'' is not unlike the chicken-and-egg problem. However, it is not possible to teach something unless the teacher knows the topic. Thus, it stands to reason that for a person to develop concepts, that person must have a content base.

It has been established that health instruction is a broad discipline that draws upon the biological and physical sciences for its content and upon the behavioral and social sciences for its process. Thus, a knowledge of anatomy, physiology, chemistry, biology, genetics, medicine, sociology, anthropology, and psychology, as well as education, is necessary. By having this knowledge, the educator will be in a much better position to select and develop both concepts and content for health education.

As stated earlier, studies of the needs and interests of learners and of society are two major sources for content selection. Three additional sources need to be considered at this point: the basic philosophy about health held by the community and the school administration, the expert advice of content specialists, and textbooks.

Philosophy

The philosophy of the community, of school administrators, and, for that matter, of individual teachers, will almost dictate what shall *not* be included in the health instruction program. This philosophy may even be manifested in specific legislative acts. For example, state law in Arizona states in part:

> Sex education shall not be taught in the common schools (K–8) of Arizona as a separate course. The common school, at the district level, may provide a specific elective lesson or lessons concerning sex education as a supplement to the State adopted health course of study, subject to the approval of the State Board. This supplement may only be taken by the student at the written request of the individual student's parent or guardian. [Arizona State Board of Education, 1978, p. 19.1]

Teachers who feel that it is important to deal with human sexuality in Arizona have a lot of work to do within their own district if they are to comply with the law in this regard. The district philosophy must reflect a broad base yet retain the basic dictates of legislative acts.

Content Specialists

Since one of the aims of health instruction is to provide the most scientifically accurate information possible, the use of persons well versed in health science content is certainly warranted. This also means that the teacher will need to develop a plan to keep abreast of the latest scientific information. Through the use of content specialists such as physicians, nurses, nutritionists, college researchers, and dentists as resource persons in the classroom as well as during the curriculum development process, it is likely that the content of health instruction will remain constant.

One must not forget that national experts have developed what should be included in a comprehensive health instruction program. As reported by the 1990 Joint Committee on Health Education Terminology (1991), comprehensive school health instruction includes but is not limited to:

- Community health.
- Consumer health.
- Environmental health.
- Family life.
- Mental and emotional health.
- Injury prevention and safety.
- Nutrition.
- Personal health.
- Prevention and control of disease.
- Substance use and abuse (p. 106).

The ten content areas listed above have been mentioned in many of the studies that were referenced earlier in this chapter. It is easy to see, given the diversity of the topics, why it is important to have an individual professionally prepared and qualified as a Certified Health Education Specialist serving in a coordination role for all curriculum planning in health education, and as the teacher of health education in the high school program. Further, the fully qualified health education specialist, according to the Carnegie Council on Adolescent Development, should serve as a health coordinator in every middle school.

In support of the Carnegie Council on Adolescent Development, the National Commission on the Role of the School and the Community in Improving Adolescent Health (1990) recently published a document entitled, *CODE BLUE: Uniting for Healthier Youth.* This Commission issued a challenge to the nation to "collectively demonstrate the political will to respond"

(National Commission, 1990, Executive Summary). In particular, one of the major recommendations of the Commission was to urge schools to play a stronger role in improving adolescent health. One of the ways that this can be done is to provide quality health education that helps students learn skills and strategies to make wise decisions and develop positive values in health matters. In order to do this, relevant and comprehensive content must be included in the health instruction program.

Textbooks

In much the same manner as just stated, textbooks are generally written by persons who are considered to be experts in a given field. In health education, these persons have usually studied the broad field of health science as well as the growth and development characteristics, maturity levels, and readiness for learning of students in different grade levels. The textbooks they produce have undergone scrutiny by others for both content accuracy and grade-level appropriateness.

Textbooks are valuable resources to use in determining content, but they should not be the sole determining factor. It is suggested that courses of study developed in other school districts (see Chapter 18) might also be examined to obtain ideas about what should be contained in a health curriculum. Schaller (1981, p. 139) suggested five major factors to consider when selecting content:

1. The physical, emotional, social, and intellectual needs of children.
2. The health interests of children.
3. The personal experiences of children.
4. The capacities and levels of comprehension of children at each age level.
5. The health needs of the nation, state, community, school, and the home.

Regardless of the source used to select health content, those responsible for selecting that content have a major task. They should use studies of learners and of society. In addition, philosophies, experts, textbooks, and courses of study developed in other school districts should be consulted. It is almost an unanswerable question whether content or concepts should be selected first. What is important, regardless of the order, is that both be flexible and adaptable to changing knowledge and social conditions.

LONG-RANGE GOALS

Long-range goals may be defined as behaviors that should be expected to be present in students at the end of the complete instructional sequence (School Health Education Study, 1967, p. 96). Since the goal of health instruction is to influence health knowledge, attitudes, and practices, long-range goals should be written in the cognitive, affective, and action domains. The frame of reference for these domains derives from learning theory and from the demands of society.

Organization of School Health Programs

Goals are written in more general terms than are behavioral objectives. As such, they do not generally contain a specification of what constitutes achievement of the goal. They are more global and provide a level to which one should aspire. Specific assessment of a long-range goal is difficult. For example, one of the long-range goals developed by the School Health Education Study writing team for the concept dealing with consumer health states that the student "is sensitive to the range of differences in health communications, products and services" (1967, p. 96). This long-range goal falls into the affective domain. Further, it is open to many interpretations of the word *sensitive*. Compounding all of this is the difficulty of defining precisely what constitutes a positive attitude. (This is one of the problems associated with criterion-referenced testing, as discussed in Chapter 19.)

> Because of their breadth and generality, goals tend to be timeless. That is, final attainment of the goal might never be fully realized. As the student grows and develops, in one way or another, throughout his or her lifetime, there is a potential for further goal attainment. Consequently, final goal attainment is elusive and thus timeless. [Fodor and Dalis, 1989, p. 48]

WRITING BEHAVIORAL OBJECTIVES

Behavioral objectives are explicit statements of the ways in which students are to be changed as a result of the educative process. If they are well written, objectives clearly specify what skills or attributes students are expected to achieve. By attaining several of the specific objectives, the student begins to move closer to the attainment of the long-range goal. As the student moves toward the long-range goal, understandings are gained. As understandings increase and become organized, concepts are developed.

Well-developed objectives make the decision on what content to emphasize quite evident. Thus, the development of good objectives becomes the foundation for designing effective instruction. According to Fodor and Dalis (1989), when objectives are properly stated, they are a guide to:

1. Specific content to be studied.
2. Specific changes in behavior that are sought in the student with respect to this content.
3. Selection of learning opportunities that best enable the learner to achieve the desired behavioral outcomes.
4. What to evaluate in terms of the health content studied and the behaviors sought in the learner.
5. The evaluation of teacher effectiveness. [Fodor and Dalis, 1989, pp. 48–51]

The importance of having clearly stated instructional objectives cannot be overemphasized. Many school districts evaluate teacher performance on how well students have met the stated objectives. In situations where no instructional objectives have been established, teacher evaluations have suffered and, in some cases, teachers have been sued.

Distinguishing Objectives from Activities

Too often the beginning teacher will confuse objectives with activities. The contrast between objectives and activities should be quite clear. An objective is a specified behavior, knowledge, or attitude, whereas an activity is a means of reaching the objective. Yet another mistake made by the novice is to confuse teacher activities with objectives. Consider the following:

- Demonstrate to students the use of the IBM personal computer.
- The student will watch a demonstration of the IBM personal computer.
- The student will be able to demonstrate three home uses for a personal computer.

The first of these statements is a statement of what the instructor will be doing. Clearly it is not student-centered. The second statement focuses on what the student will be doing in order to learn about the use of personal computers. The third statement is also student-focused, but it is an instructional objective—it communicates a skill that the teacher feels is needed. There is still a great deal of latitude in terms of the type of home situations in which the computer could be used, but it does indicate a specific behavior. The point to remember here is that the objective must be stated in terms of learning outcome, not in terms of what the teacher or student will be doing.

The educator faces a bit more difficult problem when developing objectives in the affective or attitude domain. In this instance, the objective should describe those behaviors that, in the mind of the educator, best demonstrate that the student possesses the attitude the teacher wants to instill. It is even better if the behavior is set into a specific situational context. For example, a teacher wants students to develop positive attitudes toward nonsmoking. Consider the following two objectives:

1. The student, when asked, will draw an anti-smoking poster.
2. The student voluntarily draws an anti-smoking poster.

The second objective is better because it describes a behavior the student carried out without being asked. The first objective is appropriate, but it connotes less of a commitment to nonsmoking than does the second objective. Many students may agree to do something when specifically asked, but unsolicited behavior that demonstrates the positive attribute is preferred.

How Should Objectives Be Stated?

There is some variance among educators as to how specific objectives should become. Experts such as Gronlund (1970, pp. 4–5) feel that there are two methods of stating objectives as learning outcomes. He contends that specific behaviors that should be exhibited at the end of an instructional period can be listed.

Organization of School Health Programs

1. Defines each technical term in his [or her] own words.
2. Identifies the meaning of technical terms when they are used in context.
3. Distinguishes between technical terms that have similar meanings.

The second method he purports is to list a general instructional objective first and then clarify it by listing sample behaviors that are considered to be acceptable evidence that the objective has been attained. Thus, in the example just presented, the general objective might read, ''Understands the meaning of technical terms.'' Used under this general objective, the three statements of behavior would clarify the objective and present acceptable evidence that the student did reach the general objective.

Kryspin and Feldhusen (1974, pp. 25–41) have suggested that those who write instructional objectives should remember their A B C D's:

- A—Audience (for which the objective is intended).
- B—Behavior (what the student is to do).
- C—Condition (what is required).
- D—Degree (criteria for acceptable completion).

Consider the following example: Given a list of 20 medical terms, a sixth-grade student will be able to define at least 15 of them in his or her own words.

- Audience: sixth-grade student.
- Behavior: defining terms in his or her own words.
- Condition: a list of 20 medical terms.
- Degree: at least 15 of the terms.

There is still latitude for the student who can define all 20 terms in his or her own words, and perhaps the level of specificity is somewhat loose, but the A B C D's are clearly present.

Yet another approach has been suggested by Mager (1962, p. 52). He suggests three basic criteria for writing instructional objectives:

- Terminal behavior: refers to the behavior the learner should demonstrate at the time instruction has been completed.
- Conditions: refers to the specific conditions under which the behavior is to be performed (givens or restrictions or both).
- Evaluation: refers to the criterion of acceptable performance.

The example given earlier would be stated in Magerian format as follows:

Given a list of 20 medical terms about the cardiovascular system, the student will, on a written test, be able to define at least 15 of them in his or her own words.

It is clear from this example that Mager defines the conditions more specifically than do Kryspin and Feldhusen and that all of these persons appear to be more exacting than Gronlund.

Still another approach is espoused by persons who feel that classification of objectives can follow the taxonomy developed by Bloom and his associates. Those who ascribe to this school of thought tend to pay less attention to the precision of the behavior and the criteria for acceptable performance than to the classification of the content dimension as it fits the taxonomy—either cognitive or affective (Oberteuffer, Harrelson, and Pollock, 1972, p. 60).

Those who follow the Bloom format might state our example thus:

Defines select medical terms in his or her own words.

Clearly, each of these formats has merit, and each of the examples should be relatively easy to understand. The conclusion here is that there is no single best way to state behavioral objectives. However, the objective should meet at least three criteria:

1. It is specified in terms of the learner, not the teacher.
2. It specifies a single behavior and content area.
3. It can be measured or evaluated to show that the student does have a degree of mastery of the behavior.

SELECTING METHODS AND LEARNING ACTIVITIES

It has long been recognized that the key to effective teaching is the teacher, but the appropriate use of methods and learning activities is what makes that teacher successful. Methods and activities must be appropriate for the content being covered and for the level of the students' needs and abilities. They must also stimulate the learner. Further, these methods and activities must be current and fit the teacher's style, or the chance for success is diminished.

Method and learning opportunity are combined in this section because *method* generally refers to what the teacher does, and *learning opportunity* refers to the activities students carry out to attain behavioral objectives. However, just because the teacher employs a particular method, there is no guarantee that learning will occur. For ease of discussion, the word *method* is used to refer to both method and learning opportunity.

Regardless of the method selected, it is important to involve the learner in an active, not passive, fashion. The activity should be current, provide a meaningful experience for the student, and add to the knowledge base he or she brings to the classroom.

Categorization of instructional methods is a difficult task because most educators combine several methods during any given class period. For example, the broad category *problem solving* could include almost every method imaginable, since solving a problem is the actual instructional goal. Cornacchia, Olsen, and Nickerson (1992, p. 274) proposed a relatively complete scheme that has merit in considering the broad topic of methods:

1. Problem solving.
2. Construction activities.

3. Creative activities.
4. Demonstrations.
5. Discussions.
6. Dramatizations.
7. Educational games and simulations.
8. Excursions and field trips.
9. Surveys.
10. Illustrated presentations.
11. Individual and group reports.
12. Resource people–guest speakers.
13. Show-and-tell time.

Each of these is discussed briefly in terms of the health instruction course.

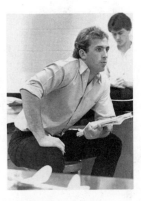

Motivation is an important part of health instruction.

Problem Solving

Many consider problem solving to be the highest form of learning that contributes to the development of positive health attitudes, behaviors, and values as well as helping the student develop cognitive powers. Problem solving connotes exactly that—apply information that has been gained for the purpose of solving a problem that has been presented. Problem solving also applies the scientific method of identification, analysis, data collection, organization of the data, analyzing possible results of what might be applied, testing the best solution that is implemented, and evaluating the results. It is an excellent method to use to develop critical thinking, and this kind of thinking is paramount to the decision-making process. To solve problems requires students to begin to sort fact from fiction, formulate hypotheses, test the hypotheses, and draw conclusions. If given rather structured problem-solving situations in the classroom, the student will be better equipped to deal with the more nonstructured problems that affect personal health. If problem solving is used as a group process, the procedure promotes cooperative work in handling mutual concerns.

It is important to remember that problem solving involves considerably more than stating a behavioral objective in question form. A great deal of care must be taken in formulating the specific problem so that the focus is limited enough to be practical, yet broad enough to allow students a degree of creativity.

Brainstorming

Brainstorming is a process used in problem solving involving what psychologists call *free association*. The students should be able to express any possible solution that comes to mind without fear of rebuke by the remainder of the group. With the establishment of a free flow of ideas, without discussion of the merits of any of them (at least initially), ideas can be generated rather quickly. When many ideas are presented and written down, students can begin to sort them into broad areas and to conceptualize about how a given problem might be solved. This method is often used as the initial stage of buzz groups.

Brainstorming enables the exchange of ideas, generates creative thinking on the part of the student, allows the student to begin to develop linkages between the thoughts of several persons, and allows the student to begin to develop models that can be applied in various problem situations. Unfortunately, the process may lead to a "rowdy" situation, especially when all students begin to talk at once. It is important that the teacher set forth specific rules for the class to follow when engaging in brainstorming activities. It is also important to understand that brainstorming works best when the group is rather small. As a result, the teacher may want to develop several different problems, all that could result in essentially the same basic solution, break the class into smaller units, and, following the brainstorming session, structure a reporting system from each group back to the larger classroom as a whole. In order to avoid having misconceptions presented, it is important that students have some basic background in the topic to be discussed prior to engaging in brainstorming activities.

Valuing

Too many people have the mistaken idea that values clarification means that the teacher intends to teach students specific values. Nothing could be further from the truth. Students bring values to the classroom, the result of many and varied experiences. Often, however, these values are in a disorganized state; values clarification strategies, when used correctly, help students sort through the maze and develop a clearer picture of what has meaning for them in their own lives.

The full ramifications of values clarification cannot be discussed in a text of this sort. However, it is important for the health educator to know that the process consists of seven basic steps under three major categories (Raths et al., 1966):

A. Choosing.
   1. Choosing freely: The individual should not be forced into a choice. There should be freedom of selection.
   2. Choosing from alternatives: A variety of alternatives should be provided.
   3. Choosing thoughtfully: Have the consequences of the various alternatives been considered?
B. Prizing.
   4. Prizing and cherishing: The choice has a positive tone and is held in high esteem.
   5. Public affirmation: If something is held in high esteem, it should be affirmed—when appropriate.
C. Action.
   6. Acting on choices: Did the person do something about the choice that was made?
   7. Repeating: Did the choice become a pattern in the life of the individual?

The inclusion of instruction in the area of values clarification is controversial in some communities. Some of the controversy revolves around the following:

- Lack of a clear-cut operational definition of values, valuing, and values clarification.
- Lack of a specific role that has been defined for the teacher in teaching values.
- Uncertainty on the part of the teacher about disclosing his or her own values.
- Uncertainty as to how accepting teachers should be of student values, especially if the student-stated values are obviously socially unacceptable.
- Uncertainty as to the depth that teachers should probe into a student's private life or feelings.
- Questions about the professional preparation for the teacher in teaching values.
- Uncertainty about the teacher's ability to select appropriate values clarification activities from the myriad of activities that have appeared in the professional literature. [Superka et al., 1976]

Further, the situations that gave rise to the development of values clarification included what might be considered by some to be negative, with less than productive behaviors that include apathy, inconsistency, overconformity or dissension, and the like. According to Eddy, St. Pierre, and Alles (1985), for teachers to successfully use values clarification, they should:

- Develop a classroom environment conducive to open communication.
- Develop operational definitions and appropriate educational objectives for values clarification exercises.
- Concentrate on the process of valuing rather than on the actual value.
- Develop a personal philosophy that can guide them as facilitators of the values clarification process.
- Adapt values clarification activities to the developmental level of the students.
- Progress from simple to complex activities.
- Avoid overuse of values clarification activities in the classroom or elsewhere.
- Avoid assessing the effect of values clarification activity on behavior change since behavior change is influenced by many factors in addition to classroom activities.

The teacher would be wise to determine local standards on this issue prior to including methods designed to teach students the seven steps suggested by Raths, Harmon, and Simon (1966).

Construction Activities

These activities involve mutual planning between the teacher and the student. Obviously, creativity is involved in developing construction activities. Such things as papier-mâché models, puppets, charts, bulletin board displays, and various safety items (traffic lights, fire alarm boxes, and so on), as well as many other things could be included. Care must be taken that the material used is safe and that students practice safety precautions, e.g., wear eye protection, if tools are involved.

Creative Activities

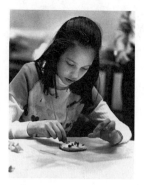

Individual projects provide creative ways for students to demonstrate their knowledge.

As with problem solving, creative activities cover a wide range of possibilities. Writing free verse, poetry of different types, skits or dramas, and developing songs are examples of creative activities that can be used in the classroom.

Open-Ended Stories

Open-ended stories allow students to create their own endings. The best success will be realized if the teacher develops stories pertinent to the group with which he or she is dealing and makes sure that the stories are plausible. It is important that all students be given the opportunity to provide endings to the stories. This should create impetus for a great deal of classroom discussion.

Learning Centers

Most classrooms will have students who have a wide variety of skills, knowledge, and attitudes. By heterogeneously grouping students and having them move from learning center to learning center, the entire group begins to look at specific problems in a different light. The creative ability of the various students begins to spring forth, and eventually one sees a group cohesiveness that will enhance the creativity of each person in the group. Use of learning centers can also be important in teaching group cooperation skills as well as leadership skills. Allowing students to rotate as the group leader for each of the learning stations provides the opportunity for them to learn about and exercise leadership skills in directing others to a mutually satisfying completion of the station.

In addition to learning group cooperation skills, students can gain skills using the newer technology such as computers, laser disks, and interactive video. Naturally, selection of the software for computer applications, and disks and tapes for the interactive techniques is important. The material that is selected should contribute to the overall goal for the lesson as well as aid students in reaching instructional objectives that have been set.

Demonstrations

Demonstrations take two specific forms: (1) teacher conducted, or (2) student conducted. For student demonstrations, the skills taught should be reinforced in practice settings, whereas teacher demonstrations give students a model to follow. When the students are conducting a demonstration, the teacher must

Organization of School Health Programs

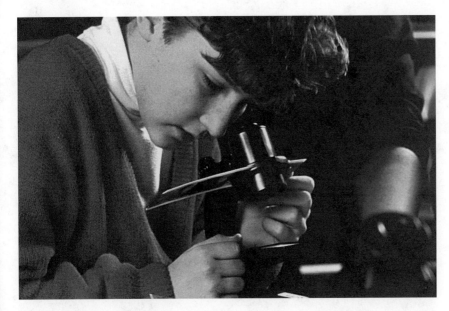

Materials centers allow students to learn through discovery.
Photo courtesy, Michigan Department of Education

plan time for them to practice before being evaluated. One advantage of demonstrations is that a wide variety of senses come into play.

However, demonstrations take planning and time. If the teacher wants all students to have the opportunity to conduct a demonstration, the time available must be carefully analyzed to be sure that each student is given equal time, depending upon the nature of the demonstration. Further, all materials for the demonstrations should be readily available so that things can move smoothly once the demonstration has begun.

Student Projects

In general, students should be given the opportunity to show or demonstrate their projects to the rest of the class. By allowing this, the teacher is assuring that each student will realize success. This has numerous ramifications for the emotional climate of the classroom. When students present their projects, offer positive comments to each student who is presenting. The teacher must be alert for possible "heckling" by other students, those who "put down" another student's project.

Materials Centers

Often materials centers are located in school libraries, but they can be located in individual classrooms. In general, these centers contain audiovisual aids the student must operate. The development of a good materials center necessitates a great deal of planning and organization. The center should contain a wide range of reference material that can be checked out on a limited basis. If equipment is included in the center, care must be taken to ensure that all students know how to operate and care for it.

Experiments motivate
students and help them
"learn by doing."

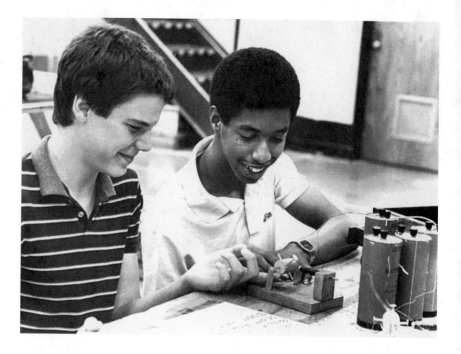

It is also important that all equipment that is returned to the media center be checked. The teacher should instill a sense of responsibility in the students who use the media center to report any equipment malfunction so that the next students also have the benefit of a working piece of equipment.

Having correct knowledge of how to use equipment in materials centers is particularly important if such items as computers, laser disks, and interactive video are included. It takes a certain amount of skill to use this equipment and students should not be allowed to use the material until they have demonstrated some degree of competence in using and caring for the equipment.

Experiments

Experiments are often combined with demonstrations. When students conduct experiments, they are learning how to use the scientific method. Experiments may be done on an individual or group basis. If they are conducted in groups, they are often set up as learning centers. Care must be taken with group experiments to assure that everyone has a chance to participate.

Discussions

Discussions provide active interchange of ideas between teacher and student and between students. By promoting group discussions, the teacher is exposing the students to a variety of viewpoints about a given topic.

It is always helpful if personal experiences can be brought into discussions. Some words of caution should be brought forth. The shy student may not participate fully. The teacher should be aware of shy students and must try to involve these students in the discussion yet not embarrass them in front

Organization of School Health Programs

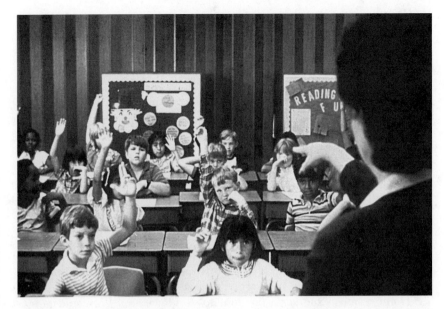

Lectures are used as a method of stimulating discussion.
Photo courtesy, American Cancer Society

of their peers. Other students like to hear themselves talk and will continue a long time if the teacher allows it. However, when the students begin to move into sensitive areas or begin "letting skeletons out of the closet," it is time to close the discussion. If students feel a need to talk about a sensitive problem, the teacher should talk with them on a one-to-one basis or refer them to someone in the school health service.

Lectures

Lectures are fine for getting specific information to a group of students. Unfortunately, lectures are primarily passive learning experiences. Most educators combine lectures with discussion and often augment them with various audiovisual aids such as slides, overhead transparencies, audiotapes, models, and filmstrips. Unless the teacher is relatively adroit at speaking, reliance on a lecture as a major method or learning activity is not advised.

Questions and Answers

Obviously, discussion will involve questions and answers. Students have numerous questions about health and health-related matters. This method is also a good way to summarize a given lesson or unit of instruction.

When discussing certain topics, it is a good idea to use a question box. Students are given pieces of paper and asked to write their questions on the paper and put them into the question box. In this way, anonymity is retained. Further, by grouping the questions, the teacher can focus responses and any ensuing discussions on specific interests of the students.

Too often quizzes are used only as a formal evaluation device. Oral quizzes and allowing other students to "rescue" a classmate serve as good discussion motivators. This type of activity also can serve as a review of material covered in various lessons.

Self-appraisals help students focus on themselves. Through such activities as self-tests, without grades, students will gain insight on what they know, feel, and do about health. These appraisals can be used as a basis for class discussions in much the same way as surveys.

Experience Charts and Records

Charts and records of this type are brief synopses of students' experiences. A question such as "Have you ever had a broken bone?" can form the basis of one of these charts. Follow-up questions might include: "What bone was broken?" "How did it happen?" "How might it have been prevented?" Through structuring the nature of the response, the discussion can be focused but can still provide a wide latitude for student responses. This is also a method that can be used to integrate health instruction into other subject areas.

Buzz Groups

In the buzz-group method, the class is divided into several small groups, generally five students. Each group is given the same problem or different aspects of a large problem and has a few minutes to brainstorm. Each student must contribute at least one idea to the group. Following the brainstorming, the group is given three to five minutes to select its best three or four responses. The responses are then presented to the class, and the main points are recorded on the chalkboard for use in additional discussion.

The buzz group has several distinct advantages over the large-group discussion method. The first of these advantages is in breadth of participation. The buzz group also allows a large question to be broken into smaller, more manageable segments. However, when each group reports, the larger problem comes into focus. This has the advantage of both showing students how to break a problem down and teaching them how to deal with the whole problem.

Panels/Symposia/Debates

It is important to remember that panels are not a series of individual reports. Rather, they are designed to allow a small group to become experts on a specific issue. A series of key problems are discussed among the panel members and eventually the audience is involved.

Symposia, on the other hand, offer the opportunity for students to present viewpoints on a variety of topics relative to a given theme. These viewpoints should be largely their own and not merely the opinions of others.

Debates combine several skills and activities including gaming strategies, detailed factual content about select issues, and communication skills. Students have the opportunity to learn about both sides of an issue and how to present one side of the issue in a convincing manner.

In all of these activities, the teacher's role is to guide the presentation and to be sure that accurate information is presented. It is important that the participants know the role they are to play and the rules they are to follow. The teacher can also act as a summarizer once the presentations have concluded.

Dramatizations

Dramatizations may take several different forms. Skits, puppet shows, role playing, sociodramas, story telling, and plays are all examples of dramatizations. This method provides students the opportunity of assuming a different character role and projecting their own feelings into that role. Often students are more apt to show their true feelings when they feel they're portraying someone else. However, this method might not be particularly appealing to shy students. Caution should also be exercised especially with sociodramas. These can get out of hand. Teachers are not psychotherapists and opponents of health education programs may use this to argue against the program. Learn the process, but be prepared if opposition arises.

Educational Games and Simulations

These are good motivators for students, particularly if the students develop the games. There are a number of ways these games can be developed. For example, following television game show formats such as in Concentration or some sort of sport-related game (baseball, football, basketball), wherein teams must answer questions to get hits, move the ball, or score baskets are fun for the students; they also foster a great deal of learning. Further, this type of activity serves as a good review. Games should only be used if they advance the cause of instruction. Don't use games as ends unto themselves.

Recently, computer-assisted instruction (CAI) has been emerging in the classroom. If the teacher is going to use CAI as a method, it will be important to make sure that all students are familiar with the use of the computers, and that the materials to be used are appropriate for the lesson being taught and the maturity level of the students. If computer games are used, it is important that they contribute to instruction, not detract from it.

In addition, new technologies are developing. Some schools already are using laser disks and interactive video. As noted earlier, when selecting materials for use with these new technologies, be sure that the educational value of the material is clear and that both the students and the teacher know how to effectively and correctly use the equipment.

Excursions and Field Trips

The community is a learning laboratory that is not used enough in the educational system. A well-planned field trip provides a realistic experience for students and can be used as a basis for class discussion. Precautions must be taken to ensure the safety of all students who go on field trips. Naturally, costs are involved in transporting students, and this must be considered. Even so, field trips add greatly to student learning.

Surveys

The use of surveys or questionnaires gives students the opportunity to apply their knowledge and to determine actual practices or knowledges of others. By helping students prepare these surveys, but letting them do the analysis, the educator is engaging in what might be termed *guided discovery*. If they present the results to the rest of the class, students are not only learning basic research skills; they are also learning how to present research to others.

Caution must be exercised if surveys and questionnaires are to be used in the classroom. It is advisable to obtain clearance from appropriate sources, such as review boards, if these types of items are going to be used in the classroom. If the teacher uses a survey that someone feels is controversial, the incident may be taken out of context, lead to controversy, and possibly to the discontinuation of the program.

Illustrated Presentations

Illustrated presentations might be included in the creative activities category. However, if done by the teacher, illustrated presentations can help provide vicarious experiences for the student. If a class cannot visit a blood bank, perhaps the teacher can take slides of a typical visit and use them in lieu of the actual field trip.

Everyone seems to like cartoons. Having children develop cartoons about a given health topic allows them to demonstrate their knowledge in a creative fashion. Having students develop captions for cartoons can also be a way to integrate creative thinking and language arts.

When using graphics, slides, charts, and so on, use information that is scientifically correct, free of bias and stereotyping, and of good quality. (See Appendixes A, B, and E for selection criteria.)

The use of illustrated presentations involves presenting numerous phases of health using various audiovisual materials. These materials may include charts, graphs, models, pictures, specimens, and the newer technologies of computers, laser disks, and interactive video. As with any of the methods discussed in this section, students should be encouraged to discuss the material they are viewing. In addition, teachers may have students develop illustrated presentations and present these materials to the rest of the class. Clearly, this type activity is not done in isolation, but rather is used as an integral part of one or several other teaching methodologies.

Individual and Group Reports

Use of this method includes both oral and written reports. The teacher can assign topics, or let the students decide the topic, within the scope of what is to be covered in the class. It is always a good idea to introduce the concept of reports and what should be included within a report. If the teacher can prepare a listing of what is expected, it assists the students by providing a generalized structure that they can follow.

If oral reports are used, students should be aware that their report may be followed by questions from other students. As a result, the teacher must be alert not to let subsequent discussions detract from the overall intent of the lesson or deteriorate into a situation wherein the student or students who deliver the report are made to feel that their report was poorly done. Periodic checks with the student or students relative to progress on the report will be useful, both to the students and to the teacher as well.

Individual and group reports have the advantage that the teacher can be reasonably sure that the student or students involved have learned something in preparing for the report. It is important that the report deal with a specific part of the lesson that the teacher is presenting. For this reason, it is important that the teacher provide guidance to those persons who wish to do individual or group reports. One thing which should be kept in mind is to avoid having a series of student or individual reports back-to-back, since the attention span of students is often limited.

Resource People–Guest Speakers

Nearly every community has individuals within it who are experts in various areas of health. Use of these individuals enriches the experiences of students when they have the opportunity to interact with the expert. However, it is important that before inviting an individual to class, the teacher should have the opportunity to meet with the guest speaker to discuss what the class has been doing, the goals for having the speaker attend the class, and what is to follow the presentation in terms of instructional outcomes. To assist the speaker, it may be useful to have students develop questions that they would like to have answered. These questions can be given to the speaker in advance of the presentation. Doing this will help in focusing the presentation on topics of relevance to the students.

Show-and-Tell Time

Show-and-tell time can present a wonderful opportunity, or turn out to be somewhat of a nightmare for the teacher. Used correctly, show-and-tell allows free discussion of health matters of interest to students. However, the teacher must be on the alert for students who may begin talking about private matters, best discussed on a one-to-one basis. Naturally, show-and-tell is most appropriate for the primary grades, but can be used effectively at the upper grade levels as well. Such things as various consumer decisions that students have made and what they purchased often provide a good basis for subsequent class discussion. Younger students who have parents in the health professions may be able to bring things such as stethoscopes, models, charts, or other equipment to class. These can be quite useful to the presentation and are of great interest to students.

Others

The preceding pages have included but a few of the myriad of methods that are available to teachers. In addition to those methods, the creative teacher will use textbooks, videotapes, films, audiotapes, laser disks, computers, exhibits, health fairs, television (especially television specials), student contracts, models, and more to provide a diversified approach to the classroom. Overreliance on any method will lead to a stagnation within the classroom.

Inhelder and Piaget (1958) have indicated that the ability of a child to understand broad concepts and abstractions depends upon that child's direct sensory experiences. Using a variety of methods and learning experiences helps ensure these experiences.

DEVELOPING UNITS

Regardless of the organizational plan used, an instructional unit is composed of all the basic ingredients necessary for the teaching process. It is what gives a more finalized organization to the curriculum. The unit contains eight major sections: (1) unit title, (2) concepts, (3) behavioral objectives, (4) content, (5) methods/learning opportunities, (6) teaching aids, (7) evaluation procedures, and (8) references.

Title

The title of the unit should be a short, concise statement that tells the reader the nature of what is contained in the unit. It should arouse interest but should not be ''cutesy.''

Concepts

As stated earlier in the chapter, concepts form the framework of the curriculum, representing the major generalizations that will be emphasized in the unit. They help to focus the rest of the unit in terms of overall learnings for the student.

Behavioral Objectives

Behavioral objectives indicate exactly what the student is expected to do and provide criteria for acceptable performance. The objective must be written in language that is not open to a wide degree of interpretation because these objectives formulate the basis for determining the worth of the program in terms of student learning and application of that learning.

Examples of good behavioral objectives would be the following:

> Given a list of 25 foods, the student will demonstrate a minimum of 80 percent accuracy in assigning each of the foods to one of the four basic food groups.

> Students will answer a 50-item multiple choice test on the benefits of exercise, attaining a minimum score of 75%.

> Students will write a 5-page paper describing the effects on the body of inhaling one puff from a cigarette.

> Students will conduct comparison shopping to determine the total price and price per ounce of six selected sunscreen products at a minimum of five local stores, and develop a chart of their findings.

Each of the above examples embodies the basic elements that should be included in a precise behavioral objective.

Organization of School Health Programs

Content

Clearly, all segments of content cannot be included. Thus, the content should be presented in a clear outline format, with a direct relationship to the behavioral objectives, concepts, and the title of the unit. Extraneous details should be omitted. Remember, the unit is proscriptive, not prescriptive.

Methods/Learning Opportunities

The methods and learning opportunities should be selected with extreme care. All the activities must be directed toward guiding the learner toward the development of behaviors that will increase his or her understandings. With increased understandings, the individual begins to achieve specific behavioral objectives, thus moving closer toward the development of concepts.

Teaching Aids

A wide variety of aids should be listed. If a limited amount of material is listed, there is a chance it might not be available or appropriate for a particular group of students. By listing a broad array of materials, the individual teacher can select from alternatives, a process that is included in the basic philosophy of health instruction. It is important that all teaching aids be previewed for appropriateness and scientific accuracy prior to their use in the classroom.

Evaluation Procedures

Evaluation will be discussed at length in Chapter 19. However, it is important that the various learning opportunities be evaluated.

The specific evaluation activities may range from informal to formal. Regardless, they should emanate from the objectives that were developed for the unit.

References

Having a set of references in addition to teaching aids provides the teacher with a resource to which he or she can refer if more content is needed. The greater the specificity of the resources (such as specific page numbers), the better. The resource list may be divided into two sections, one for the teacher and one for the student.

LESSON PLANS

Whereas the unit contains the overall information for a specific topic, the lesson plan further breaks down the unit into specifics for a given day. It may also expand on selected segments of the unit, such as the content.

Some teachers can teach quite well with an outline, whereas others need more specificity. Only experience will dictate what works best for the individual teacher. Lesson plans are, however, a "must" when teaching controversial areas.

There are numerous ways to develop a lesson plan. Regardless of the format utilized, horizontal and vertical organization must be considered. The crux of the lesson plan is that the teacher can identify what is to be done and how it is to be done. Additionally, the lesson plan, if followed, serves as a permanent record of the content and learning experiences to which a student was exposed. Having a permanent record of the content and learning experiences also provides some protection for the teacher if a parent or other individual initiates a complaint about the program.

In general, the lesson plan follows the same basic format as the unit plan:

1. The health area being studied.
2. The concept being emphasized.
3. The objective of the lesson.
4. The place of this lesson in the overall unit (for example, "This is the sixth of eight lessons on communicable disease").
5. A statement of transition from what went before.
6. A general description of the classroom organization for the lesson.
7. The amount of time for the lesson.
8. The content to be covered.
9. The specific sequence of the learning activities including opening and closing activities.
10. Suggested references and teaching aids.
11. Suggested evaluation activities, if warranted.
12. A brief description of what is to occur in the next lesson.

Although following the 12 steps presented above form a good basis for the development of lesson plans, each district may have specific content areas or experiences that must be included. Health instructors should find out if there is a standard form for lesson plans that is required within the school district or building in which they are teaching and conform to those requirements.

SUMMARY

In this chapter, various considerations for planning the curriculum have been presented. A series of five basic assumptions about curricular development from Chapter 16 was expanded so that those responsible for developing curriculum could see the applicability of those assumptions.

It was suggested that a conceptual approach to health instruction might be a preferred way to reach the goal of the health-educated individual. Principles to consider when developing concepts, selecting content, and developing long-range goals and behavioral objectives were presented and discussed. The selection of teaching methods and learning opportunities as extensions of the goals and objectives of the course was discussed, and numerous methods that could be used in the classroom were enumerated.

Finally, the basic process of developing specific units and lesson plans was presented. By following the principles set forth in this chapter, those responsible for curriculum development in a school district should be able to

Organization of School Health Programs

produce a comprehensive, articulated plan for health instruction, regardless of the specific curriculum organizations employed in any given school district.

REVIEW QUESTIONS

1. What do the authors consider to be the major building block for the development of the curriculum? Why do you think that they ascribe to that thought?

2. Why is flexibility an important aspect of any curriculum planning?

3. Why do the authors state that a conceptual approach to learning will most likely produce results superior to other types of learning? Do you agree or disagree with their reasoning? Justify your response.

4. Why is it important that the health educator have familiarity with such fields as anatomy, physiology, chemistry, biology, genetics, medicine, sociology, anthropology, psychology, and education? Do you feel that any of these fields could be omitted from the professional training of the health educator? Justify your response.

5. What are the basic sources that may be used to select the content for health instruction? Are some of these sources superior to others? List the sources in order of importance from the most important to the least important. Defend your listing.

6. Distinguish between teacher and student objectives. Why is it important to understand this difference?

7. Distinguish between the various methods presented in the text about how to write behavioral objectives. What method do you feel is best? Why?

8. What are the important things to consider when selecting methods and learning activities in health instruction?

9. Why is it important to understand the advantages and disadvantages of the various methods that can be used in the classroom?

10. How would you characterize the creative teacher?

11. If the authors do believe in a conceptual approach to learning, why do you think they provided information on how to develop units of instruction?

12. Why are lesson plans an important part of curriculum development? Who should be responsible for the development of lesson plans? Should lesson plans be checked by the school administration? Why or why not?

13. Why is it important that a professionally qualified health education specialist coordinate the curriculum development efforts in health education?

14. What do you think is the most important criterion to use when selecting a specific teaching aid for use in the classroom? Why is this the most important criterion?

15. Why do you think that many teachers, particularly at the upper grades, seem to rely on the lecture method to teach?

16. Analyze the various teaching methods that are presented in the chapter to determine which would be most useful and/or appropriate for the primary grades, the intermediate grades, and the upper grades.

17. Why do the authors indicate that seldom is one teaching method used in isolation? Present and justify your position relative to this issue.

REFERENCES

Allensworth, D., and C. Symons. "A Theoretical Approach to School-Based HIV Prevention." *Journal of School Health* 59(2):59–65, 1989.

Arizona State Board of Education. Administrative Rules and Regulations R7-2-303. *Sex Education.* Phoenix: Arizona Department of Education, December 4, 1978.

Brookbeck, M. "Logic and Scientific Method on Teaching." In Gage, N. L., ed. *Handbook of Research on Teaching.* Chicago: Rand McNally, 1965.

Byler, R., G. Lewis, and R. Trotman. *Teach Us What We Want to Know.* New York: Mental Health Materials Center, 1969.

Carter, J., and A. Lee. "Preactive Planning and Conceptions of Success in Elementary Health Education." *Journal of School Health* 59(2):79–80, 1989.

Connell, D., R. Turner, and E. Mason. "Summary of Findings of the School Health Education Evaluation: Health Promotion Effectiveness, Implementation, and Costs." *Journal of School Health* 55(8):316–321, (October 1985).

Cornacchia, C., L. Olsen, and C. Nickerson. *Health in Elementary Schools,* 8th ed. St. Louis: Times Mirror/Mosby College Publishing, 1992.

Denver Board of Education. *Health Interests of Children.* Denver: Denver Public Schools, 1954.

Eddy, J., R. St. Pierre, and W. Alles. "A Reexamination of Values Clarification for the Health Educator." *Health Education 16:* (Feb./March, 1985):36–39.

Fodor, J. T., and G. T. Dalis. *Health Instruction: Theory and Application,* 4th ed. Philadelphia: Lea and Febiger, 1989.

Gage, N. L., ed. *Handbook of Research on Teaching.* Chicago: Rand McNally, 1965.

Gronlund, N. E. *Stating Behavioral Objectives for Classroom Instruction.* New York: Macmillan, 1970.

Hayes, D., and S. Fors. "Self-Esteem and Health Instruction: Challenges for Curriculum Development." *Journal of School Health* 60(5):208–211, 1990.

Inhelder, B., and J. Piaget. *The Growth of Logical Thinking from Childhood to Adolescence.* New York: Basic Books, 1958.

Kryspin, W. J., and J. F. Feldhusen. *Writing Behavioral Objectives: A Guide to Planned Instruction.* Minneapolis: Burgess Publishing Company, 1974.

Lantagne, J. "Health Interests of 10,000 Secondary School Students." *Research Quarterly* 23 (October 1952).

Lovato, C., D. Allensworth, and F. Chan. *School Health in America: An Assessment of State Policies to Protect and Improve the Health of Students,* 5th ed. Kent, Ohio: American School Health Association, 1989.

Mager, R. F. *Preparing Instructional Objectives.* Palo Alto, Cal. Fearon Publishers, 1962.

National Adolescent Student Health Survey: A Report on the Health of America's Youth. Oakland, Calif: Third Party Publishing Co., 1989.

National Commission on the Role of the School and the Community in Improving Adolescent Health. *CODE BLUE: Uniting for Healthier Youth.* Alexandria, Va.: National Association of State Board of Education, 1990.

Oberteuffer, D., O. A. Harrelson, and M. B. Pollock. *School Health,* 5th ed. New York: Harper & Row, 1972.

Phenix, P. H. *Realms of Meaning.* New York: McGraw-Hill, 1964.

Pigg, R. M. ''Recent Developments in the Evaluation of School Health Education.'' *Health Education* 14:4 (July/August, 1983).

Raths, L. E., M. Harmon, and S. Simon. *Values and Teaching.* Columbus, Ohio: Charles E. Merrill, 1966.

''Report of the 1990 Joint Committee on Health Education Terminology.'' *Journal of Health Education* 22(2):97–107 (March/April, 1991).

Schaller, W. E. *The School Health Program,* 5th ed. Philadelphia: Saunders College Publishing, 1981.

School Health Education Study. *Health Education: A Conceptual Approach to Curriculum Design.* St. Paul, Minn.: 3M Education Press, 1967.

Sliepcevich, E. M. *School Health Education Study: A Summary Report.* Washington, D.C.: The School Health Education Study, 1964.

Sorochan, W. D., and S. J. Bender. *Teaching Elementary Health Science,* 2nd ed. Reading, Mass.: Addison-Wesley, 1979.

Superka, D., C. Ahrens, J. Hedstrom, L. Ford, and P. Johnson. *Values Education Sourcebook: Conceptual Approaches, Materials, Analysis, and an Annotated Bibliography.* Boulder, Co.: Social Science Education Consortium, 1976.

Taba, H. *Curriculum Development: Theory and Practice.* New York: Harcourt, Brace and World, 1962.

Trucano, L. *Students Speak: A Survey of Health Interests and Concerns: Kindergarten through Twelfth Grade.* Seattle, Wash.: Comprehensive Health Foundation, 1984.

U.S. Department of Health and Human Services. *Healthy People 2000: National Health Promotion and Disease Prevention Objectives.* Washington, D.C.: U.S. Government Printing Office Publication No. (PHS) 91-50121, 1991.

Woodruff, A. D. ''The Use of Concepts in Teaching and Learning.'' *The Journal of Teacher Education* (March 1964).

Yager, R., P. Kabarec, and B. Atwood. ''Assessing and Designing Statewide Comprehensive School Health Education Programs.'' *Health Education* 15(4):19 (June/July, 1985).

Current Health Instruction Curricula 18

N umerous attempts have been made to develop health instruction curricula in the United States. Those curricula have been developed not only by health educators, but also by an array of curriculum specialists; behavioral, biological, and physical science specialists; physical educators; and persons in other educational specialties. Unfortunately, these efforts have been made almost in isolation; therefore, no consistent and educationally sound philosophy of curriculum development exists. Isolated attempts often have done more damage than good.

Curriculum development is quite complicated, and few health educators totally understand all the processes involved. Basic is the ideal that it meet the needs and interests of both students and the community, while retaining the functional aspect of the instructional program. A variety of resources should be included in the development of the curriculum, including students, teachers, various community resources, and curriculum development experts who might be available from local colleges and universities. It is good to examine what others have done; too often, however, programs and curricula developed by others have been implemented without due consideration of suitabilities for the local situation, of the quality of the program, or of the impact of the program on students.

One of the pioneering efforts in the attempt to present a set of principles and procedures for the development of health education curricula was in the 1960s, under the direction of Dr. Elena Sliepcevich. A group of highly qualified health education experts generated a rather comprehensive K–12 health instruction program that employed a conceptual orientation for the organization of content. The document this group prepared has formed the basis for the development of numerous health instruction curricula across the United States. (See Chapter 15 for a detailed discussion of the School Health Education Study.) There have been many other curricula prepared, for use in a multiplicity of settings. This chapter includes examples of health instruction programs that are currently being used in the United States. It is important to understand that, of necessity, the descriptions of these programs are brief.

NATIONAL DIFFUSION NETWORK[1]

Since the passage of the Elementary and Secondary Education Act in 1965, literally millions of dollars have been spent to develop a variety of educational programs that are responsive to the needs of children. Many of these locally based programs were quite effective, but they were not disseminated to other school districts. In response to the wishes of Congress, in 1973 the U.S. Office of Education developed the National Diffusion Network (NDN).

It was recognized that if a program could be successful at the local level, perhaps it could be successful in other districts that had similar needs. Additionally, by informing school districts about programs that were successful, districts could save a great deal of money in the development stage and re-channel those resources into revising proven programs to meet the needs of the new district. All in all, the process became one of increasing cost-effectiveness by adopting high-quality education projects.

The NDN has five basic goals:

1. To stimulate positive educational change in local schools.
2. To help parents, teachers, and administrators find programs for children that match local needs.
3. To move programs quickly and cost-effectively to classrooms nationwide.
4. To help public and private schools secure information about new programs and support for their implementation in the district.
5. To ensure that nationwide communication about these programs continues among local school districts, intermediate service agencies, and state departments of education.

These goals help increase the flow of new ideas and enhance the impact of monies already spent to develop educational innovations.

Through the NDN, limited monies are available to increase local district avenues of exemplary programs; to assist schools with adoption decisions; to assist with in-service education and follow-up services; and, to a more limited degree, to assist in the purchase of instructional materials for use in the classroom implementation of programs.

The result of these efforts is that thousands of schools in every state have adopted NDN projects and in-service training. However, the true beneficiaries of NDN efforts are the students themselves.

What Constitutes an Exemplary Program?

For a program to be included on the NDN list of exemplary programs, project developers must present evidence that the project is educationally sound and cost-effective. This means that each program developer must prove, to a panel

---

1. The information contained in this section is adapted from a filmstrip and cassette on the National Diffusion Network prepared in 1979 by the U.S. Office of Education and from a pamphlet entitled "NDN, 7 Years of Helping Schools Meet Education Needs." Washington, D.C.: NDN, U.S. Dept. of Education.

of evaluation experts, that the program is effective in terms of cost per pupil; that it reaches the program's stated goals and objectives; and that it could be used in another school.

The Joint Dissemination Review Panel (JDRP)

Prior to being accepted as part of the NDN, a program undergoes close scrutiny by a panel of approximately 25 education and evaluation experts from the U.S. Department of Education. First appointed in 1972 (and originally called the Dissemination Review Panel), the Joint Dissemination Review Panel (JDRP) is specifically designed to assure that federal monies are spent only for quality programs with flexibility for use in districts other than those in which they were developed. This review also gives some national recognition to good programs. Although initially able to review only those programs developed with federal funds, the JDRP now has the latitude to review any type of educational program, regardless of the source of developmental funding. The only exception to this is that the JDRP will not review programs or products developed by proprietary concerns.

The process of attaining a program review for the possibility of joining the more than 400 NDN-approved projects is completely voluntary. Once program developers have decided to undergo JDRP review, a seven-step process is initiated.

Nomination

Depending upon the source of funding for a program, nomination for a JDRP review can occur in three ways. If developmental funding was from a federal level, the state program office that has responsibility for administering the federal funds can nominate the program. If the state program office does not institute nomination and the project developers desire review, they can request that the state program office initiate the nomination. Finally, if funds other than from federal sources were used for program development, the program developers can contact the Director of the Division of Educational Replication directly and request consideration for JDRP review.

Program Review

After nomination, the Director of the Division of Educational Replication conducts a preliminary review. This review is specifically focused upon the social framing of the program and the accuracy of the evidence that supports the effectiveness of the program. From this review a program may be rejected for further consideration, may be returned for revision of the application, or may be recommended for submission to the JDRP.

Summary of Program

Specific guidelines have been developed by the JDRP to be used in preparing a summary of a program nominated for review. This summary (a maximum of 10 pages) includes all of the basic support for program effectiveness.

Summary Review

Once the program summary has been prepared, it is again submitted to the federal program office. If all of the requirements set forth by both the federal program office and the JDRP are included in the summary, the program is sent to the JDRP. If the requirements are not met, the summary is returned for revision.

JDRP Meeting

Once three program summaries have been received by the executive secretary of the JDRP (and these programs do not have to be in the same topic area), a review meeting is scheduled. In general, this necessitates monthly meetings of the panel. The program and project staff is presented to the JDRP by an officer from the federal program office. This meeting is public, and it is advised that a person or persons familiar with the techniques employed to assess program effectiveness be in attendance to respond to questions that may arise.

JDRP Review

A minimum of seven JDRP members will review the project submission to determine if the evidence presented warrants approval of the program as educationally effective. This decision is made immediately following the review. Naturally, it is hoped that the majority decision is that the submitted program is effective, therefore worthy of dissemination. A second decision would be for nonapproval. However, nonapproval does not preclude resubmission for reconsideration at a later date.

Dissemination

If a program is given JDRP approval, it becomes eligible for NDN dissemination support, along with all other JDRP-approved programs.

Benefits of JDRP Approval

Several direct benefits accrue to any project reviewed by the JDRP, whether it is approved or not. These benefits include:

1. Assessment of the evaluation of the project by experts who can provide effective tools for subsequent evaluations.
2. Attainment of an objective view of the program, including suggestions for improvement in the evaluation component.

If the JDRP votes to approve the program, several additional benefits are realized:

1. Recognition of the program accomplishments at the local, state, and national level, bringing an affirmation of the effectiveness of the program.

Organization of School Health Programs

2. Increased possibility of winning competition for funds, since a program with proven effectiveness is less of a funding risk than an untested program.
3. Entry into a federal diffusion system that has dissemination funds available within the system.

NDN State Facilitators

The NDN consists of two major components. The first component is that of programs that are JDRP-approved. The second is that of enabling school districts to learn about and adopt JDRP, NDN-approved projects. This second component is met through a system of facilitators who are located in all 50 states, the District of Columbia, Puerto Rico, and the Virgin Islands. These state facilitators are central to the success of the dissemination of information about approved projects in a variety of curricular areas to local school district planners. These facilitators will convene awareness workshops to showcase proven programs to school districts that have expressed a need for new programs. Awareness workshops are held several times throughout the year, with no cost to the local school district.

If a local school district has a particular need in a curricular area, a representative of the district can contact the state facilitator for assistance. The facilitator can then help the district locate approved programs that match their needs. There are also limited funds available to assist school personnel who wish to visit sites of demonstration projects. In like fashion, the state facilitator can assist local program developers prepare for a JDRP review.

SELECTED SCHOOL HEALTH INSTRUCTION PROGRAMS

The next few pages contain examples of some of the more widely known elementary, junior high, and senior high school health instruction programs currently operational in the United States. It is not intended that this listing be exhaustive, since numerous school districts may have developed good programs without attaining a great deal of notoriety. It should also be noted that inclusion of a program does not connote endorsement of that program, nor does exclusion of a program connote rejection of that program.

The format of presentation of the representative health instruction programs will fall into the following broad categories: nationally validated programs (included in the NDN), state-based programs, locally based programs, programs developed by various health-related agencies, and commercially prepared programs.

Programs Included in the NDN[2]

The first health instruction program to be validated for inclusion in the NDN was a limited-focus drug education program designed for public and nonpublic school personnel who work with students in grades 1 through 6. Subsequently, one additional limited-focus program for grades 9–12, two limited-focus programs for elementary schools, and two relatively comprehensive health instruction programs for elementary schools have been approved by the JDRP.

The Me-Me Drug Prevention Education Program

The "Me-Me" program was approved by the JDRP on May 15, 1975. Initially developed for use in Appleton, Wisconsin, the project is intended to help public and nonpublic elementary school personnel to improve those conditions that seemed to be common to most teenagers who abuse drugs and alcohol. The program is based on the premise that if the conditions of low feelings of self-worth and the inability to make decisions can be improved, students will have less need to turn to drugs. Thus, the program is designed to prevent the problem before it begins.

A one-day training session provides teachers with strategies they can use to encourage positive feelings between students and teachers, gives them basic content about drug education, increases their knowledge and skills in helping students learn about themselves and how they value decisions, and helps the teachers develop an awareness of how their own feelings affect how they respond to students.

Project SCAT

Project SCAT (Skills for Consumers Applied Today) is a consumer education program in health and money management for high school students. The course is designed to acquaint students with basic economics and help them develop skills, concepts, and knowledge necessary for them to function as intelligent consumers in today's society. The six topics come in a self-contained booklet or PAL (Packaged Activities for Learning). There is also a PAL for the teacher. These booklets follow a common format throughout the six topics, are cartoon-illustrated, and contain both subjective and objective review questions. Content outlines, behavioral objectives, activities and suggested resources, and instructional aids (tests, activity sheets, film guides, and transparency masters) are contained in each of the six teacher PALs. Student competency tests, unit tests, transparency sets, and a teacher training manual are also available.

Growing Healthy

Growing Healthy is, in actuality, a combination of two programs that were approved for inclusion in the NDN. The first of the programs was the School Health Curriculum Project (sometimes referred to as the Berkeley Project),

---

2. Information in this section is adapted from *Educational Programs That Work,* a catalog of exemplary programs approved by the Joint Dissemination Review Panel, 9th ed. Washington, D.C.: U.S. Department of Education, 1983.

Organization of School Health Programs

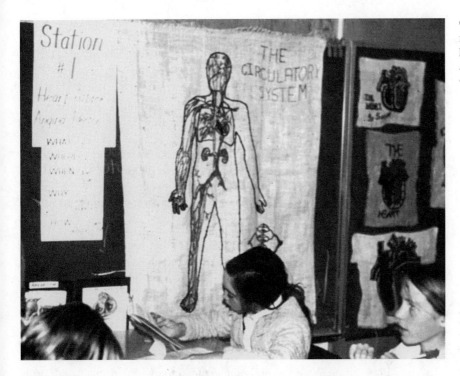

Growing Healthy is a multimedia approach to health education.
Photo courtesy, Center for Disease Control

and the Primary Grades Health Curriculum Project (sometimes referred to as the Seattle Project). The School Health Curriculum Project (SHCP) was the first relatively comprehensive health instruction program approved by the JDRP. That program was specifically developed for grades 4–6.

The companion project to the SHCP was the Primary Grades Health Curriculum Project (PGHCP). This project, specifically designed for grades K–3, was approved several years following the SHCP. These two projects have now been combined into the nationally known *Growing Healthy*—a comprehensive K–7 health education project currently being coordinated by the National Center for Health Education located in New York. The program is student-focused and is broad-based in scope.

The goals of *Growing Healthy* include:

1. Increase student knowledge and decision-making abilities about a wide range of health behaviors.
2. Help students learn how their personal health choices affect the functioning of their bodies.
3. Integrate classroom activities with other life situations.
4. Offer both students and teachers an experiential understanding of physical, mental, social, and emotional dimensions of their own health.

Growing Healthy is a broad-based, sequentially planned curriculum that employs a variety of teaching methods and uses a wide range of instructional media and aids. Central to the success of the project is an intense teacher training workshop designed to take the teachers through the planned learning activities they will be expected to replicate in their own classrooms.

Unique to the teacher training component is the nature of the team that is trained in each grade of the project. The team consists of two teachers from a specified grade level, their immediate building principal, and one or two additional support personnel (most commonly the school nurse, the district curriculum coordinator, a librarian, a health coordinator, or a departmental chairperson). This team is trained over a five- to ten-day period (depending upon where training is conducted) to become familiar with all the methods, materials, strategies, and philosophies embodied in the project.

Although the specific content of each grade-level unit varies, the general format of each unit remains constant. The basic organizational format of *Growing Healthy* is:

- Introduction: Motivational activities for the study of health.
- Awareness: The interactions between and among the body systems.
- Appreciation: A focus on the specific contributions of a given body system to overall body well-being.
- Structure and function: The specific physiology and anatomy of a given system.
- Diseases and disorders: Select health problems that affect the system being studied.
- Prevention: What the individual can do to avoid various health problems studied throughout the unit. A basic stress on wellness behavior is included.
- Culmination: A general overview of the entire unit of instruction, designed by students and presented to their parents at a special parents' night.

The project is designed primarily as a direct method of teaching, but integrative activities are interwoven throughout the curriculum. It has been referred to as a multi-media, student-centered, hands-on approach to health education.

The program at the various grade levels was developed around several themes as follows:

Kindergarten:	Happiness Is Being Healthy.
Grade 1:	Super Me.
Grade 2:	Sights and Sounds.
Grade 3:	The Body: Its Framework and Movement.
Grade 4:	About Our Digestion and Our Nutrition.
Grade 5:	About Our Lungs and Respiration.
Grade 6:	About Our Hearts and Circulation.
Grade 7:	Living Well with Our Nervous System.

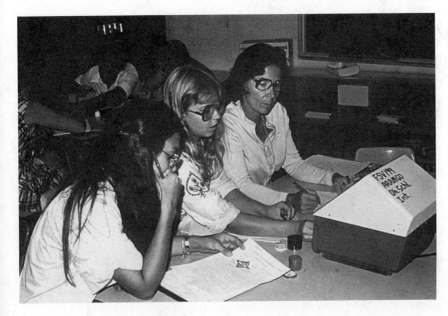

Inservice training is an important part of many health education programs.

As mentioned previously, each of the units of instruction follows the same basic pattern. However, new material that is developmentally appropriate is introduced in each unit. The units are designed to last approximately eight to ten weeks and for best results, should be taught daily for approximately one class period per day.

At present, *Growing Healthy* is the most widely disseminated health instruction program in the United States. Over 8000 school districts in 41 states and several international sites are currently using the project. The upper grade levels of the project (grades 4–7) were part of the nationally recognized School Health Education Evaluation (SHEE) conducted by Abt Associates of Cambridge, Massachusetts (Connell, Turner, and Mason, 1985).

The American Lung Association has been conducting an ongoing program of research relative to the effects of *Growing Healthy*, particularly on the smoking practices and the attitudes of students exposed to the program. The focus of this research has been within four selected demonstration centers from four school districts across the United States. Reports of these evaluation efforts are available from the national office of the American Lung Association.

Have a Healthy Heart

The fourth of the health instruction programs approved by the JDRP for inclusion in the NDN, *Have a Healthy Heart,* was developed in Bellevue, Washington and has been included in the NDN since 1980. The program is a heart health curriculum and aerobic fitness program designed for use in grades 4 through 6 in a physical education program, in science class, or in health education class. The course is designed as a supplement to existing curriculums and consists of separate fitness and life-style units, each with its own set of student materials. The project was developed by model classrooms and in cooperation with sports medicine physicians and members of the Heart Health and the Young Committee of the American Heart Association. The program combines aerobic activities and life-style mastery (including the effects of smoking, overweight, stress, heredity, exercise, cholesterol, and hypertension on heart disease) as central themes.

The materials contained in the project are designed for use by students for approximately 30 minutes, two or three times a week, over a three-month period. The aerobic segment of the program is designed to put students at a specified target heart rate for approximately 20 minutes three times per week. The basic goal of the program is to help students begin to learn the importance of exercise and fitness in preventing cardiovascular disease.

Incorporated into the program is a special teacher training component. The American Health Association and the Red Cross often participate in these training programs and provide follow-up services to school districts that adopt the program.

The results of various evaluations of the program have indicated that student knowledge about risk factors associated with cardiovascular disease improves, and the performance of students on general tests of physical fitness increases with involvement in the program.

A teacher's manual, a fitness program kit, four videocassettes, and various resource/enrichment packets are also available. These are obtained when teachers, for a nominal fee, attend the one-day training workshop, usually at a regional site.

Learning for Life

This project is designed specifically for grades 2 and 5. It is a nutrition and fitness program designed to help children learn how to make healthy, informed choices about food and fitness. The basic philosophy of the program developers is that early positive experiences with good food and good physical activity will lead to lifetime commitment to good health.

The second-grade program builds on a series called "The Doofus Stories." This 10-week, daily program is a story that contains a lot of nutrition information. It is accompanied by 52 student worksheets, as well as by many nutrition and fitness activities designed for use in the classroom, the home, or physical education classes.

For the fifth grade, the program combines factual nutritional information with challenging and fun activities. It is designed to take place on a daily basis over a 16-week period of time. It is partially adapted from the program *From the Inside Out*.

Specific teacher training is not required, but a teacher's guide and resource manual are available at nominal cost.

State-based Programs

Although the education codes in 43 states specify that health instruction be a part of the public school curriculum, it is seldom defined in terms of time allotments or the scope of that health instruction. In general, the teaching of drug, alcohol, and tobacco misuse is the most commonly mandated topical area. Seven states (California, Colorado, Florida, Illinois, New York, North Carolina, and Vermont) have gone a step further and have more sweeping legislation that defines health instruction and recommends specific topics to be included in the curriculum.

The Illinois legislation is called enabling legislation. This legislation enables the Superintendent of Public Instruction to develop specific guidelines for health instruction. The legislation further states that "instruction shall include but not be limited to. . . ." In this way, a great deal of latitude was provided individual school districts in developing health instruction curricula that were responsive to local needs.

Rather detailed frameworks for health instruction have been developed in North Carolina and California. A progression chart for health instruction was developed in Pennsylvania, and the State Board of Education in Arizona has recently revised their list of essential skills or competencies in health instruction for students in grades 1 through 8. Arizona has also added a 9–12 component.

In the fifth edition of *School Health in America* (Lovato et al., 1989, p. 10) recently published by the American School Health Association, it was noted that the state boards of education or the legislatures in 43 states have addressed some form of health instruction in policy or position statements, resolutions, administrative regulations, or bylaws. Additionally, 32 states require health education to be taught sometime during K–12; 13 additional states require a combination of physical education and health education. A total of 19 states require health education to be taught sometime during grades 1 through 6, and 3 additional states combined the health education requirement with physical education. Forty-four states have an administrative office at the state level that has specific responsibility for directing and supervising health education in the public schools, but no such office is present for private schools.

Pennsylvania Health Curriculum Progression Chart (PHCPC)

In 1982, the Pennsylvania Department of Education provided funds to the Pennsylvania Association of Health, Physical Education, Recreation and Dance for the purpose of developing a health curriculum progression chart. The final product was the result of many hours of work by dedicated professionals who drew extensively upon previously developed materials, especially those curriculum progression charts from the School Health Education Study (1967), the Health Education Curricular Progression Chart (National Center for Health Education, 1980), and from the Pennsylvania Department of Education *Project 81 Student Outcome Statements* (1981).

Although not intended to be a state-mandated guideline, the *Pennsylvania Health Curriculum Progression Chart* does provide local school districts with a well-developed scope and sequence of health instruction objectives that could be accomplished by a student. By drawing upon previously developed and proven scope and sequence charts, the developers of PHCPC have been able to pull the strongest elements from those prior works and have focused on objectives that facilitate life-style development and healthy behaviors in grades K through 12. This chart is being reviewed for possible revision.

California Framework

The *Framework for Health Instruction in California Public Schools* (1972) was originally published in 1970 and reviewed in 1978 by the California State Department of Education. The purpose of the framework was to assist local school district personnel to plan a sequentially based program of health instruction for grades K through 12.

The framework evolved from an assessment of the health needs of school-age children in California and incorporated a conceptual approach involving three multidisciplinary goals. These goals were self-awareness, decision making, and coping action. The scope of the framework contains ten basic topical areas (personal health, family health, nutrition, mental–emotional health, use and misuse of substances, diseases and disorders, consumer health, accident prevention and emergency health services, community health, and environmental health).

The framework includes an overview, major concepts, specific grade-level concepts, and suggested level behavioral objectives and content for each of the ten topic areas. The concepts or generalizations form the major points that should be the focus of the health instruction classroom. Since the framework's original development, it has been widely distributed throughout the United States and forms the basis for many health instruction programs at the local level. At present this framework is being revised and may be available in late 1992.

North Carolina Framework

The North Carolina Department of Public Instruction's *A Framework for Health Education* (1985) uses process, concept, and topic concept interaction as a base for developing specific behavioral objectives and classroom activities in health instruction. Values clarification, decision making, and self-actualization are the major process areas contained in the 13 content topics. Each of the content topics contains grade-level concepts directly related to the various topic areas. Basic activities, which were written specifically in order to integrate topic and process, have been developed for each of the behavioral objectives.

Arizona Comprehensive Health: Essential Skills

As mentioned in Chapter 15, in 1983 Arizona drafted an initial set of competency-based skills that all students who graduate from grade 8 should have. In 1989 these skills were reassessed and revised and a component for high school students (grades 9–12) was added. The skills that were specified were termed ''essential skills'' that a student should have when he or she graduates from high school in Arizona. Unfortunately, health education is only required at the elementary level, thus the high school skills may not be evaluated in

Organization of School Health Programs

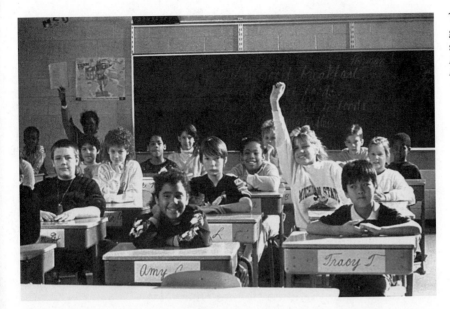

The *Michigan Model* generates a great deal of student enthusiasm.
Photo courtesy, Michigan Department of Education

any systematic fashion. Examples of selected skills and key indicators from the *Arizona Essential Skills* framework were presented in Chapter 15.

Michigan Model

The *Michigan Model* is another example of a state-based program that evolved from the efforts of many individuals over a 10-year time period. Sometimes referred to as the "Wellness Curriculum," the *Michigan Model* is a combination of many components of existing programs tempered with local reality. The purpose of the model is to aid in the avoidance of the fragmentation of health education in terms of the many projects in health education that are available.

The curriculum consists of about 60 lessons per grade level for the elementary grades, and 50 lessons each for grades 7 and 8. Included in the model are the ten basic content areas suggested by most health education experts. Also included is a teacher training component that requires a minimum of 30 hours of training, designed to acquaint teachers who will be implementing the model with the philosophy, content, process, and materials contained in the curriculum.

Locally Based Programs

Many local school districts have developed either broad or limited-focus health instruction curricula. Many of these efforts have been recognized as exemplary health education programs by the Metropolitan Life Foundation *Healthy Me Initiative* from programs that applied for such recognition. There are programs that may be exemplary, but did not apply for recognition. However, some of the programs that were recognized include the Decatur City

Schools (Decatur, Georgia), Apache Junction Unified School District (Apache Junction, Arizona), Clovis Unified School District (Clovis, California), Suffield Public Schools (Suffield, Connecticut), Horace Mann School for the Deaf and Hearing Impaired (Allston, Massachusetts), Grafton School District No. 3 (Grafton, North Dakota), and Western Albemarle High School (Crozet, Virginia). The descriptions of these programs are adapted from the Compendium of Award Winning Programs (Metropolitan Life Foundation, 1990). *The Sunflower Project* in Shawnee Mission, Kansas is also a program that has received widespread acclaim.

Decatur City Schools

The program developed in Decatur is called *My Best Me* and is designed for grades K–5. The program used creative motivational techniques to develop a feeling of wellness in children. Included in the activities portion of this multimedia health program are field trips, making models of parts of the body, growing plants, participating in community-wide science fairs, and conducting fund-raising drives for health campaigns.

Apache Junction Unified School District

This is a program that supplements the state's more basic essential skills that have been developed. Included in the program is training for self-protection, desert survival, and coping skills. Also included are drug abuse prevention and AIDS education. The curriculum is designed to be flexible so that the individual needs of the schools in the district can be included. The program is designed for K–12.

Clovis Unified School District

Designed as a preschool–grade 12 program, the goal of the program is to provide knowledge and decision-making skills for the development of positive, life-changing health habits for all students in the district. Activities in the program go beyond the classroom to the cafeteria as well as on the various school campuses. Special efforts are expended to reach high-risk adolescents such as teenage parents and their infants, and Southeast Asian refugees who have settled in the area.

Suffield Public Schools

Also designed as a K–12 program, this unique health education program incorporates weekend trips and community meetings into its format. *Life Education* is designed to assist students acquire self-knowledge, improve self-esteem, gain health knowledge, and develop decision-making skills. The program is also incorporated into the physical education program and involves classroom teachers, physical educators, nurses, guidance counselors, local medical professionals, the clergy, personnel from the fire department, as well as other community health resources. Key elements of the program include sexuality, love, prejudice, substance abuse, nutrition, stress management, environmental health, and the medical system.

Organization of School Health Programs

Horace Mann School for the Deaf and Hearing Impaired

This may be the only program of its kind. This curriculum concentrates on human growth and development with special education about AIDS. It provides physically challenged students a foundation for decision making, responsibility for behavior, and the importance of self-esteem. An integral part of the program is an after-school program which provides an alternative to high-risk behavior, and a peer education program. The peer education component is designed to let students help each other, particularly younger students being helped by older students. Community health organizations assist in the program by providing exhibits and materials at health fairs and demonstrations, both in the classroom and in the community setting.

Grafton School District 3

This is an integrative program designed for grades K–12. The program is designed to raise student consciousness in health matters, even outside of classes specifically devoted to the topic. Health content is integrated into all subject matter in the curriculum. For example, presentations on AIDS may be developed for a speech class and material on drug abuse may be incorporated into a typing class. A broad spectrum of content is included—mental health, decision making, disease prevention, community health, environmental health, drug abuse, safety, exercise, sexual responsibility, and stress management. There is a special annual teacher in-service training in teenage pregnancy, stress, discipline, suicide, chemical abuse, and AIDS education.

Western Albemarle High School

The major goals of this 9–12 program are to increase students' knowledge about good health, foster decision-making skills, and provide enriching activities beyond the classroom. Contemporary health issues are the focus of instruction. Many professionals from the community participate in the myriad of classroom activities which include use of health assessments, simulations, games, behavioral contracts, a CPR course, as well as community-based efforts such as "Jump Rope for Heart" and the "Great American Smokeout."

Sunflower

The Sunflower Project has brought together many health agencies in the Shawnee Mission school district in addition to drawing upon personnel from the University of Kansas Medical School and UK's Department of Health, Physical Education, and Recreation. Project developers refer to the project as "a working model of cooperation."

The project consists of four major units of instruction. These include units on nutrition, fitness, cardiovascular health, and respiratory health. The goals of the program are as follows:

1. To teach children fundamentals of good health and fitness.
2. To create a positive attitude within students about themselves, their nutrition, and their life-style that will carry over into later life.

3. To provide each student with a positive experience that will demonstrate the feeling associated with good personal health and fitness.

The program was specifically developed for grades K through 6 and has teaching modules that include basic content for each subject, test materials, and suggested teaching activities. It is designed to supplement the district's already comprehensive health instruction program.

Programs Available Through Health-Related Agencies

A number of voluntary health agencies have developed health instruction curricula that, in general, are designed to supplement existing health instruction programs. Examples of these include the American Heart Association, the American Cancer Society, the National Society to Prevent Blindness, and the National Dairy Council.

Putting Your Heart into the Curriculum

This K through 12 cardiovascular health instruction program, developed by the American Heart Association, consists of a resource guide and teaching modules to be used to supplement the regular health instruction program. The activities are designed to affect the health behaviors of students. The following areas are included:

1. Choosing not to smoke.
2. Making informal and healthful food choices.
3. Developing a habit of regular physical exercise and weight control.
4. Maintaining a blood pressure within normal limits.
5. Having a good knowledge of the risk factors associated with the development of cardiovascular disease.
6. Knowing how to make effective and intelligent use of the health care system.

Specific instructional modules have been developed for the following:

1. Cardiac physiology.
2. Risk-factor education.
3. Nutrition.
4. Antismoking.
5. Emergency procedures.

These modules have been developed for grades K through 2; 3 through 5; 6 through 8; and 9 through 12. Local chapters of the American Heart Association make available much of the material needed for the program. Depending upon the quantity of material ordered, there may be a slight charge.

An Early Start to Good Health

This program, developed by the American Cancer Society, is a four-unit program designed for grades K through 3. The program is self-contained and includes teacher guides, filmstrips, posters, phonograph records, and student activity sheets. The major concentration of the program is on tobacco, alcohol, and drugs. The four units of instruction are:

Unit 1: My Body—Designed to help students understand that the body functions best when all its systems are cared for and remain healthy.

Unit 2: Myself—Teaches the concept of self and helps students understand the difference between inner and outer selves.

Unit 3: My Health—Covers what is necessary to maintain health and a vital body, including good health habits, nutritional needs, exercise, and emotional outlets.

Unit 4: My Choice—Shows students that they control their lives and their futures through the various choices that they make.

Health Network

The continuation of the previous program was also developed by the American Cancer Society for use in grades 4, 5, and 6. The three units of instruction are as follows:

Unit 4: Special People—Cigarettes don't enhance self-image and a person need not be a ''star'' to be valuable.

Unit 5: Health News—A simulated television broadcast that reports on how the respiratory system uses oxygen in the process of respiration.

Unit 6: Starga's World—A girl from outer space visits earth and learns how to make decisions about herself and her health.

Each unit consists of a filmstrip and either a phonograph record or audio-cassette that provides a story about the unit. The program is designed to supplement existing health instruction curricula.

Nature of Cancer

The American Cancer Society has developed two limited-focus programs, one for junior high school and one for senior high school, on the nature of and the problems associated with cancer. These two packets consist of a teacher introduction, student activities background information for the student, student activity sheets, vocabulary lists, review tests, and transparencies.

As with the other American Cancer Society programs, the program is designed to supplement existing health instruction programs. Appropriate audiovisual aids, filmstrips, and booklets may be obtained free of charge from the local affiliate of the American Cancer Society.

An Option to See

This is a program of vision health and safety education for grades 7 through 12. The program was developed by the National Society to Prevent Blindness to encourage students to use safety eyewear whenever it is needed. It is particularly appropriate for students in lab and shop classes.

A 17-minute 16mm film is included with the program. This film shows dramatically how safety eyewear can prevent serious eye injury. Also included is a resource guide that contains duplicating masters, tests, attitude surveys, first aid information, overhead transparencies, a poster, and a medicine cabinet first aid sticker. Parental letters in English and Spanish are also included.

Food: Your Choice

The National Dairy Council designed this program as a nutrition education program in grades 1 through 10. (There is also a kindergarten program entitled *Food: Early Choice*, which will not be discussed in this text.)

The program is sequential and activity-oriented. The three purposes of the program are to:

1. Foster an understanding of the lay concept of nutrition.
2. Convey the importance of nutrition in preventing health problems.
3. Encourage maintenance of a healthy body.

The four levels obtained in the program are as follows:

Level 1: This is designed for use in grades 1 and 2. Hands-on experiments and meal preparation are stressed.

Level 2: Designed for use in grades 3 and 4, the concepts in Level 1 are expanded. The role of food in society and the consequences of poor food selection and eating patterns are explored.

Level 3: This level, designed for grades 5 and 6, focuses on a study of nutrients in food, as well as an analysis of factors that influence eating patterns, and food selection and advertising.

Level 4: This level actually contains four separate kits designed to integrate nutrition education with health, home economics, social studies, and science at grades 7 through 10. Specific integrative activities for each specialty area are available.

Most state dairy council offices have staff members who conduct teacher training workshops designed to acquaint school personnel with the program. Evaluation components are also included in the program.

Commercially Prepared Programs

Numerous school districts rely upon commercially prepared health instruction programs as a basis for local curriculum development. In general, these programs are based upon textbooks written for a specific grade level. Several elementary school health instruction textbook series are available, as well as separate high school health instruction textbooks. Sources for these textbooks are listed in Appendix C.

Commercial companies prepare various types of instructional media; however, the programs they develop are self-serving. The curricula they develop generally incorporate the various material aids that they also manufacture.

Two such programs are the *Health Activities Project,* distributed by Hubbard Scientific Company, and *Health Skills for Life* developed in Eugene, Oregon.

Health Activities Project (HAP)

Initially developed by personnel at the Lawrence Hall of Science at the campus of the University of California, Berkeley, the project has now been turned over to Hubbard Scientific Company. HAP relies on the active involvement of students and is designed as a series of activities to supplement existing health instruction programs. A basic assumption of the program developers is that by learning how the human body functions, students will realize how to improve their health.

A total of 58 different activities are included in the HAP. A teacher's guide supplements the program and contains a description of each activity, the health background for that activity, the amount of space needed, and what materials are needed. The main purpose of HAP is to make students more aware of the control they have over the health of their own bodies.

Health Skills for Life

This is a K–12 program which is a skill-based program originally funded by the Oregon State Department of Education as part of a Title IV C grant. Developed in the Eugene, Oregon public schools, it is now available through a private, commercial company that carries the same name as the project. Consisting of 118 units of instruction, the project encompasses all of the major content areas that are considered to be a part of the comprehensive health education curriculum. For each K–8 grade level, 7 to 12 units of instruction have been developed. For the high school level, 35 units of instruction are available. Because each grade level is packaged separately, a school system can select those units that are responsive to the specific needs within the system. Each unit is a self-contained entity, so the flexibility is maximized.

The goal of the program is to enable students to practice health behaviors in the dimensions of physical, emotional, mental, and social health. The basic units were designed as competency-based units so the student should be able to demonstrate the various behaviors that are included. This process also facilitates the evaluation of the various units of instruction. Also included are performance indicators, health content, and a set sequence of activities that assist the student develop skills that lead toward the terminal skill in the unit. There are suggestions offered relative to ways that the material can be integrated into other curricular areas such as mathematics, reading, and writing.

A 3½-hour teacher training component is an integral part of the program, as is a detailed scope and sequence chart. This chart allows teachers to "track" what occurred prior to a given unit, as well as what is to follow. Optional resource materials that could be included in the program are also mentioned. There is also a 2-hour administrator training program that is offered by the project developers.

This program has been validated by the Oregon State Department of Education and was selected in 1985 as one of the first exemplary health education programs awarded the "Healthy Me" certificate by Metropolitan Life Foundation.

SUMMARY

As stated at the outset, the programs described in this chapter represent the tip of the iceberg in terms of health instruction programs. If local school personnel are planning to develop a health instruction program, they would be wise to examine programs that have been previously developed very carefully. However, the critical elements in each program must be identified to see if they are consistent with local needs and interests. Further, each program should be assessed for flexibility, ease of implementation, and comprehensiveness. Districts should seek the assistance of persons familiar with both the concept of curriculum development and the content materials of health instruction. This assistance may be obtained from the state facilitator, the state department of education, or health educators who are based in universities and colleges. Dale W. Evans has developed a short poem that summarizes the dilemma of anyone involved in developing health instruction curricula:

OH, CURRICULA, PLEASE ANSWER MY PRAYERS

Dale W. Evans

Before the 1960s life seemed so simple:
Most curricula were based on the knowledge principle.
Few worried about skills, let alone behavior,
Although such curricula had not much flavor.

During the '60s education discovered
Some new ideas not previously covered.
Objectively speaking, Bloom made a great find,
Krathwohl's attitudes opened our minds.

The School Health Education Study provided a quirk,
Something entitled a conceptual framework.
That overhead projector became a useful tool,
Hundreds of transparencies for each grade in school.

On the West Coast—you know, where everything begins—
The Berkeley Project was born with hopes for a win.
It started slowly and changed its name;
Today 32 states know of its fame.
Values clarification seemed like an answer to a prayer;
The way of dealing with attitudes seemed fair.
Affective-Humanistic Education soon followed
Although some questioned whether such ideas were hallowed.

Now it's drugs, health promotion, and STDs;
Thoughts of all these bring me to my knees!
To whom can I turn to reduce my fear
When thousands of curricula suddenly appear?

This help seems confusing, boggling the mind.
Oh, curricula, please tell me, what I can find?
Those letters you use really confuse me:
There's HECG, KYB, and, of course, HAP.

Oh, wait just a minute, before I'm consumed.
Are those curricula for me—what shall be presumed?
Forget not the *students,* their *ideas* and *needs,*
Should become the health educator's personal creed!

REVIEW QUESTIONS

1. Why do you think that the authors gave examples of health instruction curricula in this text?
2. What is the National Diffusion Network? Why is this an important ally for the schools?
3. Why is the Joint Dissemination Review Panel important? What is the process they follow in examining a program for possible inclusion in the National Diffusion Network?
4. What are some of the benefits a program receives as a result of becoming a part of the National Diffusion Network?
5. Obtain local courses of study in health instruction and examine them for completeness relative to the principles that have been set forth for curriculum development.
6. What words of caution would you offer a school district whose board of education wishes to adopt an existing health instruction curriculum? How would you convince them of your wisdom in making these suggestions?
7. What commonalities do you see in the various locally developed health education programs that are contained in the text?

REFERENCES

California State Department of Education. *Framework for Health Instruction in California.* Sacramento: The Department, 1972.

Connell, D., R. Turner, and E. Mason. "Summary of Findings of the School Health Education Evaluation: Health Promotion Effectiveness, Implementation, and Costs." *Journal of School Health 55* no. 8 (October 1985): 316–321.

Evans, D. "Oh Curricula, Please Answer My Prayers," *Health Education* 14(2) (Mar/Apr, 1983), p. 35.

Evans, N. "Advancing School Health Education via the National Diffusion Network." *Health Education* 11(5):10 (Sept/Oct, 1981).

Metropolitan Life Foundation. *Compendium of Award Winning Programs.* New York: Met Life, 1990.

National Center for Health Education. *Health Education Curricular Progression Chart* (from the PGHCP and the SHCP). San Bruno, Cal.: NCHE, 1980.

North Carolina Department of Public Instruction. *A Framework for Health Education.* Raleigh: The Department of Public Instruction, 1985.

Pennsylvania Department of Education. *Project 81: Student Outcome Statements.* Harrisburg: Pennsylvania Department of Education, 1981.

Pine, P. *Promoting Health Education in Schools—Problems and Solutions, Critical Issues Report.* Arlington, Virginia: American Association of School Administrators, 1985, pp. 42–51.

School Health Education Study. *Health Education: A Conceptual Approach to Curriculum Design.* St. Paul: 3M Company, 1967.

State Advisory Council on Health Education. *Planning Health Education Programs in Oregon Schools—Administration.* Salem, Ore.: Oregon State Department of Education, 1978.

University of the State of New York, State Education Department. *Suggested Guidelines for the Development of Courses of Study in Health Education.* Albany: The Department of Education, 1970.

Organization of School Health Programs

Evaluation of the School Health Program

19

E valuation—the very word makes students quake, gives teachers headaches, and causes administrators to develop ulcers. Everyone is sure that the "vulture public" is waiting to leap on the "carrion school," laid bare as a result of the evaluative process. Accountability is a watchword in today's society, and rightly so. Parents have entrusted a great deal to teachers; it is only appropriate that this trust be proved to be warranted.

Evaluation is important to teachers. Teachers want to know if they have had an effect on students' learning. They want to know what they did well and what they did not do well. They want to improve their art. They want to improve the science of teaching.

Evaluation is important to school administrators. They have been societally designated the responsibility of making sure that the nation's children have the opportunity to learn at an optimal level. As knowledge expands, this responsibility expands.

There is yet another concern. The school-age child spends six or more hours in school each day. When parents send their child to school, they expect that the child will learn, and that this learning will occur in an atmosphere free of unnecessary hazards. Further, these parents expect to be notified if their child experiences a health problem that could be detrimental to that child's learning.

Evaluation is important to the school-age child. For some, the only thing that truly matters is getting the "A" in a class. But what of the student who has the potential for the "A" but never seems to reach that potential? What if that potential is thwarted because of a health problem? It is the responsibility of everyone involved with the school system to be constantly aware of what is happening in the school. This too is evaluation.

Evaluation is so important to the overall functioning of the school that most educators probably believe they are living in an "evaluation generation" (Popham, 1975, p. 1). Willgoose (1972, pp. 389–390) exemplifies this when he states:

> The concept of accountability links student performance with teacher performance; it relates precise educational objectives; and it brings improved measurement techniques and evaluation practices to bear on educational programs and subject matter areas. Very specifically, it means that schools are being judged on how well they perform, not on what they promise.

Participation in health fairs helps students develop an appreciation of positive health and serves as a method of evaluating student achievement.

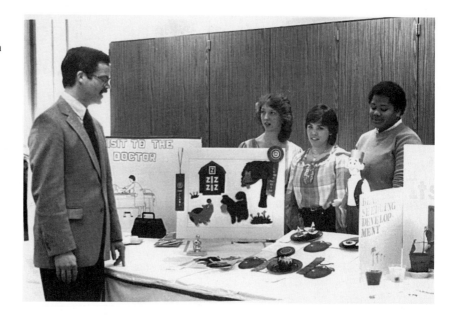

There is a very vocal movement to go back to basics in the nation's schools. This means the schools are having to do some serious introspection to determine what skills are needed to function effectively in today's society. The only way the school has of determining its effectiveness is to evaluate.

Evaluation is a very complicated process, particularly in the area of the school health program. This problem is compounded by the fact that extremely precise measurement instruments are not available. Additionally, efforts in behavior change might not manifest themselves until years after the student has left school. According to Combs (1979, p. 72):

> It is possible . . . that the means we choose to achieve accountability may boomerang to destroy or impede the goals of education.

One should also keep in mind that regardless of the precision of the measurement tool, if the objective being measured is not well developed, or is "off the mark," the precision of the evaluation will not correct the poor objective. Rather, the evaluation may support the fact that imprecise objectives are being attained. If the objectives being measured are not appropriate, for whatever reason, the evaluation will not be very useful in determining the strengths and weaknesses of the program. It should also be clear that if the objective is too idealistic (e.g., promising or guaranteeing behavior change), educators may be setting themselves up for failure, from an evaluation standpoint, as well.

For example, the purpose or objective of a program in the area of drug education—to change student behavior so that no student experiments with illicit drugs—may be unattainable. The objective of a school services program—to identify every child who has a health defect that might impact on

Organization of School Health Programs

his or her learning—also may not be attained since screening may produce some false negatives. If the objective of the healthful school environment program is to eliminate all accident hazards, the basic tenet of safety that the potential for accidents exists, regardless of the environment, has been forgotten. As a result, the mere impreciseness of possible measurement instruments should not be discouraging. Educators should continue to strive to make evaluation instruments as precise as possible, but efforts should also be made to state realistic objectives. Clearly, evaluation is a challenge to everyone involved in the school health program, teachers, medical personnel, administrators, students, staff, and parents.

It is unfortunate that school health programs have been under a great deal of fire over the past few years. The general public has the mistaken idea that the school health program should show immediate results. Regardless of the preciseness of measurement techniques, it is questionable whether anyone will ever be able to say, ''Johnny never had a heart attack because he had a health instruction course in grade six, where he learned the risk factors associated with the development of cardiovascular disease.'' Educators would like to think that the sixth grade program may have affected Johnny in such a manner that he opted to engage in healthful rather than unhealthful practices. We can measure the effect of the program on his knowledge and, to a lesser degree, on his attitudes. From this, it can be suggested that his behavior was affected. The bothersome thing here is that we cannot compare the health of Johnny to an ''identical Johnny'' who did not have the health program. Environmental conditions, new advances in medical science, the maturity of the individual, and a myriad of other factors may impede or expedite a behavior change.

In this chapter, some basic information about the application of evaluation to the total school health program is discussed. It should be noted that the suggestions offered are not meant to be all-inclusive. Rather, they are an attempt to develop a concept of evaluation that those in the schools might apply to their own situation.

EVALUATION DEFINED

Evaluation differs from measurement. Measurement is the part of evaluation wherein a particular attribute is counted or enumerated. The number of items a student answers correctly on a knowledge test is an example of measurement. It is a process used to quantify—assign numbers to ''objects.''

Evaluation uses measurement to determine the value of an attribute relative to a stated objective or purpose. It is subjective, since it represents value judgments derived from a compilation of measurements. Its purpose is for assessment and improvement.

The Joint Committee on Evaluation of School Health Programs of the American Public Health Association, in 1955, stated that evaluation was appraising something according to a set of values or criteria (1955, p. 2). These values or criteria generally emanate from two sources. The first is the set of objectives that has been developed at the local level. Obviously, the objectives represent what local planning committees feel is important within the school structure. The second source has a broader base, which is the recommended practices or standards as developed by professional organizations, agencies, joint committees, and the like. Both sets of criteria must be used if evaluation is to be meaningful.

Evaluation must be both quantitative (How much?) and qualitative (How well?). Such things as test scores, the number of food service or health service personnel, the number of visits to the school nurse, the number of health instruction classes, and the number of cartons of milk served at the school lunch counter are all quantitative data.

Qualitative data, on the other hand, are much more subjective. It is through qualitative data that we try to determine how effective we have been with our efforts. If a child visits the school nurse, was the nurse efficient and effective in handling the child's problem? Is the nutritional value of the meals served worth the cost and effort of preparing them, and do the meals truly benefit the child in terms of promoting health? The daily observations of teachers are also a source of qualitative data.

Evaluation may be both subjective and objective. Subjective data may be gathered using anecdotal records of teachers and staff, administrators, parents, or students; by using observational techniques and by asking "opinion" questions of a variety of people. Objective data may be obtained with tests, checklists, surveys, inventories, or by merely counting events.

Even though a particular technique for collection of data may be termed objective, it is important to remember that, for the most part, the object being measured and the way that object is being measured, may be subjective in nature. For example, when a teacher decides what items to include on an examination, the teacher most likely uses subjectivity to select items. The item may be "objective" in that it is associated with a particular behavioral objective, but the nature through which the item was developed may have been subjective. In the case of essay examinations, it is often quite difficult to remove personal bias when reading the response of a student; so is the resultant evaluation subjective or objective? Herein lies part of the dilemma of preciseness of measurement.

Whoever is conducting an evaluation must keep in mind two important concepts of evaluation—validity and reliability. Validity refers to preciseness of measurement. Is a particular question, observation, or checklist a "true" representation of the attribute in question? Are we evaluating what we want to evaluate? On the other hand, reliability refers to consistency of measurement. If the same instrument were to be used by the same individual again, would the results be the same? Further, if the same attribute were to be observed by two different evaluators or observers, would the two individuals "see" the same thing? As an example, if you ask a student to tell you how old he or she was on March 1, 1991 on three different occasions, the student most likely will give the same response each time. This is a reliable measure. If, however, you ask a student what he or she had for breakfast today and three months later you ask the same student what he or she had for breakfast three months ago, the results might be quite different. The reliability of the measurement is suspect. The results are not consistent. These concepts are discussed in greater depth later in the chapter.

Clearly it is beyond the scope of this text to discuss all of the nuances associated with evaluation. It is recommended that students enroll in a specific course that deals with measurement and evaluation. Regardless, there are some general considerations that must be discussed so that the individual becomes aware of some of the overarching issues associated with the evaluation of the school health program.

Oberteuffer, Harrelson, and Pollock (1972, p. 418) stated that once the decision to evaluate has been made, it is important to develop principles for the evaluative effort. They have suggested seven principles that have proven worthwhile:

1. Evaluation should be continuous and concurrent with program activities.
2. Evaluation should embrace all the important functions of the school health program, including instruction, services, and activities.
3. Evaluation should be concerned with outcome, process, and structure.
4. Evaluation should be cooperative. All who are affected by the evaluation should participate. This includes administrators, teachers, pupils, parents, physicians, nurses, hygienists, nutritionists, and community representatives.
5. Evaluation should be focused upon the important values that underlie the health program of the school. Those values are best expressed in terms of program objectives and goals stated during the program planning period.
6. A long-range evaluation program should be planned so that no one year will involve a complete study of every aspect of school health education.
7. Data gathering and record keeping should be performed to aid in the evaluation of the functions of school health education and not as ends in themselves.

These seven principles, though worthy, omit the school environment, a factor many people feel has a major impact on the overall learning of the school-age individual. What is high-lighted in these seven principles are the two major beneficiaries of the evaluation, the program and the student.

Creswell and Newman (1989, pp. 429–430) have set forth five purposes for program evaluation and five purposes for product or pupil evaluation. These ten points are as follows:

In the area of program evaluation, the following purposes are served:

1. To determine the present status of the school health program.
2. To assess progress made toward achievement of program objectives.

3. To provide information about program strengths and weaknesses.
4. To provide data that can be used as justification for seeking additional support and funds for the program.
5. To provide information about program activities as a basis for modifying the program in order to improve it.

Important purposes of pupil health evaluation are:

1. To determine pupil health status as well as individual health education status.
2. To provide information that will enable students to make self-evaluations and adjustments in their study programs in order to improve their progress.
3. To inform parents of their children's health status.
4. To provide data on students' learning achievements from the health instruction program that can serve as a basis for grading students.
5. To enable teachers and school officials to adapt school programs in order to meet the health and educational needs of children.

It is obvious that evaluation is both a process and a product. The method of evaluation, what is evaluated, who does the evaluation, when it is done, how it should be done, and how it is used are all important to consider. Regardless of all the various factors that are used to make decisions regarding the evaluation, it must be systematic. It must be carefully planned and conducted as part of the total educational effort within the school system.

USES OF EVALUATION

It would be nearly impossible to list all the specific uses of evaluation. However, Cornacchia, Olsen, and Nickerson (1992) have set forth ten major uses for evaluation:

1. To use as a diagnostic device. By knowing what students know prior to beginning a unit of instruction, or what they don't know, progress and increases in knowledge can be assessed.
2. To determine progress toward objectives and to appraise the changes in understandings, attitudes, and practices that result from learning experiences in health education.
3. To motivate pupils by stimulating their curiosity about specific health issues.
4. To identify students who may be in need of special health guidance or counseling.
5. To provide data useful in the continual revision of course and curriculum content.
6. To provide a basis for grading.
7. To provide a basis for meaningful parent education and involvement during parent–teacher conferences.

8. To provide information useful for program planning.

9. To improve instruction by providing feedback on teaching, methods, and instructional aids.

10. To develop good public relations for the health instruction program. [pp. 405–406]

This final use for evaluation could be expanded to include developing good public relations and support for the total school health program, not merely the instructional phase. This is particularly important if one subscribes to the expanded concept of the school health program as including school and community cooperative efforts (Lovato et al., 1989). It is also important to remember that in addition to the ten points above, parents should be kept informed and, in many cases, involved in the evaluation process. By doing this, parents may become more aware of the efforts of school personnel and actually alter what is done at home, thus reinforcing positive concepts being developed in the school setting. The importance of recognizing the impact of the sociocultural settings in which students interact cannot be underestimated when assessing changes in student behaviors. Parents are in a very advantageous position to assist in conducting evaluations of changes in student health behavior.

STEPS IN EVALUATION

Clearly, some parts of the school health program get more evaluative attention than others. However, regardless of how much attention is paid to each part, it is important to have a set plan for the conduct of the evaluation. Suffice it to say that there is no absolutely correct plan. One should also realize that evaluation does not occur as an isolated event. As it is completed, it exerts an impact on all who participate in the process.

In general, the steps to be followed in planning systematic evaluation include:

1. The objectives of the program must be clear to all persons who will be involved in the evaluation, and these objectives must be written in specific terms.

2. Specific criteria for determining success, derived directly from the objectives, must be stated.

3. A great deal of care should be taken to determine what data need to be collected, and a systematic plan for the recording and storage of those data must be developed.

4. Appropriate instruments that have reliability, validity, and objectivity must be identified. If these instruments cannot be located, appropriate instruments must be developed.

5. It must be determined if outside expert assistance is required to ensure that the evaluation is done objectively.

Availability of appropriate and sufficient amounts of equipment is important for good health instruction.

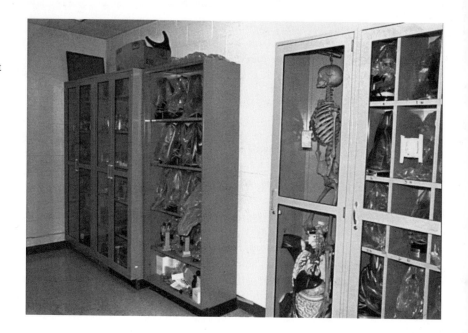

6. Conduct the data collection. Who will collect the data, how the data will be collected, and who will be responding to the data collection instruments should be identified. A pretest of the process will be quite useful.

7. Conduct a preliminary analysis of the data to determine if the necessary types and amounts of data have been collected. It may be necessary to go beyond the confines of the school to determine program impact.

8. Determine if additional data will have to be collected, what type data are needed, and how those data will be collected.

9. Develop a format for presenting the final report.

10. Present the results of the evaluation, following the format that was developed.

11. The strengths as well as the weaknesses of the program should be pointed out.

12. Offer recommendations for revising the program to maintain or enhance strengths while alleviating weaknesses. These recommendations might be such simple things as revising a few objectives. In other cases, major conceptual changes may be suggested. At any rate, be sure the recommendations are feasible and that they incorporate adaptability and flexibility into the program.

Whenever one attempts to evaluate the total school health program, it is important to identify instruments that can be used to assist in this endeavor. A rather comprehensive instrument was developed by the state of Ohio (Ohio

Department of Education, 1966, 35 pages). Consulting this instrument (see Appendix D) should help anyone who is either evaluating an existing school health program or developing a new school health program, for it contains most of the elements that should be contained if the program is to be comprehensive.

More recently an extremely comprehensive document that was designed to assist in the evaluation of the school health program was developed by Steven Nelson of the Northwest Regional Educational Laboratory (1984). This 240-page manual contains numerous checklists that can be used in determining the health-related activities that are carried on in any school. It is pointed out in the document that evaluation of the total school health program is most likely a team task since total evaluation is rather formidable for one individual. Complete evaluation of the total school health program generally will occur over a period of time rather than all at once.

WHAT SHOULD BE EVALUATED?

As presented throughout this text, the school health program consists primarily of three major facets: health services, school environment, and health instruction. Each of these segments should be evaluated separately as well as in combination with the other facets. For those who subscribe to the expanded, eight component school health program, suggestions for evaluations of all components will be included within the context of the more traditional school health program of services, instruction, and environment. It must also be remembered that the evaluation can be formal or informal. Although the following discussion focuses primarily on formal evaluation, the importance of informal evaluation must not be overlooked.

Evaluating School Health Services

Many individuals feel that evaluation of the school health services component of the health program is rather simplistic. In general, their basic question is, "Are the services available, yes or no?" This may be carried a bit further into various components of the school health service, but it is still an overly simplistic view.

Schaller (1981, pp. 193–194) has set forth nine objectives to be attained from the evaluation of school health services:

1. To appraise the health status of pupils and school personnel.
2. To counsel pupils, teachers, parents, and others for the purposes of helping students obtain health care and arranging school programs in keeping with their needs.
3. To help prevent and control communicable diseases.
4. To provide emergency care for injury or sudden illness.
5. To promote and provide optimum sanitary conditions and safe facilities.
6. To protect and promote the health of school personnel.

7. To provide concurrent learning opportunities that are conducive to the maintenance and promotion of individual and community health.
8. To maintain safety measures that will protect the health of pupils.
9. To plan services that will provide a healthy environment.

Since the three major components of school health services involve health appraisal, prevention of health problems, and follow-up or remedial aspects including health guidance and counseling, any evaluative effort should reflect those three components. Areas that should be rated include frequency of health appraisals, including health examinations and screening procedures for visual, auditory, dental, and mental health; growth and development assessment; preventive and control measures for communicable diseases; emergency care, including transportation and the presence of written emergency procedures; equipment; record keeping; teacher appraisal of the health of the pupils; health guidance and counseling; and the follow-up or remedial aspect of school health services.

Checklists will quickly lead to the conclusion that medical, dental, and guidance personnel are the key elements of a school health services program. However, the teacher spends far more time with the students than does any individual traditionally considered a part of the school health services program; thus, the teacher's role in the school health service should also be carefully evaluated. Cornacchia, Olsen, and Nickerson (1992, pp. 36, 49–50) suggest four areas where teachers have considerable responsibility in terms of the health services component: (1) observation for health problems, (2) emergency care, (3) follow-up programs, and (4) educational programs that complement some of the health services.

Teacher Observation

It is critical for the teacher to become a ''suspectition.'' The teacher should suspect that something may be wrong when a child continually rubs his or her eyes, squints, scratches his or her head, continually is thirsty, or has an unusual number of requests to go to the lavatory. This information must be given to the nurse or whomever is in charge of the school health program. To aid in training teachers in observational techniques, Metropolitan Life Insurance Company has developed a 16mm film entitled *Looking at Children*. We suggest that every prospective teacher view this film.

Emergency Care

All teachers will at some point in their careers be faced with an emergency situation. It may range from a simple bruise or scratch to a seizure, an asthma attack, a broken bone, or a major accident on the playground or in a crosswalk. The teacher must know the proper procedures to follow, thus avoiding the possibility of a lawsuit or, worse yet, the death or disabling of a student. Emergency care procedures should be written, distributed, and interpreted for everyone in the school. All teachers should be trained in first aid, or at least one person with these skills should be on duty whenever students are at school.

Follow-up Procedures

Whenever a child is referred for a health problem or is absent from school for a prolonged period, the teacher must be a part of the follow-up for that child. The teacher and nurse should have a conference to determine what should be done to help the student return to an optimal health state as quickly as possible. If a child has been absent for a prolonged period, teacher observation becomes even more critical. The teacher should know the signs of possible recurrence of the initial health problem and, if these symptoms begin to appear, referral should be immediate.

Educational Programs

During the course of the school year, a number of health-screening procedures such as vision and hearing testing may be performed. It would reinforce the procedures if the teachers could plan an educational program dealing with the same topic at the same time. The teacher can also serve as an interpreter of the results of the various screening procedures conducted in school and can assist in the conduct of the procedures. Thus, the teachers should also be familiar with basic principles of health guidance.

Evaluating the Healthful School Environment

The physical school environment is evaluated relatively easily with a checklist, especially since the school is expected to meet certain environmental, safety, and construction standards, as set forth by the local building authority. Such factors as the number of washbasins per 100 students, the student-to-commode ratio, the location and number of drinking fountains, and other quantitative attributes, such as ramps for the handicapped, are included in this category. Regular inspections of emergency equipment such as fire alarms and extinguishers must be made. Procedures to follow in case of fire, earthquake, tornado, hurricane, or civil defense problems should be written, understood, and practiced by all teachers and students on a regular basis. Having school disaster-preparedness drills should be a standard item when evaluating the school health environment.

Much more difficult to assess is the emotional environment of the school. This type of evaluation is qualitative and cannot be reduced to a checklist format; it may entail conducting interviews with administrators, teachers, other school staff, students, and parents.

Since children are required to be in school from ten to twelve years, it is an ethical responsibility to be sure that the environment is safe and free from unnecessary exposure to disease.

Evaluating Health Instruction

The health instruction component of the school health program will be the primary area of responsibility for the teacher. Evaluation of the health instruction component of the school health program should focus on two planes: process variables and product outcome variables. Process evaluation includes

Subjective evaluation
may involve assessing
student projects.

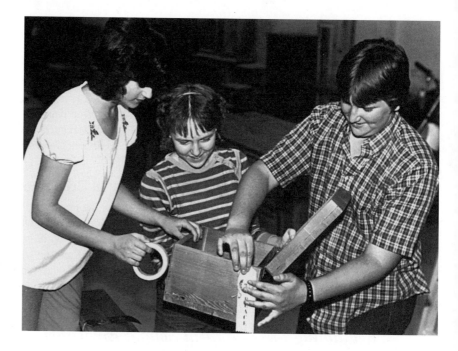

teaching methods or strategies used, teaching aids used, how objectives are
being met, the adequacy of instructional objectives in meeting student and
community needs and interests, how the curriculum guide (if one is available)
was developed and implemented, what content is included, and the total scope
and sequence of the curriculum.

Product or outcome evaluation is focused on the impact of the program
in terms of student knowledge, attitudes, and practices. It relates to specific
program objectives, as well as the impact of the program on teachers, administrators, other facets of the school program, parents, and the community.

The process of evaluation of health instruction should incorporate both
subjective or clinical techniques and objective or statistical techniques. Subjective techniques require the evaluator or the respondent to make a judgment
about the specific criterion in question. Specific techniques used in subjective
evaluation include observations, checklists, questionnaires, surveys, records,
interviews, self-appraisals, discussions, sociodramas, and informal
autobiographies.

Objective evaluations generally concentrate on student outcome measures. In general, these evaluations employ the use of pencil-and-paper tests,
either standardized or teacher-constructed. The results of the administration
of either type of instrument are subjected to one or more statistical analyses.

Subjective Evaluation

As was stated earlier, subjective evaluative techniques involve someone
making a value judgment relative to a given criterion. Therefore, subjective evaluation is often less precise than objective evaluation. Although

Organization of School Health Programs

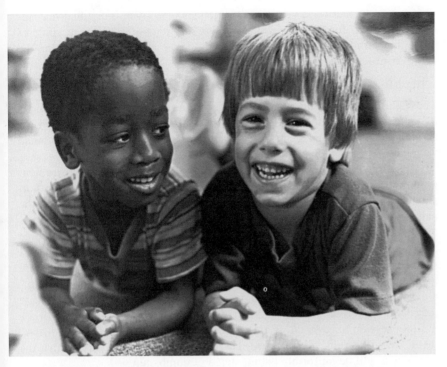

relatively objective instrumentation exists for appraising such things as student vision and hearing, subjective interpretation of how any deficiency might affect the health and learning of the student is necessary.

At present there are no fully objective measures available to assess student attitudes and practices across all grade levels.[1] Therefore, more subjective techniques from both a formal and informal standpoint are often used to ascertain the effect of the health instruction program.

Observations

Observations may be formal or informal. Such procedures as those used in scoliosis screening are formal procedures. However, to evaluate the impact of the health instruction program, observation of students in more "natural" surroundings is desirable. Such behaviors as the choices students make in the school lunchroom; how they dispose of waste paper; safety practices of students on school grounds, in crosswalks, or in other community settings; how students get along and interact with their peers; how they handle property that is not theirs; their activity levels in free periods such as lunch or recess; and how they respond to various suggestions from peers and teachers are all observable events. The teacher must be cautioned, however, against making a value judgment based upon a single observation of an event. Continual

---

1. It should be noted that several instruments are available that assess facets of both attitudes and practices. Further, Abt Associates, Inc. of Cambridge, Massachusetts, has developed a valid and reliable series of instruments in these domains for use in grades 4, 5, 6, and 7.

observation of untoward behavior or practices of a given individual may indicate the need for referral. Collective observations of a group of students engaging in unhealthful practices may necessitate altering or refocusing the health instruction program.

Checklists, Surveys, and Questionnaires

These particular techniques can cover a broad range of topics in the three areas of knowledge, attitudes, and practices. In addition, they can be used in assessing process outcomes. In many cases, use of these instruments is combined with direct observation of behavior.

It is important to remember that the wording of this type of instrumentation is critical, especially if the instrument is to be used in a peer-report situation. If those expected to respond to the instrument do not understand the nature and intent of the item, they may respond in an inappropriate manner, thus putting the utility of the results in serious jeopardy. To help overcome this, any instrument of this sort should be pretested, or tried out with a small sample population that is representative of the population in which you are interested. This should also be done in checking the reliability of the instrument. If two independent observers see the same behavior, will they indicate that behavior the same way on the evaluation instrument? Only by having a training session for evaluators, designed to show them how to use the instrument, will it be somewhat assured that all items are understood and that the instrument will be uniformly administered or completed.

Records

Records appear in schools in several forms, but the ones with which teachers should be most familiar are the school health records (including attendance records) and anecdotal records. The school health record was discussed in Chapter 8. It is important that this record be current and contain complete information about the health status of the student. When a member of the school staff enters something into the student's health record (or academic record), the entry should be based on fact and not on conjecture. Such things as "Johnny is a slow learner" or "Billy is a troublemaker" or "Suzie is very bright and a fast learner" truly have no place in the student's record. By introducing these comments into the record, a teacher is altering the perception of subsequent teachers relative to the "worth" of the individual student.

Anecdotal records are short statements of observations people have made with respect to a child's behavior. Again, care must be taken in interpreting these records. They should be factually based and not contain conjecture as to why a particular behavior occurred. Precipitating factors, if factually based, do have a place in such records. These are time-consuming to develop and would probably only be completed for children who begin to exhibit altered behavior, either positive or negative. Too often, educators prepare these records only to report negative behaviors. Positive behaviors, continually noted, are equally important when evaluating the health instruction program.

Interviews and Conferences

As with the preparation of records, interviews and conferences take time. They must be scheduled and structured if much is to be gained. These techniques may be used when obtaining information from students, staff, parents, and other community members. A great deal of insight can be gained by the discerning teacher who interviews a parent or guardian. In many cases, the interview is combined with a survey form that contains a series of open-ended questions.

Self-appraisals

Self-appraisal can be particularly useful as both an evaluation instrument and a teaching tool. Too often students will not look objectively at their current health status. However, by stressing the importance of the assessment and taking care in wording the various items, the evaluator can gain a great deal of insight about how the student perceives his or her health status. By using open-ended questions, one can also gain some insight into the attitudes of the student about health in general and the health course in particular. Use of this type of evaluation can also serve as a motivational device for classroom instruction. Specific health practices such as food intake; exercise; and personal health habits, such as tooth brushing and flossing, can also be assessed in the self-appraisal process.

Sociodramas and Discussions

If properly prepared, sociodramas and discussions, both formal and informal, can provide the teacher with a wide variety of information. By listening carefully to what is being said by the students, teachers will be able to discern the type of information that is being retained. If health misinformation is present, the teacher can then plan educational programs to correct the misinformation.

If the teacher observes how students react in role-playing situations, a great deal can be learned, not only about the child's health knowledge, but also about the child's interpersonal relationships. The situation should be structured in such a way that the child believes the purpose of the drama is to show how that child feels his or her peers would react. This is the realm of projective techniques of psychological assessment. In this type of assessment interpretation becomes quite important and should only be done by someone trained in the skill.

Informal Autobiographies

By having the student develop an autobiography, especially if it is designated as a health assignment, the teacher gains a valuable cross reference for the more formal school health record. This will also help the teacher gain insight as to the needs and interests of the students.

The teacher should also be aware that students may write suicide notes in autobiographies. If a student begins to disclose information that raises suspicion on the part of the teacher (suicide, abuse, depression, or other problems) the teacher should go to the guidance counselor and express concern for the health of the student. Naturally, follow-up from the referral should be undertaken by all concerned.

Objective Evaluation

Objective measures generally refer to either standardized or teacher-constructed paper-and-pencil tests. These are particularly appropriate when assessing students' knowledge, and they often form the basis for issuing a grade. Unfortunately, this type of measurement is probably the most misused of the evaluation procedures; teachers often do not or will not take the time necessary to develop a valid and reliable evaluation instrument. Part of the reason for this is historical. The traditional reason students were subjected to tests was for the purpose of grading.

> When pupils took tests in earlier times, there was a rather common purpose underlying that test-taking; the kids were going to be graded. Oh, of course there were some teachers who employed tests as diagnostic instruments or as aids in instructional decisions. And every few years pupils could expect to be given a battery of intelligence type tests; the results of which would find their way into each student's permanent record. But in the main, teachers gave tests in order to assess students' academic progress. That just isn't the way it is any more. [Popham, 1978, p. 2]

Today, educational tests are being used as a means of assessing the efficacy of various programs and as a basis to make curricular decisions. Because of this, the form of tests should be taking on a new look. It is increasingly difficult to locate tests that serve more than one specific purpose. Thus, one must understand norm-referenced and objective-based evaluation instruments, as well as criterion-referenced evaluation instruments.

Norm-referenced items are based upon the specific objectives of a course. They are designed to determine the particular status or standing of a given person in relation to another person or group of persons who have completed the same measurement instrument.

Criterion-referenced testing is designed to determine the relative performance of an individual against an absolute measure. Either the person does or does not possess the attribute in question; there is no "gray area" or variance produced, as is the case with norm-referenced measurements. Popham (1978, pp. 176–184) states that there are six characteristics of a well-constructed criterion-referenced test:

1. An unambiguous descriptive scheme. This refers to the procedure used to describe absolute performance. The purpose is to make an unequivocal description of what a test score truly means.
2. An adequate number of times per measured behavior. In general terms, five to twenty items per measured behavior will suffice.
3. Sufficiently limited focus. One can't measure all facets of the program with a single instrument. Somewhere in the neighborhood of five to ten measured behaviors per subject per year is probably reasonable.

4. Reliability. It must assess whatever behavior is being measured, in a consistent manner.
5. Validity. The results of the use of the instrument do serve the purpose for which it was developed.
6. Comparative test data. There should be some sort of field trial of the instrument that indicates how other persons perform on the same set of items.

Persons who will be involved in a thorough evaluation of the instructional phase of the school health program should be well versed in both norm-referenced and criterion-referenced testing. However, few absolutes exist in the field of health science, so it is questionable whether criterion-referenced testing will assume a major posture in the basic classroom evaluation scheme.

VALIDITY, RELIABILITY, PRACTICALITY, AND OBJECTIVITY

Before discussing specific measurement techniques, the four concepts of validity, reliability, practicality, and objectivity need to be reviewed.

Validity

If an instrument measures what it is supposed to, it is considered valid. Validity assumes three major forms: content validity, construct validity, and criterion-related validity.

Content Validity

Content validity of an instrument is based upon a judgment of the relevance of the set of items contained in the instrument compared to the specific objectives for the part of the school health program being assessed. For example, in the area of health instruction, you may ask, ''Does this test actually sample the specific attributes and content specified in the objectives?'' Often an outside review of both the instrument and the objectives, by someone other than those involved in developing either of the two, is a more satisfactory means of establishing content validity.

Construct Validity

Construct validity is a difficult concept and often is not considered in evaluation schemes. Construct validity refers to the foundational elements upon which a given piece of knowledge, an attitude, or a practice is built. To ascertain construct validity, three steps are required. The first of these steps is to identify what foundational elements or constructs underlie or account for a given test performance. Second, if we know how the foundation element should influence test performance, a hypothesis is generated. Finally, empirical evidence, using the test instrument, is gathered to test the hypothesis. For example, we may be interested in an individual's attitude about cigarette smoking. Our hypothesis might be that persons who do not smoke cigarettes have more negative attitudes toward cigarette smoking than those who smoke cigarettes. Using a population of cigarette smokers and a comparable population of nonsmokers, the test instrument that is to be validated is given to both groups. Upon analysis—it is found that the nonsmokers have less positive attitudes toward cigarette smoking than the smokers—evidence has been provided that the hypothesis was correct and that the test instrument can measure that hypothesis. If the evidence fails to support the original hypothesis, either the hypothesis was wrong initially, the test was not well developed, or there is a combination of both a wrong hypothesis and a faulty test instrument.

Criterion-Related Validity

Criterion-related validity entails two elements—concurrent validity and predictive validity. To establish concurrent validity in the area of health instruction, a student's score on a particular test is correlated with that same student's score on some other intellectual measure. Predictive validity involves a time delay between initial data collection and gathering the criterion data, for example, predicting future cigarette smoking behavior from a score attained on an attitude inventory administered several years previously. Another example of predictive validity would be comparing a group's scores on a test measure given to them while they were in elementary school with their grade point average in high school. If the correlation is high then predictive validity for the test instrument has been established. Both concurrent and predictive validity involve a criterion measure and both should be considered part of criterion validity. The distinguishing feature between concurrent and predictive validity is the time lapse between taking the test instrument and obtaining the criterion measure.

Reliability

Reliability refers to consistency of measurement. The test should measure the same attribute in the same way each time that the same person takes the test. In actual practice, reliability represents a statistical relationship between a series (it may be as few as two) of scores on a given test instrument. There are three major ways to determine the reliability of an instrument. They are test–retest, equivalence, and internal consistency. The test–retest procedure involves giving the same instrument to a group of respondents at two different times and then calculating a correlation coefficient between the two sets of scores.

Equivalence is a less-used form of reliability determination for most classroom teachers because of the time factor involved in developing the instrument and the relatively small number of students in the classroom. Equivalence means that if two instruments with equal standard deviations and difficulty ratings are given to the same individual or group, the scores will remain relatively equal.

Internal consistency is an estimate of instrument reliability using data gathered from only one administration of the test instrument. The test is then treated as two tests. That is, the scores on the even-numbered items are

Organization of School Health Programs

correlated with the scores on the odd-numbered items. The closer the scores are to being the same for both even- and odd-numbered items for any individual, the greater the internal consistency of the instrument.

Practicality

Obviously, the teacher or other evaluator does not have an unlimited amount of time or money available to develop, administer, and analyze a test instrument. Most teachers will rely on past experience to predict just how long a test will take and how long it will take to analyze the data collected. The teacher must have alternative methods available or must revise the instrument until it is acceptable. To expect a child to pay attention to a test that is twice as long as could possibly be completed in the time allotment is to turn one's back on practicality. Further, the information that is gathered must be relevant. If nothing is to be done with the information that is gathered, the question arises whether or not the information should have been gathered initially.

Objectivity

Tests must be factually, not judgmentally, based. This is objectivity. There should be but one correct response to any given item, unless the directions specify that more than one response might be correct. The correct response to an item should not be based upon the particular interest of the teacher. Such items as "True or false—Red is a better color than brown" lack objectivity and should not be included on subjective measures.

MEASURING HEALTH KNOWLEDGE

Clearly, the easiest facet to measure of the triumvirate of knowledge, attitudes, and practices is knowledge. We have pointed out the importance of having a knowledge of both subjective and objective evaluation measures; each teacher will have to decide what type of measure will best serve the specific goals of evaluation for the attribute under consideration. In order for teachers to make these decisions, they must know something about the various testing modalities that are available.

Testing modalities will be either objective or subjective tests. Objective tests may consist of true–false items, multiple-choice items, matching items, or completion items. Subjective tests will include essays, written reports, and sometimes performance tests. However, one must keep in mind that even though a test may contain objective items, the selection of the content of the item and the format into which that item is placed are clearly subjective processes by the teacher.

Kime, Schlaadt, and Tritsch (1977) have developed an abridged form of a more lengthy document to indicate the relative strengths and weaknesses of each of the three types of subjective items (see Table 19.1).

TABLE 19.1

Relative Comparison of Strengths and Weaknesses of Evaluation Modalities*

Type of Test	Strengths	Weaknesses
Objective	1. Gives an extensive test.	1. Frequently neglects measurement of higher thought processes.
	2. Can be made highly reliable.	2. Overemphasizes rote learning.
	3. Can be graded objectively and quickly.	3. Promotes poor study habits.
	4. Eliminates bluffing.	4. Encourages guessing.
	5. Can be subjected to item analysis and further refinement.	5. Is difficult to prepare.
	6. Can be adapted to several teaching objectives.	6. Costs more than essay to prepare and reproduce.
	7. Can be made highly valid for some teaching objectives.	7. Not applicable to all teaching objectives.
Essay	1. Is applicable to measurement of writing, organizational ability, and creativeness.	1. Gives a limited test sample.
	2. Is easy to construct.	2. Is difficult to grade.
	3. Promotes proper type of study.	3. Favors the verbally inclined student.
	4. Is adaptable to several subject fields.	4. Has low reliability.
Performance	1. Stresses application of knowledge.	1. Is not adaptable to many fields of learning.
	2. Can be used as a learning device.	2. Is difficult to construct.
	3. May give a truer achievement picture for the verbally handicapped pupil.	3. Is often difficult to grade.
	4. Measures some skills and abstract abilities not measured by other conventional test forms.	4. Is often time-consuming.

*From R. E. Kime, R. G. Schlaadt, and L. E. Tritsch: *Health Instruction: An Action Approach,* op. cit., pp. 282–283.

Objective Tests

True–False Items

A major problem with the true–false item is that the respondent has a fifty percent chance of getting the item correct merely by guessing. A great deal of ambiguity often creeps into this type item. Too often the teacher knows what the question means, but it is interpreted differently by students. Students who possess a great deal of insight may find responding to this type item somewhat difficult because of situational differences that may arise. The statements should be simple and precise. They should not contain qualifiers such as ''all,'' "never," "none," "every," "usually," "several," "often," "sometimes," and so on. True–false items are completed quickly by students; thus, a broad range of content can be covered in a relatively short period of time. It is estimated that a true–false item can be answered by most students in thirty seconds or less.

Multiple-Choice Items

Multiple-choice items are generally considered the most flexible and the most used of the objective tests. It has also been suggested that multiple choice is probably more effective in evaluating student learning than is the true–false item. The item itself consists of two parts, a stem and a series of foils or distractors.

There are several advantages and disadvantages to using multiple-choice tests. As noted, these are the most versatile of the objective-type test items; there is less tendency for students to correctly guess the answers; and they are very easy to score. Disadvantages of the multiple-choice test include the difficulty of writing good items at a higher level of learning; they take more paper since they are longer; they take longer for a student to answer than true–false items; and although guessing is minimized, it is not totally eliminated. Students who are "test wise" may have an advantage in multiple-choice tests, particularly if the basic principles of item development are not followed by the teacher who constructs the test.

McGarry (1989) reviewed the work of 15 recognized test development experts to ascertain if there were basic principles to which the majority of them ascribed in writing multiple-choice test items. He found that there were seven basic principles that seemed to have a great deal of consensus. These are:

- The item stem should have a clear, definite, explicit, and singular problem.
- The options should be grammatically parallel with the item stem.
- Negatively stated item stems should be avoided if possible.
- Verbal cues as to the correct answer should be avoided in the item stem.
- As much of the incomplete statement as possible should be included in the item stem in order to avoid repetition of words or phrases in the distractors.
- The relative length of each distractor should not provide a clue to the correct answer; they should be nearly equal in length.
- The use of inclusive options such as "More than one of the above," "All of the above," or "None of the above" should be avoided.

In general, multiple-choice items should contain at least four distractors. Care should be taken to avoid writing opposites as distractors, for that effectively eliminates one of them for further consideration. A longer stem with shorter distractors is preferred to a short stem with relatively lengthy distractors. Care must be taken to ensure grammatical consistency between the stem and the distractors, and there should not be any clues in the stem about the correct response. If qualifiers such as "not," "best," "does," "does not," and so on are used, they should be highlighted by either underlining them or capitalizing them. The teacher is not trying to trick the student; he or she is trying to ascertain if the student knows the content covered in the health instruction course.

Matching Items

If properly constructed, matching items are well suited to measuring student recall and identifying relationships. Some feel that matching items may be as effective as multiple-choice items in this regard. If matching items are used, it is generally better that each set of items be homogeneous, covering only one subject per set, not several subjects. There should always be more responses available than there are premises. This does not allow the student to eliminate several responses that he or she knows and then guess about the remaining ones.

The list of premises should not exceed ten in any one set, since the number of comparisons that must be made is equal to the number of premises times the number of responses. Thus, if a set of matching items contains ten premises and twelve responses, the student may be required to make as many as 120 comparisons in order to answer the items!

Completion Items

These items begin to move toward more subjective types of evaluation. In some cases, lists of possible response words or phrases are provided. More often, a series of sentences is developed and the student must fill in a key word or phrase that has been omitted from the sentence. A major problem with the completion item is that more than one response to a given item might be correct. An example of this problem would be the following: "Exercise will generally result in an increase of _____ development." Obviously, at least three responses could be correct: "muscular," "organic," or "cardiovascular." If the possibility of more than one correct response exists, these alternatives must be included in the scoring key.

Another common pitfall in writing completion items is that so many blank spaces are left that the item loses meaning. Sentence construction in this type of item is also a major concern, since the syntax of the statement to be completed must not give a hint as to the correct answer.

Subjective Tests

Essays and Written Reports

Unfortunately, most essay questions and written report assignments have too broad a focus. It is almost like asking a student to write down everything he or she knows about health. When an item is too broad, confusion is the natural result, for the student will not know how much to write. This problem is compounded if the space for the response is quite small.

It is important to phrase the question or assignment in such a way that the student will have to apply knowledge to solve one particular problem. If the student is given too many problems to address, the question or assignment becomes a modified form of short-answer test, just slightly beyond sentence completion.

Performance Tests

Performance tests or demonstrations of acquired skills are yet another type of testing. This type of testing would be particularly appropriate for such categories of learning as first-aid skills, wherein the student is faced with a hypothetical situation and must demonstrate, in order, the procedures to be followed in effecting successful rescue of the victim. This type of situational testing could be developed in an essay format as well; however, performance of skills is probably more important than being able to verbalize what should be done.

These evaluations take a bit longer to administer, but they form a good basis for classroom motivation and provide the less verbal learner the opportunity to show that he or she has learned certain skills.

APPRAISING HEALTH ATTITUDES

Attitudes have been defined in many different fashions. To some, they form the basis of one's belief system. To others, they are precursors to action. If nothing else, attitudes are personal and are affected by many things.

Because of the personal and somewhat imprecise nature of attitudes, construction of specific inventories to assess them is extremely difficult. It has been suggested that direct observation of pupil behavior in health matters is indicative of attitudes. The problem here is that most health behavior is not amenable to direct classroom observation; the behavior that would indicate a favorable attitude may not manifest itself until long after the child has graduated from school.

Since attitudes represent feelings, one way of assessing student feelings is to ask students how they feel. This may or may not reveal the student's true feelings, depending upon who is doing the asking, the setting in which the question is asked, and the desirability, in the student's mind, of making his or her true feelings known. One of the more common techniques is to have a student population, comparable to the one in which you are interested, respond to a series of open-ended questions. Examples of this type of question are:

- People who smoke cigarettes are _____ .
- With respect to cigarette smoking, I wish _____ .
- If parents smoke cigarettes, they should _____ .
- I think smoking cigarettes is _____ .

Once responses to these and similar items have been obtained, the evaluator has an idea of the universe of possible responses. This universe of responses can then be analyzed in a variety of ways, using various statistical techniques.

The group of statements can be subjected to various analyses.[2] The purpose of analysis is to develop a set of items that, when responded to by a given population group, yields a quantifiable score indicative of their feeling toward the attribute in question.

It is important to realize that attitudes held by students should *not* form a basis for issuing a grade. If this happens, it is quite doubtful that any of the data collected, if students know that it will become the basis for a grade, will stand the tests of validity or reliability discussed earlier in the chapter. It is also advisable to seek clearance through proper channels, before this type instrument is used. Securing this clearance may help the teacher avoid possible problems if some persons in the community object to the type item or the content of the items included on the instrument.

APPRAISING HEALTH PRACTICES

If assessing attitudes is difficult, the problem of assessing health behavior becomes formidable at best. Too often students know what they should do but do not do it. We all know we are safer if we wear seat belts when riding in an automobile, but how many of us actually wear them on a regular basis?

Certain direct observation of behavior, over time and in informal settings, will provide a great deal of insight into the behavioral patterns of the student. Various practice inventories have been developed for health behaviors, such as the one by Olsen and Baffi (1982, pp. 97–102), to determine drug and alcohol use in a Native American population (see Table 19.2).

Countless other inventories of this type have been developed. The problem here is that if the evaluator wants true responses, the specific identity of the respondent must not be made known to the evaluator. This does not detract from the evaluation because its purpose is to help determine the effect of the instruction program on the health practices of students, not to issue grades. Again, to avoid possible problems with this type evaluation, proper approval should be secured prior to initiating the evaluation.

STANDARDIZED TESTS

To call a test standardized means that large numbers of persons have taken the test under similar testing conditions. In health instruction, these tests tend to be norm-referenced tests pertaining to specific programs that have been developed in local situations. The problem in using tests of this nature is that they do not measure the specific objectives that have been developed for a particular program. Too often, a standardized test is selected simply because a lot of data are available about the test and about the students who took it; thus, a school can compare the scores obtained by their students in relation to the "norms" developed by those who took the test earlier or who took it

---

2. For the student who is interested in pursuing the specifics of attitude instrument construction, see A. L. Edwards, *Techniques of Attitude Scale Construction.* (New York: Appleton Century Crofts, 1957).

Organization of School Health Programs

TABLE 19.2

Sample Practice Inventory

Check All That Apply:	Experiment Only	Monthly	Weekly	Daily
I use:				
Alcohol	_____	_____	_____	_____
Marijuana	_____	_____	_____	_____
PCP	_____	_____	_____	_____
Heroin	_____	_____	_____	_____
Glue (sniffing)	_____	_____	_____	_____
Cigarettes	_____	_____	_____	_____
Other	_____	_____	_____	_____

Source: L. K. Olsen and C. R. Baffi: ''A Descriptive Analysis of Drug and Alcohol Use Among Selected Native American High School Students,'' *Journal of Drug Education,* Vol. 12(2), 1982, pp. 97–102.

in a different situation. Unfortunately, the norm group may be considerably different from local students, which makes the comparison invalid. For the comparison to be valid, select demographic characteristics, such as the boy–girl ratio, ages represented in the classroom, socioeconomic status, and the like would have to be determined for the target population. Then, using the same demographic characteristics represented in the target population, a norm group possessing these demographic characteristics can be generated or constructed from the group of students who took the standardized test one wishes to use. These scores can then be compared with the target population.

It should be recognized that standardized tests have generally been developed over a much longer period of time than is available to the classroom teacher. Further, they are developed by persons with a great deal of knowledge of test construction; the tests have also been submitted to rather rigorous psychometric analysis. Therefore, use of a standardized test as a guide for developing local tests is certainly warranted.

Fodor and Dalis (1989, pp. 139–140) suggest that the advantages and disadvantages of standardized tests are as follows:

Advantages of standardized tests:

1. The content of the items is generally accurate, so there is a high degree of validity.
2. Norms have been developed for the test, thus allowing comparisons.
3. Reliability coefficients have been established.
4. They can be used as learning opportunities because students can learn from reviewing and discussing test items.

Disadvantages of standardized tests:

1. They do not always relate to your specific course objectives.
2. Instruction may be directed toward the test rather than course objectives.
3. They generally emphasize a low level of cognitive, primarily factual, recall.
4. The tests may be obsolete owing to the rapid advances in the health sciences.
5. It is doubtful they specifically measure attitudes and practices. Rather, they measure knowledge about the attitudes or practice desired.

As stated at the outset, all teachers and prospective teachers should develop good evaluation skills. It is suggested that they take specific coursework in the area of evaluation and test construction. The suggestions that are contained in the preceding paragraphs are merely the "tip of the iceberg" in terms of evaluation. Regardless, teachers should strive for validity, reliability, and objectivity in any test that they develop. To do less is to lose a valuable part of the comprehensive school health instruction program.

ASSESSING HEALTH INSTRUCTION MATERIAL AIDS

Instructional aids are any materials or resources used in the conduct of the health instruction program, including textbooks, photographic slides, films, filmstrips, phonograph records, videocassettes, laser disks, computers, models, and resource persons. In select instances, computer programs or programmed learning texts may form the basis for the entire health instruction course.

Too often, teachers will utilize a material aid in the classroom without knowing much about it. This is particularly true with respect to films. A title in a film catalog catches the teacher's eye, and that film is immediately ordered for classroom use. Although the teacher usually has every intention of previewing the film prior to using it, when the film does arrive, the time to preview it never seems to materialize, and the teacher dutifully shows the film to the class—totally ignorant of what material, factual or nonfactual, it contains. These same problems will confront the teacher who uses any of the other types of resources just enumerated (see Appendixes A and E).

Most teachers will at some time be confronted with the selection of a textbook. It is important that this decision not be taken lightly. There are several textbook series available that have been developed for the elementary school. Additionally, there are few texts that are designed for the junior high and senior high school level (see Appendix C). It is important to evaluate any textbook in light of the specific objectives that have been developed for the health instruction program. Several checklists for evaluating textbooks have been developed by those who are involved in this process (see Appendixes E and F).

When selecting teaching aids, care must be taken to ensure that sexual, ethnic, or racial stereotyping, as well as other such biases, are avoided (see Appendix B).

Resource speakers are yet another classroom aid. The teacher must be familiar with the presenter prior to inviting the individual to the classroom. Naturally, if a speaker is referred by a colleague, personal knowledge of the individual is less important than knowing what he or she will present. It is critical that a thorough orientation be given any guest speaker prior to the classroom appearance. Providing the guest in advance with specific questions from students is always a helpful tactic. It is also a good idea to tell the guest what subjects have been covered, what should be covered in the presentation, and what will be covered subsequently. This gives the guest a better idea of how his or her presentation fits into the total educational package.

EVALUATION OF HEALTH INSTRUCTION METHODS

The specific methods used in health instruction, as well as the learning opportunities provided, are critical to the success or failure of the educational program. Teachers must continually assess the methods they use in the classroom.

Selection of feasible and appropriate instructional objectives helps dictate choice of methods and learning opportunities.

Cornacchia, Olsen, and Nickerson (1992, p. 416) suggest five rather simple techniques to assist in assessing the effectiveness of health instruction methods:

1. Teachers observe pupils' reactions and check their own internal feelings of effectiveness. Experienced teachers know when instruction is going well and when a method or activity is going flat.
2. Teachers ask students to respond orally or in writing to these questions: "What did you learn today about (topic)?" "How did you feel when we (method/activity)?" "If you were going to teach today's lesson to your friends, how would you do it?"
3. Use a tape recorder to capture the dialogue and tone of the class during the lesson. Then analyze the tape.
4. Videotape the lesson if feasible. Analyze the tape.
5. Ask the principal, nurse, coordinator, or another teacher to attend the class to evaluate a specific lesson or lessons.

ISSUING GRADES IN HEALTH INSTRUCTION

It is the authors' contention that the only way for anyone to fail health is to expire. Unfortunately, students, parents, and society demand that some sort of quantifiable assessment be attached to what might be considered a qualitative subject matter.

Rather than issue a specific grade to a student, it might be more appropriate to engage in some in-depth discussions with the student and the parents about the student's health status, including his or her apparent understandings of health concepts. This then becomes a formative or qualitative evaluation.

If a grade must be issued in health instruction, it should be based upon the collection of a variety of data, instead of merely reflecting student performance on one evaluation instrument that may have been developed rather quickly. In addition to such traditional measures—tests, projects, written assignments, and daily classroom activities—student self-assessments should be included. It is our firm belief that the student should be involved in the evaluative process. In this way, the process of evaluation becomes yet another learning experience for the student.

WHO SHOULD EVALUATE?

Anyone involved in any aspect of the school is automatically involved in the evaluation process. Granted, many persons are not consulted in formal evaluation, but they certainly are concerned in an informal way. The custodian who selects a nonslip wax or repairs a broken stair; the food service worker who alters the menu because the ingredients needed for the planned meal are not available; the secretary who contacts a parent to ascertain where an ill child should be taken; the bus driver who refuses to start the bus until all children are seated and wearing seat belts; the crossing guard who insists that bicycles be walked, not ridden, across the highway—all these persons and more are involved in evaluation of the school health program.

However, the person most involved in evaluation is the classroom teacher. The assessment of the instructional phase of the program rests squarely on the teacher's shoulders. Naturally, there is help available from a variety of sources, particularly school administrators, board members, nurses, other teachers, parents, community members, and perhaps evaluation specialists from nearby colleges or universities. The teacher should draw upon these sources as needed.

Obviously, evaluation is not an easy task. It entails a conscientious and time-consuming effort on the part of all persons if it is to be completed effectively and efficiently. It would certainly behoove teachers to learn as much as they can about the evaluative process, for it is through evaluation that instruction can improve.

WHEN SHOULD EVALUATION BE DONE?

Evaluation is a continuous process. It is not done only after completing an instructional endeavor or after initiating a service program. It is as important as any other facet of an educational program and should be planned concurrently with all the other elements. If evaluation is included in the total planning process, it is quite likely that some of the pitfalls mentioned throughout this chapter will be avoided. By making evaluation continual throughout the implementation and conduct of a program, problems will be identified and corrective measures instituted before the problems become barriers to efforts in the future.

EVALUATION OF THE EVALUATIVE PROCESS

Whenever evaluation is conducted, the underlying question ''Was this a proper way to do the evaluation?'' must be asked. Were correct and appropriate procedures utilized? Were valid and reliable instruments used? Did the process involve a variety of measures, or did it rely on a single measure? Were both subjective and objective methods employed? Were a variety of appropriate data sources utilized? Were the appropriate people involved in the evaluation process? Will the evaluation be used in a constructive manner so that everyone benefits? It is important that any evaluation be used to improve the overall program.

The answers to the preceding questions will provide the accountability that the public desires. It will also help ensure that evaluation is a continual and positive process.

SUMMARY

Evaluation is an extremely important part of the school health program, since any educational program should demonstrate that it is effective. Evaluation uses measurement to quantify attributes felt by educators to be important in terms of knowledge, attitudes, and practices. Evaluation serves many purposes including improving the program through analyzing the strengths and weaknesses of all components of the comprehensive school health program; ascertaining if any gaps exist; issuing student grades; determining the value of various screenings; helping students and parents correct any remedial defects so the student gains the most from the educational experience; and planning for the most healthful environment possible.

It is important to understand that evaluation is a continuous process and not something that is undertaken when a program has been completed. The purpose of this continual evaluation is to provide feedback about the impact of the program so that if problems are identified, immediate steps can be initiated to correct the problems. Systematically planned and conducted evaluations can also be used as a basis for planning and conducting in-service education programs for school personnel.

Although there is no single form of evaluation that could be considered best, there are several steps that should be followed if the evaluation is to be meaningful. One of the critical components in evaluation involves the selection of measurement instruments. If the instruments used to assess the school health program are not valid and reliable, the evaluation will have little meaning. In order to help overcome problems associated with validity and reliability, some standardized instruments are often utilized. Although the standardized instruments do provide good guidelines for the evaluation process, they should be examined carefully to be sure that they do measure the objectives of the program to which they are applied.

Evaluations take many forms including formal and informal observations; checklists, surveys, and questionnaires; interviews, conferences, and self-appraisals; and such specific tests as knowledge tests, attitude inventories, and practice inventories.

Instructional materials and aids should be evaluated carefully to be sure that they are appropriate for the student population and the lessons with which they are being used. The actual classroom methods that are employed should also be evaluated.

All persons who are involved in the school could be involved in some part of the evaluation process. However, classroom evaluation of student progress is generally left to the individual teacher. For this reason, all teachers should be familiar with basic concepts of measurement and evaluation as well as test development and should continually upgrade their skills in this area.

In order to be sure that evaluations are being conducted properly, the evaluation process itself should be assessed. However, a good evaluation process can be conducted and serve no purpose if it is not used to improve the existing school health program and provide the accountability that is desired and demanded by the public.

REVIEW QUESTIONS

1. Distinguish between measurement and evaluation.
2. Why should teachers, schools, parents, and the community be held accountable for the successes and failures of the school health instruction program?
3. Why should the school health program be evaluated?
4. You have been put on a committee charged with developing an evaluation program for your school's health program. Discuss your viewpoints with respect to the following questions:
   a. What should be evaluated?
   b. Who should be evaluated?
   c. When should evaluation be done?
   d. How should evaluation be done?
   e. Who should conduct the evaluation?

5. What problems are associated with the use of standardized test and/ or instruments as evaluative devices?
6. Do you feel that grades should be issued for the health instruction course? Justify your response.
7. Distinguish between norm-referenced testing and criterion-referenced testing.
8. If you were to develop an evaluative instrument for a health instruction class, what considerations would you use in developing that test? What type items (format) would you use? Why would you use that (those) format(s)?
9. What are the major problems associated with assessing health knowledge? How might some of these problems be overcome?
10. What are some of the major problems associated with assessing health attitudes? How might these problems be overcome?
11. What are some of the major problems associated with assessing health practices? How might these problems be overcome?
12. Why is it important to evaluate the evaluative process?
13. Examine some tests that you have written to see if any of the basic principles of test construction presented in this text have been violated. How might you revise the items to make them ''better?''

REFERENCES

Combs, A. W. *Myths in Education.* Boston: Allyn and Bacon, 1979.

Cornacchia, H., L. Olsen, and C. Nickerson. *Health in Elementary Schools,* 8th ed. St. Louis: Times Mirror/Mosby College Publishing, 1992.

Creswell, W. Jr., and I. Newman. *School Health Practice,* 9th ed. St. Louis: Times Mirror/ Mosby College Publishing, 1989.

Fodor, J. T., and G. Dalis. *Health Instruction: Theory and Application,* 4th ed. Philadelphia: Lea and Febiger, 1989.

Joint Committee on Evaluation. *Evaluate Your School Health Program.* A report of the Joint Committee on Evaluation of the School Health Section of the American Public Health Association. Washington, D.C.: The American Public Health Association, 1955.

Kime, R., R. Schlaadt, and L. Tritsch. *Health Instruction: An Action Approach.* Englewood Cliffs, New Jersey: Prentice-Hall, 1977.

King, K., M. Taylor, and M. Dignan. ''Health Education Evaluation: Improving the Product.'' *Health Education* 12(5):19 (Sept/Oct, 1982).

Lovato, C., D. Allensworth, and F. Chan. *School Health in America: An Assessment of State Policies to Protect and Improve the Health of Students,* 5th ed. Kent, Ohio: American School Health Association, 1989.

McGarry, R. *An Analysis of Introductory Health Education Textbook Multiple Choice Test Item Files.* Unpublished M. Ed. project. University Park, PA: The Pennsylvania State University, 1989.

Nelson, S. *How Healthy Is Your School? Guidelines for Evaluating School Health Promotion.* New York: National Center for Health Education Press, 1984.

Oberteuffer, D., O. A. Harrelson, and M. B. Pollock. *School Health Education,* 5th ed. New York: Harper & Row, 1972.

Ohio Department of Education. *A Self-Appraisal Checklist for School Health Programs.* Columbus: The Department, 1966.

Olsen, L. K., and C. R. Baffi. "A Descriptive Analysis of Drug and Alcohol Use Among Selected Native American High School Students." *Journal of Drug Education* 12: 2(1982).

Pigg, R. M. "Recent Developments in the Evaluation of School Health Education." *Health Education* 17(4):29 (Jul/Aug, 1983).

Popham, W. J. *Criterion-Referenced Measurement.* Englewood Cliffs, N.J.: Prentice-Hall, 1978.

Popham, W. J. *Educational Evaluation.* Englewood Cliffs, N.J.: Prentice-Hall, 1975.

Schaller, W. E. *The School Health Program,* 5th ed. Philadelphia: Saunders College Publishing, 1981.

School Health Education Evaluation. *Journal of School Health,* Special Issue, 55(8) (October 1985).

Solleder, M. K. *Evaluation Instruments in Health Education,* 3rd ed. Washington, D.C.: The American Alliance for Health, Physical Education, Recreation, and Dance, 1979.

Stone, E. "Challenges and Directions in Research and Evaluation Training: A Focus on School-Based Settings." *Health Education* 16(6):34 (Oct/Nov, 1986).

Willgoose, C. E. *Health Teaching in Secondary Schools.* Philadelphia: W. B. Saunders, 1972.

Current Status of School Health Education

20

It is difficult to predict what will happen in the future with respect to health education, partly because of the lack of a united front dedicated to bringing about legislation for the inclusion of health education in the K through 12 school curriculum and perhaps beyond into the college years. Getting legislation passed requires a great deal of work, since numerous political, social, and economic forces are involved in shaping what occurs not only in schools, but also in the whole society, and school health is often considered a controversial issue. However, numerous groups and individuals are working hard to try to convince Congress to fund the Office of Comprehensive School Health Education currently located within the U.S. Department of Education. By the time this textbook is available, it is possible that funding legislation will have occurred and the office may be fully operational.

Although, as mentioned elsewhere in this text, there is a great deal of support for health education throughout the United States as demonstrated by the fact that health education is specifically included in educational codes and legislative mandates in 43 states, health education is *mandated* in only 36 of these states. Further, although 36 states mandate health education, it appears that comprehensive school health education is not present in many school districts across the nation. Pollock and Hamburg (1985) aptly summarized the situation when they indicated that in situations where school health education programs exist, the programs vary a great deal in their quality and comprehensiveness.

Unfortunately, the lack of comprehensive school health instruction programs may be traced to several critical factors. There appears to be a lack of administrative support and leadership, as well as a lack of qualified teachers. Further, although numerous national statements in support of health education have been published and circulated, these statements do not seem to have had a great deal of impact at the local level (Pollock and Hamburg, 1985).

Some of the basic findings reported in *School Health in America* (Lovato et al., 1989) are grim testimony to the lack of comprehensive health instruction programs in the nation's schools:

- Only 17 states allocate state funds for health education in addition to basic salaries for state personnel.
- Only 40 states have any type of curriculum guide to assist local districts plan health instruction programs, most of which were published between 1973 and 1987 (however one-half of the states reported that revisions were underway).

- Only 17 states reported having conducted an evaluation of their health education programs.
- Only 25 states require a course in health education for high school graduation.
- Only 32 states require that health education be taught sometime during grades K–12, and an additional 13 require a combination of physical education and health education.
- Of the 21 states that offer certification for elementary health education teachers, only 18 offer separate certification in health education.
- Of the 49 states that offer certification for secondary health education, 42 offer separate certification.
- Only 39 states require a teacher to be certified in health education to teach the subject in secondary school.
- Only 26 states require health education teachers to complete additional course work or attend in-service programming to maintain their certification.

In 1985, Metropolitan Life Foundation, as a part of their "Healthy Me" initiative, conducted a survey of school superintendents across the nation. This survey revealed that only approximately one-third of the nation's children received comprehensive health instruction and that in grades 1 to 6, 81 percent of the health education is taught by teachers who have no health education training. Further, in secondary schools, only about half of the classes in health education are taught by certified health education teachers.

In 1988 Metropolitan Life Foundation contracted with Louis Harris and Associates to survey public school students and their parents, and teachers about the quality and quantity of school health education. The major findings from this were:

- Eighteen percent of the students reported having health education in only one grade.
- Four percent of the students reported having no health education.
- Sixty-seven percent of the teachers reported that their schools had adopted comprehensive health education programs in which multiple topics were covered over a period of years.
- Thirty-two percent of the students indicated that their health classes were more interesting than other classes they took.
- Ninety-one percent of students who had three or more years of health education indicated that they had learned things that helped them to live a healthier life compared to 86 percent of those with only one year of health education, and 79 percent of those with no health education.

The findings of the above studies show that there have been some positive results that have occurred over the years. However, clearly there is a long way to go if we are to reach the stated goal of having quality K–12 health education in 75 percent of all schools by the year 2000. As noted in the 1989 Carnegie Foundation report for the advancement of teaching, "Clearly, no knowledge is more crucial than knowledge about health. Without it, no other life goal can be successfully achieved. Therefore, we recommend that all students study health, learning about the human body, how it changes over the life cycle, what nourishes it and diminishes it, and how a healthy body contributes to emotional well being."

Society is undergoing rapid change; it follows that the school will be affected by these changes. As technology advances, new problems will confront us. We already see that there is an increased emphasis on study of the aging process, of chronic diseases and, most recently, of HIV/AIDS. The advancement of artificial joints and the artificial heart appear to be bringing the age of bionics closer and closer.

There is an increased awareness of life-style and how life-style affects total well-being. However, it is somewhat disheartening that, with all the effort that has been put into providing meaningful health instruction, not a great deal appears to have been accomplished.

In 1983 Pigg indicated that the following trends were in evidence:

1. American children and young adults continue to know little about health.
2. The levels of health knowledge in young adults and children do not seem to be increasing.
3. The majority of teachers providing health instruction still are not prepared to perform completely.
4. School administrators, though supportive of health education in principle, seem to be unaware of the true nature and purpose of health education.
5. As a discipline, health education isn't receiving the same treatment as other disciplines, in terms of facilities, equipment, budget, scheduling, and staffing.
6. State laws and regulations about school health education are generally inadequate.
7. Existing state requirements are only passively enforced, if enforced at all.
8. The trends seen today mirror those of the School Health Education Study some 20 years ago. [p. 33]

Although these trends and those noted by Lovato et al., (1989) certainly are not encouraging, it should be remembered that 20 years ago there was very little support for health instruction on a national basis. There has been an increased awareness on the part of national, state, and local officials that health education is one of the basics. If one closely examines the health goals for the year 2000 (*Healthy People 2000*, 1991), of the nearly 300 goals that are specified, nearly 100 of them can be positively influenced by school health programs. The importance of health education to the total field of education is beginning to gain more notice, and it is critical that there be professionals prepared to deal with potential increased demand for qualified health educators. The Education Commission of the States in 1981 indicated:

> There seems to be a high level of interest in school health education in many states although program support and resources committed to the program vary. [p. 27]

It must be pointed out that specific behaviors relative to learning are not always easily observable. In addition, educational experiences may produce increased awareness of a health problem to the extent that the problem may appear to get worse rather than better. Take, for example, the individual who decides to lose weight. Unfortunately, the person may exercise hard, diet faithfully, but still not lose much weight. In these cases, the fat tissue has been replaced by muscle tissue; since muscle tissue has a higher density than fat tissue, the person may actually gain weight.

Another example might be the case in which there is an increase in reported instances of sexually transmitted diseases (STDs). Upon first glance, the school that has a unit on STDs as a part of the health instruction program might be said to be at fault—if these topics were not taught, students would not get curious and experiment. However, increased reporting of STDs might well mean that, because of the health instruction, students are more aware of signs, symptoms, and possible harmful effects of the diseases. Thus, they are more apt to visit physicians or clinics. Prior to the educational program, many of these people would have ignorantly continued to spread disease.

Even though qualified health teachers appear to be in short supply, it should also be pointed out that, for the first time in history, those who teach health on a secondary level are persons who have had undergraduate and perhaps graduate preparation in health education. Further, these persons were most likely trained by professors who also went through baccalaureate, masters, and often doctoral programs in health education (Rash and Pigg, 1979, p. 256).

A FEDERAL FOCUS

It was not until the President's Committee on Health Education focused on public and community health that a great deal of discussion and even action on health occurred at the federal level. As a direct result of the President's Committee, the federal Bureau of Health Education was formed in 1974 within the bureaucratic structure of the Centers for Disease Control. The mission of the Bureau of Health Education (1974, p. 186)—subsequently named the Center for Health Promotion and Health Education, now the Centers for Chronic Disease Prevention and Health Promotion—was to provide leadership and direction to a comprehensive national health education program for the prevention of disease, disability, premature death, and undesirable and

Organization of School Health Programs

unnecessary health problems. Since its inception, the center continues to oversee many of the health education programs and wellness promotion programs of the nation.

Also as a result of the President's Committee on Health Education report, a private sector organization, the National Center for Health Education, was formed. Funded initially by the government through a grant to the National Health Council, the National Center for Health Education became a reality in October 1975. Although funded at a minimal level, the center became a focal point for health education and was instrumental in getting the School Health Curriculum Project and the Primary Grades Health Curriculum Project (now called *Growing Healthy*) approved by the Joint Dissemination Review Panel for inclusion on the National Diffusion Network. At present the center is located in New York City, where it continues to serve as a coordinator for the revisions of *Growing Healthy* (see Chapter 18).

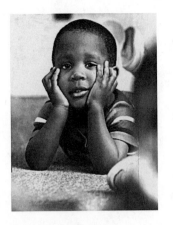

There are 47 million reasons school health programs are important. *Courtesy Centers for Disease Control*

In 1976, the former U.S. Department of Health, Education and Welfare (now the U.S. Department of Health and Human Services) established the Office of Health Information and Health Promotion in the Office of the Assistant Secretary for Health under Section 1706, Title 1 of the National Health Promotion and Disease Prevention Act of 1976 (PL 94–317). Although the name of the office has subsequently changed to the Office of Disease Prevention and Health Promotion, its primary functions remain the same:

1. Coordinate health information, health promotion, preventive health services, and education within the department and the private sector.
2. Facilitate coordination among Public Health Service Components and other federal agencies, professional organizations, and citizens' groups having common interests in health.
3. Coordinate the operation of a national clearinghouse on health information, promotion, and prevention activities. [Dept. of HEW, 1976, p. 2]

Further, within the Centers for Chronic Disease Prevention and Health Promotion, a new division (Division of Adolescent and School Health) has been created and given the specific responsibility as a focal point within the Centers for Disease Control for school health. The Division of Adolescent and School Health has entered into cooperative agreements with numerous professional associations and societies to produce guidelines and materials specifically dealing with school health issues. One particular agreement with the American School Health Association has resulted in the development of a book entitled *School-Based HIV Prevention: A Multidisciplinary Approach* (Kerr, Allensworth, and Gayle, 1991). This book contains strategies for HIV/AIDS education for schools and communities and is available from the American School Health Association. Similar cooperative agreements have been developed with other professional associations as well.

Although much has been done at the federal level in terms of promoting school health, it should be pointed out that there have been major setbacks as well. In 1978, Congress passed S544 and HR2600, which established an Office of Comprehensive School Health within the U.S. Office of Education. These two bills were designed to establish a system of grants for teacher training and pilot demonstration projects and to encourage the development of comprehensive school health education programs. Under this program, the U.S. Commission of Education was to be able to make direct grants to state education departments, to higher education facilities, and to other appropriate agencies to:

1. Develop and conduct training programs for elementary and secondary education teachers who will work in comprehensive health education programs in the schools.
2. Develop curricula and demonstrate projects and methods for evaluating their effectiveness, develop materials and other training aids, and develop preservice and inservice training programs such as institutes, workshops, and seminars to train personnel.
3. Develop comprehensive programs in elementary and secondary schools in health education and health problems and assist local education agencies in the implementation of such programs. [Galli, 1978, p. 70]

Unfortunately, although an appropriation bill was passed, the monies to enact this broad program were never appropriated. Thus, there remains an Office of Comprehensive School Health within the U.S. Department of Education that has no personnel or operating budget. At present, efforts are underway to secure fundings for this office.

PROFESSIONAL PREPARATION

As has been pointed out in numerous sections of the preceding chapters, if health education is to be successful, it should be taught by qualified health educators who have been professionally trained in the discipline. It is also important that teacher training institutions provide basic training for teachers who will not become professional health educators, but who will have a role in the health instruction program.

Just what constitutes a well-developed professional preparation program is open to a great deal of debate. Just because all the right courses are in place does *not* necessarily mean that those who manage to pass the courses are "qualified."

Preparation of Elementary School Teachers

As stated earlier, 43 states have a legal basis for health education as a part of the school curriculum. Thus, all teachers should be exposed to basic concepts of health teaching. However, as noted earlier, in some states, only one health

Organization of School Health Programs

course must be taken by all prospective elementary school teachers. Some states that **require** health as a part of the curriculum do not require a course in health *instruction* for the prospective elementary school teacher.

According to Fodor and Dalis (1989, p. 153), if health content is to be included in the curriculum of the elementary school, all elementary teachers should have preparation in:

1. Health problems of elementary school-age children.
2. Teaching of health at the elementary school level.
3. The function, purpose, and organization of the school health program.

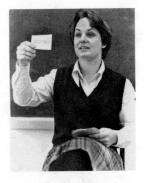

Teacher enthusiasm is important if health education is to be effective.

The point is that if teachers are required to teach any topic, they should be able to do it with accuracy, effectiveness, and efficiency. The only way to begin to do this is through at least a minimum of formal training.

Most recently, a Joint Committee of the Association for the Advancement of Health Education and the American School Health Association developed a document in which the minimum standards for the professional preparation of elementary teachers in the area of health education was specified. The specific responsibility of the Committee was to suggest minimum standards that should be instituted in all elementary teacher-education professional preparation programs. The Committee recommended that all elementary teachers enroll in a minimum of one three-credit (semester hours) preservice course designed to help them understand their role and the role of health education in the elementary school, and develop skills to implement a health education curriculum into the elementary school program. The proposed course would supplement another required three-credit semester course in personal health that would provide the basic content background for the elementary teacher. The recommendations of the Joint Committee are presented in Table 20.1. It is anticipated that the recommended guidelines will be sent to all elementary teacher professional preparation programs in the nation and will be widely publicized in the media. It is hoped that the guidelines will become part of the NCATE standards for approving programs in elementary education.

Preparation of Secondary School Teachers

The secondary school teacher is often more of a specialist in a specific content area than is the elementary school teacher. However, in a number of schools, there is no specific health course; if health is taught at all, it is through integrating health with another school subject. If this is the case, as was stated in Chapter 15, integration is the quickest way to do nothing but pay lip service to health instruction. As a minimum, teachers in these schools should meet the same requirements as elementary teachers, except that the health problems of secondary school students should be included.

TABLE 20.1

Health Instruction Responsibilities and Competencies for Elementary (K–6) Classroom Teachers

Responsibility I—Communicating the concepts and purposes of health education

Competency A: *Describe the discipline of health education within the school setting.*

Sub-Competencies:

1) Describe the interdependence of health education and the other components of a comprehensive school health program.
2) Describe comprehensive school health instruction, including the most common content areas.

Competency B: *Provide a rationale for K–12 health education.*

Competency C: *Explain the role of knowledge, skills, and attitudes in shaping patterns of health behavior.*

Competency D: *Define the role of the elementary teacher within a comprehensive school health education program.*

Sub-Competencies:

1) Describe the importance of health education for elementary teachers.
2) Summarize the kinds of support needed by the K–6 teacher from administrators and others to implement an elementary school health education program.
3) Identify available quality continuing education programs in health education for elementary teachers.
4) Describe the importance of modeling positive health behaviors.

Responsibility II—Assessing the health instruction needs and interests of elementary students

Competency A: *Utilize information about health needs and interests of students.*

Competency B: *List behaviors and how they promote or compromise health.*

Responsibility III—Planning elementary school health instruction

Competency A: *Select realistic program goals and objectives.*

Competency B: *Identify a scope and sequence plan for elementary school health instruction.*

Competency C: *Plan elementary school health education lessons which reflect the abilities, needs, interests, development levels, and cultural backgrounds of students.*

Competency D: *Describe effective ways to promote cooperation with and feedback from administrators, parents, and other interested citizens.*

Competency E: *Determine procedures which are compatible with school policy for implementing curricula containing sensitive health topics.*

TABLE 20.1   Continued

Responsibility IV—Implementing elementary school health instruction

Competency A: Employ a variety of strategies to facilitate implementation of an elementary school health education curriculum.

Sub-Competencies:

1) Provide a core health education curriculum.
2) Integrate health and other content areas.
3) Incorporate topics introduced by students into the health education curriculum.
4) Utilize affective skill-building techniques to help students apply health knowledge to their daily lives.
5) Involve parents in the teaching/learning process.

Competency B: Incorporate appropriate resources and materials.

Sub-Competencies:

1) Select valid and reliable sources of information about health appropriate for K–6.
2) Utilize school and community resources within a comprehensive program.
3) Refer students to valid sources of health information and services.

Competency C: Employ appropriate strategies for dealing with sensitive health issues.

Competency D: Adapt existing health education curricular models to community and student needs and interests.

Responsibility V—Evaluating the effectiveness of elementary school health instruction

Competency A: Utilize appropriate criteria and methods unique to health education for evaluating student outcomes.

Competency B: Interpret and apply student evaluation results to improve health instruction.

Source: Joint Committee of the Association for the Advancement of Health Education and the American School Health Association. *Journal of School Health* (February 1992), Vol. 62, No. 2, p. 77.

When health instruction is a separate course, there is a consensus that three primary areas of professional preparation are needed. These three areas are:

1. Common personal and community health needs.
2. Related areas (social, behavioral, and biological sciences).
3. Structure and process of school health programs and modern concepts of health instruction. [Fodor and Dalis, 1989, pp. 154–155]

TABLE 20.2

Suggested Minimum Requirements for the Professional Preparation
of Health Educators

	Semester Hours	Quarter Hours
I. Content Areas		
A. Direct Health Content	12–16	18–24
B. Related Health Content	15–20	22–30
II. Educational Skills	8–12	12–18
III. Orientation to the Profession	8–12	12–18
IV. Demonstration of Skills and Knowledge	8–14	12–21
TOTAL HOURS	51–74	76–111

Reprinted from C. E. Bruess and J. E. Gay: *Implementing Comprehensive School Health,* New York: Macmillan Publishing Co., Inc., 1978, p. 189. By permission.

As noted previously, 49 states offer certification for secondary health teachers. A total of 24 states offer both separate and dual certification in health and physical education, and 18 states offer separate certification in health education. Five states offer only dual certification in health and physical education.

It is generally agreed among health professionals that, at minimum, an individual should have a college minor in health education in order to teach health education at the secondary school level. Unfortunately, even in states where certification in health education is required in order to teach health, there are ways to circumvent the process (Lovato, Allensworth, and Chan, 1989). If health education is going to attain a rightful place in the school curriculum, it will be important to identify these problems and work to alleviate them by having professionally qualified health education specialists available.

The minimum requirements suggested for the professionally prepared health educator are presented in Table 20.2.

The direct health content areas should include a minimum of personal health and a community health course. All of the other standard content courses fall under this 12- to 16-semester-hour block.

Related health content areas should include a basic biology course. Additional biological science courses should be taken to complete the 15- to 20-semester-hour requirement.

The educational skills should include courses on tests and measurements, methods in school health, and educational psychology (including learning theory).

Professional orientation should include the school health program, the community health program, and organizing and administering a school or community health program.

The demonstration of skills and knowledge should occur throughout the professional preparation program and culminate in student teaching.

Fodor and Dalis (1989, p. 155) suggest a 60-semester-hour program:

	Introductory Health	2
	Human Physiology	3
	General Biology	4
Lower Division	Introductory Chemistry	3
	College Algebra or Statistics	3
	Introductory Psychology	3
	Introductory Sociology	3
	Biology (elective)	2
	Biostatistics	4
	Health Behavior	3
	Solving School/Community Health Problems	3
	School Health Education	3
Upper Division	Teaching Strategies in Health Education	3
	Epidemiology	3
	Community Health Education	3
	Intercultural Communications	3
	Electives	12
	TOTAL	60

These two suggested professional preparation schemes are quite similar. It should be noted that the Fodor and Dalis scheme does not contain the education courses. However, this does not mean that they should not be required. Fodor and Dalis focused on the health education component of professional preparation rather than on the total scope. They would certainly agree that the basic education courses, including the student teaching experience, are necessary components for training the prospective teacher.

ROLE DELINEATION PROJECT

In 1978, the Bureau of Health Professions of the Health Resources Administration provided funding under a contract with the National Center for Health Education for a study that would specify the appropriate roles and responsibilities, together with the requisite skills and knowledges, for entry-level health educators.

Representatives of eight professional organizations, patient education specialists, health educator employers, and health education consumers comprised the advisory committee of 12 persons. A nine-person working committee was drawn from the memberships of the Association for the Advancement of Health Education; the American College Health Association; the American School Health Association; the Public Health Education and the School Health Education sections of the American Public Health Association; the Society for Public Health Education; the Society of State Directors of Health, Physical Education and Recreation; and state and territorial directors of Public Health Education (National Center, 1980, p. 2).

After numerous meetings, a document that delineated the skills that should be held by entry-level health educators was developed. These skills are far too numerous to include in this text; however, the Working Committee and the Advisory Committee decided that the second step should be verification that what had been developed was representative of what was occurring in the field.

Analysis of the data collected during the verification study did indicate that there were generic health educators—all health educators in all settings who are considered entry level and use the same basic set of skills. The only difference between them is the degree of emphasis on the various skills and knowledges they possess.

As a result of the role delineation and verification efforts, a curriculum guide (National Task Force, 1983) was developed in which a competency-based framework for the professional preparation of health education specialists was developed. This framework was distributed to all professional preparation programs in the nation and comments were received from various program heads and chairpersons relative to the document. Based upon the comments that were received, the document was revised and redistributed in 1990 (National Task Force, 1990). The document was developed specifically to serve as a guide for the development of the professional preparation of the generic, entry-level health education specialist.

Within the document that was developed, three themes are clearly in evidence:

- Health education process and methodologies,
- Health topics and issues,
- Professional socialization of the health educator. [National Task Force, 1990, p. 6]

Additionally, seven basic areas of responsibility and the competencies and subcompetencies needed in order to demonstrate abilities in each of the seven areas of responsibility are presented. The seven areas of responsibility that should be demonstrated by all generic, entry-level health educators are as follows (National Task Force, 1990, p. 26):

1. Assessing individual and community needs for health education.
2. Planning effective health education programs.
3. Implementing health education programs.
4. Evaluating the effectiveness of health education programs.
5. Coordinating provision of health education services.
6. Acting as a resource person in health education.
7. Communicating health and health education needs, concerns, and resources.

If one were to examine the suggested program of study for health educators presented previously it is rather clear that the seven basic areas of responsibility contained in the National Task Force document are included. It should also be noted that the basic responsibilities presented above have been adopted as the basic criteria that are used by the Association for the Advancement of Health Education and the Society for Public Health Education, to accredit baccalaureate-level health education programs in colleges and universities. Further the National Council for the Accreditation of Teacher Education (NCATE) has included these responsibilities as one of the criteria for the national accreditation of teacher education programs in health.

One additional innovation has emerged as a result of the Role Delineation Project (National Center for Health Education, 1980). As of September 1990, a national test has been available for individuals who wish to become certified health education specialists (C.H.E.S.). This is an entirely voluntary certification, but does indicate to prospective employers that the individual does possess the basic competencies and understands the basic areas of responsibility for a generic, entry-level health education specialist. It is the feeling of the authors that individuals who wish to work as health education specialists should possess the C.H.E.S. designation.

SUMMARY

This chapter contained three major foci: the status of health education and how the federal government fits into the picture; professional preparation of elementary and secondary school teachers; and an explanation of the Role Delineation Project and the impact of that project, particularly with reference to the accreditation of baccalaureate-level health education programs, and the newly developed process for certified health education specialists.

In closing this text, we feel it is particularly appropriate to make reference to a landmark report recently published by the National Commission on the Role of the School and the Community in Improving Adolescent Health (1990) entitled *Code Blue: Uniting for Healthier Youth.* This commission was a joint effort of the National Association of State Boards of Education (NASBE) and the American Medical Association to call national attention to dangerous trends in adolescent health so that action could be recommended to reverse the trends, particularly in the spread of human immunodeficiency virus (HIV) and to avoid other health problems. This commission was formed in August 1989 and consisted of educators, health professionals, clergy, advocates for children, and leaders from business, entertainment, and the political and civic arenas. The basic objective of the commission was to identify linkages and "common grounds and institutional opportunities for schools, health service providers, and communities to address the adolescent health crisis" (Preface).

As a result of numerous meetings, conversations, and interviews, the commission developed four recommendations that could form the basis for a national dialogue across many professions and agencies to meet the current adolescent health crisis. The four broad recommendations are:

- Guarantee all adolescents access to health services regardless of ability to pay.
- Make communities the front line in the battle for adolescent health.
- Organize service around people, not people around services.
- Urge schools to play a stronger role in improving adolescent health.

Although all of the recommendations by the commission could be impacted by a comprehensive school health program, the last recommendation has particular importance. If adolescents are to reach their full potential, educators, parents, and community members must recognize that adolescents have special emotional, physical, social, mental, and spiritual needs. These young people are seeking answers to a myriad of questions that arise as a result of growing up in a fast-moving technological society. Schools "should offer students a new type of health education that provides honest, relevant information and teaches skills and strategies to make wise decisions and develop positive values. They should assure schools are smoke free, drug free, and violence free, and promote the emotional and physical wellness of students and staff. They should make arrangements for students to receive needed services, increasing their own service capacity and establishing collaborative relationships with external agencies" (National Commission, 1990, Executive Summary).

If one carefully examines the above statement, it becomes readily apparent that by following the guidelines presented in this textbook and implementing a comprehensive school health program, we will go a long way in attaining the goal of improving and promoting the health of the most valuable resource we have, our children.

REVIEW QUESTIONS

1. How would you characterize health programs in the schools of today? Do you think that this is a realistic characterization? Why or why not?
2. What factors in today's society may give impetus to the planning of comprehensive school health programs?
3. What do you feel is the federal focus with respect to school health?

4. What is the importance of the National Center for Health Education?
5. What are the key issues in the professional preparation of health education specialists?
6. Briefly discuss the Role Delineation Project for health educators. What impact do you think this project will have?
7. Some persons have suggested that health educators should not have a licensing or credentialing process. What are your thoughts on this issue?
8. Why do your authors feel that *Code Blue* is a landmark document? What do you think might be the long range impact(s) of this document?

REFERENCES

Bureau of Health Education. *Federal Register 139.* Washington, D.C.: Government Printing Office, 1974.

Education Commission of the States. *Recommendations for School Health Education.* Denver: Education Improvement Center, 1981.

Fodor, J. T., and G. T. Dalis. *Health Instruction: Theory and Application,* 4th ed. Philadelphia: Lea & Febiger, 1989.

Galli, N. *Foundations and Principles of Health Education.* New York: John Wiley & Sons, 1978.

Joint Committee of the Association for the Advancement of Health Education and the American School Health Association. ''Health Instruction Responsibilities and Competencies for Elementary (K–6) Classroom Teachers.'' *Journal of School Health 62* (2), 76–77, 1992.

Kerr, D., D. Allensworth, and J. Gayle. *School-Based HIV Prevention: A Multidisciplinary Approach.* Kent, Ohio: American School Health Association, 1991.

Lovato, C., D. Allensworth, and F. Chan. *School Health in America: An Assessment of State Policies to Protect and Improve the Health of Students,* 5th ed. Kent, Ohio: American School Health Association, 1989.

Metropolitan Life Foundation. *Healthy Me: 1985 School Health Education Survey.* New York: Author.

Metropolitan Life Foundation. *An Evaluation of Comprehensive Health Education in American Public Schools.* New York: Author.

National Center for Health Education. *Initial Role Delineation for Health Education, Final Report.* San Francisco: The Center, 1980.

The National Commission on the Role of the School and the Community in Improving Adolescent Health. *CODE BLUE: Uniting for Healthier Youth.* Alexandria, Virginia: National Association of State Boards of Education, 1990.

National Task Force on the Preparation and Practice of Health Educators, Inc. *A Framework for the Development of Competency-Based Curricula for Entry Level Health Educators.* New York: National Commission for Health Education Credentialing, Inc. 1985. Reprinted in 1990.

National Task Force on the Preparation and Practice of Health Educators, Inc. *A Guide for the Development of Competency-Based Curricula for Entry Level Health Educators.* New York: The Task Force, 1983.

Pigg, R. M. ''Recent Developments in the Evaluation of School Health Education.'' *Health Education* 14:4 (July/August 1983).

Pine, P. *Promoting Health Education in Schools—Problems and Solutions: American Association of School Administrators, Critical Issues Report.* Arlington, Virginia: American Association of School Administrators, 1985.

Pollock, M., and M. Hamburg. ''Health Education: The Basic of the Basics.'' *Health Education 16* no. 2 (1985): 105–109.

President's Committee on Health Education. *Report of the President's Committee on Health Education.* Washington, D.C.: Government Printing Office, 1973.

Rash, J. K., and R. M. Pigg. *The Health Education Curriculum.* New York: John Wiley & Sons, 1979.

U.S. Department of Health, Education and Welfare (HEW), Bureau of Health Education. *Focal Points.* Washington, D.C.: U.S. Government Printing Office, November, 1976.

U.S. Department of Health and Human Services. *Healthy People 2000: National Health Promotion and Disease Prevention Objectives.* Washington, D.C.: Superintendent of Documents, DHHS Publication No. (PHS) 91–50212, 1991.

Appendix

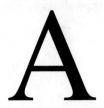

Audiovisual Aids Evaluation Form

Audiovisual Aids Evaluation Form

Title _____ Produced by _____

Running Time _____ min. Filmstrip _____ Slides _____

B & W _____ Color _____ Previewer _____ Date _____

A. Technical Qualities

	Excellent	Good	Fair	Poor
1. Quality of camera work	____	____	____	____
2. Organization and development of content	____	____	____	____
3. Sound accompaniment	____	____	____	____
4. Condition of print or slides	____	____	____	____
5. Presents subject clearly	____	____	____	____

B. Instructional Qualities

1. Accuracy of information	____	____	____	____
2. Correlation with course of study	____	____	____	____
3. Importance of subject matter	____	____	____	____
4. Develops desirable attitudes	____	____	____	____
5. Objectionable or irrelevant elements				

None _____ Few _____ Excessive _____

C. Other Considerations

   1. How will the film be used?

     Introduce a unit   _____

     Summarize   _____

     Cover a specific concept   _____

     Other   _____

   2. Will the film require a lengthy class preparation before it is shown?

     Yes _____ No _____

   3. What follow-up activities will be necessary after the class has viewed the film?

     Discussion _____ Projects _____

   4. At which grade levels would the film be most appropriate?

     _____   _____   _____   _____
     K-3   4, 5, 6   7, 8, 9   10, 11, 12

   5. General rating of film: Excellent _____ Good _____ Fair _____ Poor _____

D. Comments: Use reverse side of form.

From: C. Wilgoose: *Health Teaching in Secondary Schools* (Philadelphia: W. B. Saunders, 1977), p. 361.

Appendix

B

*Guidelines for Sex-Fair Vocational Education Materials**

A CHECKLIST FOR EVALUATING MATERIALS

Language

- Is the generic *he* used to include both males and females when sex is unspecified (e.g., the carpenter . . . he . . .)?
- Is the generic *she* used where the antecedent is stereotypically female (e.g., the housekeeper . . . she . . .)?
- Is a universal male term used when the word is meant to include both sexes (e.g., mankind, forefathers)?
- When referring to both sexes, does the male term consistently precede the female (e.g., he and she, the boys and girls)?
- Are occupational titles used with man as the suffix (e.g., chairman, businessman)?
- When a woman or man holds a nontraditional job, is there unnecessary focus on the person's sex? (e.g., the woman doctor, the male nurse)?
- Are nonparallel terms used in referring to males and females (e.g., Dr. Jones and his secretary, Ellen; Senator Kennedy and Mrs. Gandhi)?
- Are the words ''women'' and ''female'' replaced by pejorative or demeaning synonyms (e.g., girls, fair sex, chicks, ladies)?

*Developed by Women on Words and Images; Princeton, New Jersey.

The research reported herein was performed to a contract No. 300760460 with the Office of Education, U.S. Department of Health, Education, and Welfare. Contractors undertaking such projects under Government sponsorship are encouraged to express freely their professional judgment in the conduct of the project. Points of view or opinions stated do not, therefore, necessarily represent official Office of Education position or policy.

Reprinted by permission of The Office of Education, USDHEW.

- Are women described in terms of their appearance or marital and family status while men are described in terms of accomplishments or titles (e.g., Senator Kennedy and Golda Meir, mother of two)?
- Are women presented as either dependent on, or subordinate to, men (e.g., John took his wife on a trip and let her play bingo)?
- Does a material use sex-fair language initially and then slip into the use of the generic he (e.g., A worker may have union dues deducted from his pay)?
- Is the issue of sexual equality diminished by lumping the problems of women, 51% of the population, with those of minorities (e.g., equal attention will be given to the rights of the handicapped, blacks, and women)?

A CHECKLIST FOR EVALUATING MATERIALS

Roles Occupational/Social

- Are all occupations presented as appropriate to qualified persons of either sex?
- Are certain jobs automatically associated with women and others associated with men (e.g., practical nurse, secretary—female; construction worker, plumber—male)?
- Are housekeeping and family responsibilities still a prime consideration for females in choosing and maintaining a career (e.g., flexible hours, proximity to home)?
- Is the wife presented as needing permission from her husband in order to work (e.g., higher income tax bracket)?
- Is it assumed that the boss, executive, professional, etc., will be male and the assistant, helpmate, "gal Friday" will be female?
- In addition to professional responsibilities, is it assumed that women will also have housekeeping tasks at their place of business (e.g., in an assembly plant with workers of both sexes, the females make the coffee)?
- Is tokenism apparent, in an occasional reference to women or men in nontraditional jobs, while the greatest proportion of the material remains job stereotyped (e.g., one female plumber, one black woman electrician)?
- Are men and women portrayed as having sex-linked personality traits that influence their working abilities (e.g., the brusque foreman, the female bookkeeper's loving attention to detail)?

Omissions

- Does the text deal with the increasing movement of both men and women into nontraditional occupations?
- In historical and biographical references are women adequately acknowledged for their achievements?
- Are quotes and anecdotes from women in history and from important living women used as frequently as those from men?
- Is there acknowledgement of the limitations placed on women in the past (e.g., Women couldn't attach their names to literature, music, inventions, etc.)?
- Are women identified by their husband's names (e.g., Mme. Pierre Curie, Mrs. F. D. Roosevelt)?
- When a historical sexist situation is cited, is it qualified, when appropriate, as past history no longer accepted?

A CHECKLIST FOR EVALUATING MATERIALS

Audio/Visual Materials

- Are male voices used consistently to narrate audio material?
- Are female voices used only when dealing with traditional female occupations, such as child care?
- Do illustrations of males outnumber those of females?
- Do the illustrations represent mainly young, attractive and preferred-body types both in composite pictures as well as in the body of the material?
- Is the text inconsistent with the illustrations (e.g., a sex-fair text illustrated with sexist graphics)?
- Are the illustrations stereotyped (e.g., male mechanics and female teacher aides)?
- Are women shown caring for the home and children while men earn the income?
- When children are illustrated in role rehearsal, are their behaviors and aspirations stereotyped?
- Are women and men commonly drawn in stereotyped body postures and sizes with females shown as consistently smaller, overshadowed, or shown as background figures?
- Does the artist use pastel colors and fuzzy line definition when illustrating females and strong colors and bold lines for males?

- Are women frequently illustrated as the cliché dumb broad or child-woman?
- Are graphs and charts biased, using stereotyped stick figures?
- Are genderless drawings used in order to avoid making a statement or to appear to be sex-fair?
- Are bosses, executives, and leaders pictured as males?
- Is only an occasional token woman pictured as a leader or in a non-stereotyped role?
- Has the illustrator missed opportunities to present sex-fair images?

A CHECKLIST FOR EVALUATING MATERIALS

Physical Appearance

- Are females described in terms of their physical appearance and men in terms of accomplishment or character?
- Is grooming advice focused only on females and presented as a factor in being hired (e.g., advice to secretaries—*proper girdles to firm buttocks*)?
- Is a smiling face considered advisable only for a woman in many occupations?
- Are only men presented or described in terms of accomplishment or character rather than appearance?
- Are only men presented as rarely concerned with clothing and hairstyle?
- Are men shown as taller and more vigorous, women as smaller and more fragile?
- Are women presented as more adroit with a typewriter than a saw?
- Are men presented as dexterous and at ease with tools and machines and baffled when confronted with a filing cabinet?

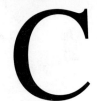
Selected Sources of Textbooks for Health Instruction

This listing is not meant to be all-inclusive. It represents but a few of the textbook sources that are available.

Elementary School

Charles E. Merrill Publishing Company
1300 Alum Creek Drive
Columbus, Ohio 43216
(*Health Focus on You,* grades 1 through 8)

Harcourt, Brace, Jovanovich, Inc.
Orlando, Florida 32887
(*Being Healthy,* grades 1 through 8)

Laidlaw Brothers
Thatcher and Madison
River Forest, Illinois 60305
(*Good Health For Better Living,* grades K through 8)

Scott, Foresman & Company
1900 East Lake Avenue
Glenview, Illinois 60025
(*Health for Life,* grades 1 through 8)

Steck-Vaughn Company
Box 2028
Austin, Texas 78768
(*Choosing Good Health,* grades K through 8)

Junior High School

Scott, Foresman & Company
1900 East Lake Avenue
Glenview, Illinois 60025
(*Health for Life*)

McGraw-Hill Book Company
1221 Avenue of the Americas
New York, New York 10020
(*Health & Safety for You*)

J. B. Lippincott Company
East Washington Square
Philadelphia, Pennsylvania 19105
(*Living in Safety and Health*)

Laidlaw Brothers
Thatcher and Madison
River Forest, Illinois 60305
(*Health and Your Future*)

Houghton Mifflin
1 Beacon Street
Boston, Massachusetts 02108
(*Modern Health Investigations*)

Senior High School

Harcourt, Brace, Jovanovich, Inc.
757 Third Avenue
New York, New York 10017
(*Your Health & Safety in a Changing Environment*)

Houghton Mifflin
1 Beacon Street
Boston, Massachusetts 02108
(*Investigating Your Health*)

Laidlaw Brothers
Thatcher and Madison
River Forest, Illinois 60305
(*Health Today and Tomorrow*)

Steck-Vaughn Company
Box 2028
Austin, Texas 78768
(*Focusing on Health*)

Scott, Foresman & Company
1900 East Lake Avenue
Glenview, Illinois 60025
(*Health and Safety for You; Health: A Way of Life*)

Appendix

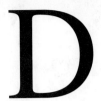

*Criteria for Evaluating the School Health Program (Ohio)**

A SELF-APPRAISAL CHECKLIST FOR SCHOOL HEALTH PROGRAMS

Foreword

In 1966, The Ohio Association for Health, Physical Education and Recreation, in cooperation with the State Department of Education, the State Department of Health, and The State Planning Committee for Health Education in Ohio, developed and distributed the Evaluative Criteria manual for use in Ohio's schools.

This instrument was useful in surveying and comparing actual practice with ideal practice. It included the three major areas:

School Health Services
Healthful School Environment
Health Instruction

This appraisal checklist was well received. In answer to the many and continuing requests for the ''Self-Appraisal Checklist,'' this new revised edition has been developed.

Additional copies may be requested by writing to:

Ohio Department of Education   or   Ohio Department of Health
Health, Physical Education and   Health Education
Recreation Section   P.O. Box 118
65 South Front Street   Columbus OH 43216
Columbus OH 43215

*Reprinted from *A Self-appraisal Checklist for School Health Programs,* Ohio Department of Education, Ohio Department of Health, the Ohio Association for Health, Physical Education and Recreation, and the State Planning Committee for Health Education in Ohio.

Introduction

The School Health Program is designed to maintain and enhance the health of students, school personnel, and the community. It should be a foundation for action programs in the community by providing a health oriented school population. Students will be equipped to deal wisely with their own and their families' health problems and should provide a potential source of adult leadership for future community health problems. The program supplements and reinforces home and community programs. It utilizes the resources of official agencies, professional associations, voluntary organizations, and other community groups, including civic clubs.

Four interrelated parts make up the School Health Program: (I) Administration of the School Health Program, (II) School Health Services which strive to determine the total health status of the student and seek remedial action for health problems, (III) Healthful School Living which designates the plans, procedures and activities which provide a school environment conducive to optimum physical, mental and social health and safety, and (IV) Health Education which provides formal classroom experiences for favorably influencing knowledge, attitudes, habits, values, and skills and behavior pertaining to individual and group health.

This guide can be useful in surveying what a school is doing in terms of health and comparing this to what is considered good practice. As a result, desirable changes can be undertaken to improve the school health program as the needs are indicated.

How to Use this Guide

It is recommended that an evaluation team be organized which includes representatives from school administration, teaching staff, medical and dental professions, nursing, health departments, parents, community groups, etc.

The team should review and discuss the guide prior to its utilization and formulate a plan of action to help insure that techniques and resources are available to appropriately complete the study. The team can then proceed to evaluate its health program by answering the questions and comparing the existing program with the recommended practices.

The third column of the form provides space for comments, priorities, proposed plans and time schedules.

Shortcomings should be prioritized upon consideration of how critical they are and what resources are needed to correct them. A thorough plan of action will include deficiencies subject to immediate and easy correction as well as a timetable and methodology for the correction of problems requiring larger amounts of resources and time (may take one to two years). Follow-up is encouraged to see that corrections are being made according to the specified plan of action.

The study group should not hesitate to request help from specialists or consultants from agencies listed, in addition to local community resources.

Also, this checklist could serve as a valuable tool to school personnel to point out strengths and weaknesses of their respective areas or responsibilities.

Organization of School Health Programs

PART I

Administration of the School Health Program

A successful school health program involves understanding and leadership by the School Administrator in his role as top-ranking coordinator and liaison with the Board of Education, his [her] staff members and the community. He [she] must be able to present school health needs to his board and utilize all resources and facilities in the community for fostering the health of the school children. He [she] is responsible for the enforcement of the state laws regarding school health, including immunizations. The school experiences of students in our school health programs will largely determine their knowledge and their attitudes about health. It is the responsibility of every school to offer a comprehensive and effective health education program taught by adequately prepared instructors. This effort should be supported by all groups in the community. The administrator sets the keynote for effective working relationships with school personnel, students and the community. A school should be responsive to and involve the community in planning, developing, implementing and evaluating programs in a variety of ways, including the establishment of and/or the participation in school-community health committees.

Standards and Recommended Practices	What are We Doing	Comments, Priorities, Proposed Plans, Time Schedule

Program Organization and Administration

A. A well organized school health program should be planned jointly by the schools, the health department, educational and health professional associations and other responsible community groups.

   A. What methods are used to provide for joint planning of the school health program?
     1. on a community-wide basis?
     2. on an individual school basis?

B. Both the Board of Health and Board of Education may be charged with specific responsibilities. If this is so, the administration of the duties should be the result of joint planning, and roles and responsibilities of personnel clearly defined.

   B. List the responsibilities of the:
     1. School
     2. Department of Health

C. A school health program is best integrated when a well qualified school person is appointed to coordinate it.

   C. 1. The person responsible for the coordination and administration of the school health program is:
     a. Superintendent   _____
     b. Health Coordinator   _____

c. Principal _____
d. School Medical Advisor

_____

e. School Dental Advisor

_____

f. School Nurse _____

2. The person responsible for the development of the health curriculum is:
   a. Superintendent _____
   b. Curriculum Director _____
   c. Health Coordinator _____
   d. Principal _____
   e. Nurse _____
   f. Supervisor, Health, Physical Education and Recreation _____
   g. Other (list): _____

3. The person responsible for Health Services is:
   a. Superintendent _____
   b. Health Coordinator _____
   c. Nurse _____
   d. Supervisor, Health, Physical Education and Recreation _____

D. Administrative objectives are:
   1. To develop sound school health policies and to facilitate and make more effective the work of teachers, school health service personnel, and other related non-teaching staff (cafeteria workers, bus drivers, custodians).

D. 1. Does the school have written policies that:
   a. Clearly define agency responsibility including legal.
      Yes _____ No _____
   b. Clearly define roles of personnel, e.g., nurses, administrators, teachers, etc.
      Yes _____ No _____
   c. When were the policies last reviewed?

Standards and Recommended Practices	What are We Doing	Comments, Priorities, Proposed Plans, Time Schedule
2. To provide for special in-service education programs to be conducted for the personnel directly involved in the school health program.	2. Special in-service education programs are conducted for these personnel? Yes _____ No _____ How often? These in-service education programs are evaluated to determine their effectiveness? Yes _____ No _____	
3. To provide for periodic evaluation and improvement to help keep the program in step with changing needs and trends.	3. Periodic evaluations and improvements are provided in the program? In what ways? How often?	
4. To define and develop sound and effective working relationships among agencies directly concerned with the school health program, and to communicate school health concerns to the community-at-large.	4. There are sound and effective working relationships between those involved in the school health program and agencies? Yes _____ No _____ If not, what plans are being made to improve these relationships? Check ways the school health concerns are communicated to the community: P.T.A. or P.T.O _____ School Health Committee _____ School Communications_____ Official Agencies _____ Voluntary Health Agencies _____	

| | The person responsible for helping to insure sound and effective working relationships is:
 a. Superintendent _____
 b. Principal _____
 c. Health Coordinator _____
 d. School Nurse _____
 e. Supervisor, Health, Physical Education _____
 f. Other (list): _____ | |
| E. Well prepared personnel, in all phases of the school health program are essential for its effective and successful implementation. | E. Qualifications of school health personnel.
 1. Check the qualifications and experience of the school health coordinator:
 a. Certificated _____
 b. 3 to 5 years experience in health education or school health programs _____
 c. Recent courses or workshops related to school health _____
 d. Other (list):

 2. What percent of the school nurses are:
 a. Registered in the State of Ohio? _____
 b. Certificated? _____
 c. Have had post-baccalaureate courses in school health? _____

 3. How many elementary teachers have background (a minimum of three semester hours) in health education and/or health science? _____

 4. Are the secondary teachers assigned to teach health certificated in health education? Yes ____ No _____ | |

Standards and Recommended Practices	What are We Doing	Comments, Priorities, Proposed Plans, Time Schedule

5. The school provides an in-service education program for:

a. Teachers?

Yes _____ No _____

Date:

One-half day or less _____

One day or more _____

College Credit _____

b. Nurses?

Yes _____ No _____

Date:

One-half day or less _____

One day or more _____

College Credit _____

c. Administrative Personnel? Guidance counselors, social workers, etc.

Yes _____ No _____

Date:

One-half day or less _____

One day or more _____

College Credit _____

d. Non-teaching (non-certified) personnel?

Yes _____ No _____

Date:

One-half day or less _____

One day or more _____

College Credit _____

F. The school administration promotes the integration of health and safety in all curricular and extracurricular activities of the school.

F. The school administration promotes the integration of health and safety in all curricular and extracurricular activities of the school by:

Leaving to individual teachers

_____

Combined efforts of teachers/coordinators _____

Suggestions in teachers' guides

_____

Written policies and procedures

_____

Standards and Recommended Practices	What are We Doing	Comments, Priorities, Proposed Plans, Time Schedule
G. If available, schools utilize their community directory of health services.	G. The directory is readily available to all school personnel? Yes _____ No _____	
H. Schools should know what health resources are available in the community and how they can be utilized effectively.	H. The school utilizes the following community resources: Health Department _____ Other official agencies _____ Medical Society/Auxiliary _____ Dental Society/Auxiliary _____ Voluntary Agencies _____ Civic Groups _____ Other (list):	

First Aid for Sudden Illness and Accidents:

A. State law (Sec. 3313.712) requires that an emergency medical treatment authorization form be annually filled out on each student by his parent or legal guardian before October of each year. This form is to be kept on file in the school.	A. Emergency medical treatment authorization forms for all students are filled out annually and are on file in each school? Yes _____ No _____	
B. First aid and sudden illness procedures agreed upon by administrator and staff are written and disseminated to all staff.	B. 1. Are policies agreed upon by administrators and staff? Yes _____ No _____ 2. Are written copies of first aid and sudden illness policies made available to all staff? Yes _____ No _____	
C. Persons (other than nurses) trained in first aid procedures should be available for administering first aid or providing direction in cases of sudden illness.	C. 1. How many persons with current first aid preparation are available? _____	

Organization of School Health Programs

Standards and Recommended Practices	What are We Doing	Comments, Priorities, Proposed Plans, Time Schedule
	2. Are all teachers working in high risk areas qualified in first aid, such as: Science Labs _____ Shops _____ Home Economics _____ Physical Education _____	
D. First aid procedures should be briefly written for quick reference and posted in special areas, such as science labs, shops, home economics rooms, school health clinic, and physical education areas.	D. Check areas posted: Science Labs _____ Shops _____ Home Economics Room _____ Health Clinic _____ Physical Education _____	
E. First aid equipment/supplies should be kept in stock and readily accessible. All medicines, compounds, bandaging materials should be clearly labeled for use. A designated person should be responsible for ordering supplies.	E. 1. In what locations are first aid supplies stored? 2. All supplies are clearly labeled? Yes _____ No _____ 3. Check the person responsible for ordering and restocking supplies? Superintendent _____ Principal _____ Nurse _____ Supervisor, Health, Physical Education, and Recreation _____ Health Coordinator _____	

Accident Reporting System

A. Written policies and procedures (developed by administration and faculty, outlining a system for reporting school accidents) should be available to all school personnel.	A. Policies are written and made available to all staff: Yes _____ No _____	

Standards and Recommended Practices	What are We Doing	Comments, Priorities, Proposed Plans, Time Schedule
B. The Ohio Department of Health has an Accident Reporting Form, No. 4966.32. They may be utilized if the schools will report the statistical data to the Accident Prevention Program at the end of the year.	B. Does your school use the Ohio Department of Health Accident Reporting Form? Yes _____ No _____	

C. The reporting system should:
1. define a ''reportable accident''
2. indicate the time lapse in reporting the accident
3. record information to include: who, what, where, when, why
4. include follow-through on treatment or referral
5. indicate who is responsible for recording and reporting accidents
	C. Does the reporting system include:
	1. definition of a reportable accident _____
	2. time lapse in reporting accident _____
	3. who-what-where-when-why _____
	4. follow-up-
	  a. number of days lost from school _____
	  b. determining cause of accident _____
	  c. possible action in future to avoid or eliminate future occurrences _____
	5. who is responsible for recording accidents? _____	

D. School personnel should be familiar with school accident forms and should complete or use them uniformly.	D. School personnel are informed regarding the use of accident forms by: 1. Staff conferences _____ 2. News bulletin _____ 3. Teacher handbooks _____ 4. Other (list):	
E. At the end of each school year, all accident data should be reviewed, analyzed, and compared with last year's records to determine the needs for next year's program.	E. List recommendations as a result of reviewing this year's records.	

Standards and Recommended Practices	What are We Doing	Comments, Priorities, Proposed Plans, Time Schedule
F. A safety committee is recommended to provide leadership for planning a comprehensive safety education program. It should include such people as: administrator, safety specialist, teacher, driver education teacher, physician, school nurse, sanitarian, custodian, student, parent, etc.	F. 1. Do you have a safety committee? Yes _____ No _____ 2. Who is on the committee? 3. List the name of the Specialist in Safety.	

PART II

School Health Services

In order to meet the educational and health needs of students, it is essential to secure data concerning their physical, mental and emotional condition. Thus, school health services are an important part of the school health programs. These services are planned to protect the health of the students and to help each pupil reach and maintain good health. Also, the school health service program serves as a learning experience for students, teachers, and parents, thereby helping to insure positive health practices.

The school health program is influenced by local customs, the types of professional manpower, the resources available, the understanding and cooperation of the community.

Standards and Recommended Practices	What are We Doing	Comments, Priorities, Proposed Plans, Time Schedule
Teacher Observation A. To teach effectively it is important that the teacher keep informed of the health needs of all her pupils. 1. Teachers should receive in-service education in the health observation of school children so that they may refer children who they suspect as having a health problem to appropriate health service personnel. This should be a year round program.	A. What type of in-service education is provided teachers to improve their skills of observation and referral procedures? 1. Teacher/Nurse Conferences Yes _____ No _____ Health Education Workshops Yes _____ No _____ College/University Credit Courses Yes _____ No _____ Other (list):	

Standards and Recommended Practices	What are We Doing	Comments, Priorities, Proposed Plans, Time Schedule

2. "A Teacher Worksheet for Student Health Observation" would be useful to familiarize teachers with signs and symptoms of health and emotional problems. This may be ordered from the Ohio Department of Health. (No. 3611.13)

2. Do teachers use "A Teacher Worksheet for Student Health Observation"?
Yes _____ No _____

Health Screening

Hearing

A. The following should be screened annually:
  1. all children in grades K through 3
  2. all teacher referrals
  3. all children new to the school system
  4. all children in grades 6 and 9

  These tests should be administered with the individual pure tone audiometer.

A. Check grades you are screening with the pure tone audiometer:

	No. Screened	No. Failed 1st Screening	No. Failed 2nd Screening	Failed Threshold Test and Referred
K				
1st				
2nd				
3rd				
Other Grades				
Referrals				
New Students				
Total				

B. All students failing the first screening should be re-screened within two weeks.

B. The number of children who failed to pass threshold screening tests represents _____ percent of all children screened.

C. Refer all children who fail to pass the threshold screening test to appropriate resources as: medical or audiological.

C. What percentage of the children referred for follow-up care are known to have received it? _____

Standards and Recommended Practices	What are We Doing	Comments, Priorities, Proposed Plans, Time Schedule

D. Assure that follow-up care has been obtained for each person referred for care.

D. Procedures used to secure follow-up care
_____ Visit to home
_____ Telephone call (by teacher or nurse)
_____ Note sent home
_____ Other (list):

Vision

E. Ideally, all children (Kindergarten through grade 12 and all teacher referrals) should be screened annually with a Snellen chart. Minimum: K and grades 1, 3, 5, 7, 9.

E. Check grades you are screening with the Snellen eye chart:

	No. Screened	No. Failed 1st Screening	No. Failed 2nd Screening and Referred
K			
1			
2			
3			
4			
5			
6			
7			
8			
9			
10			
11			
12			

F. Screen all children for ocular muscle imbalance, excessive farsightedness, and near acuity in grades one or three, and screen for color deficiency in either elementary or junior high grade.

F. Are you screening all children in grades 1 or 3 for:
Ocular muscle imbalance
Yes _____ No _____
Excessive farsightedness
Yes _____ No _____

Standards and Recommended Practices	What are We Doing	Comments, Priorities, Proposed Plans, Time Schedule
	Near acuity Yes _____ No _____ Color deficiency Yes _____ No _____ (elementary or Jr. High grade. Please indicate which grade ___).	
G. Refer all children who fail a screening test to a vision specialist.	G. How many children were referred for eye care after last screening? _____ This represents _____ percent of the children screened.	
H. Determine that follow-up care has been obtained for each child referred for eye care.	H. What percentage of the children referred are known to have received follow-up care? _____ %	

Health Room (Clinic)

A. A health room or clinic should be provided and adequately equipped to carry on essential school health services: examinations, tests for vision, hearing, speech, psychological, and private conferences.	A. Does your school have a room where the school physician, school nurse and other specialists can perform: Examination Yes _____ No _____ Vision testing Yes _____ No _____ Hearing testing Yes _____ No _____ Psychological testing Yes _____ No _____ Speech therapy Yes _____ No _____ Private Conferences Yes _____ No _____ 1. Does it have a place where pupils who are injured or who become suddenly ill can wait until someone can transport them home? Yes _____ No _____ 2. Does it have space for use by health service personnel for individual or small group conferences? Yes _____ No _____	

3. Is there adequate space for storing first aid supplies, school health records, etc.?
Yes _____ No _____

Medical Examinations

A. "School Health: A Guide for Physicians," American Academy of Pediatrics, suggests that the priority of medical appraisal should be:
1. children identified as having problems
2. children entering school
3. children in mid-school (6–7 grades)
4. children before leaving school (11–12 grades)

Medical examinations should be done by a physician in his [her] office or in a clinic. Parents of elementary children should be present. These examinations should be comprehensive and any abnormal findings of the school screening tests should be provided to the physician. The results of the physician's examination should be reported to school personnel.

A. Do pupils receive a medical examination upon entrance to school?
Yes _____ No _____
1. Are they examined at mid-school?
Yes _____ No _____
2. Are referrals with special problems examined?
Yes _____ No _____
3. Are they examined at senior high school?
Yes _____ No _____

B. Arrangements should be made for children of low income families to receive examinations. Plans should be formulated whereby school and physicians share necessary information.

B. Is this examination done by:
Health Department
Yes _____ No _____
School Health Service
Yes _____ No _____
Other (list):

If there are no arrangements for this examination, give reason:

Standards and Recommended Practices	What are We Doing	Comments, Priorities, Proposed Plans, Time Schedule
C. Medical examinations should be given to students enrolled in athletic programs. Consideration should be given to students enrolled in other groups, such as, marching bands, intramural and inter-scholastic sports, etc.	C. Are boys and girls in the athletic program provided medical examinations? Boys Yes _____ No _____ Girls Yes _____ No _____ By whom? _____ When? _____ Other groups such as: Marching Band Members Yes _____ No _____ Drill Teams Yes _____ No _____ Intramural Sports Yes _____ No _____ Interscholastic Sports Yes _____ No _____	
D. All families receiving ADC should be enrolled in the Early Periodic Screening Diagnosis and Treatment (EPSDT) Program.	D. How many children are enrolled in EPSDT Programs in: Elementary _____ Secondary _____	
E. Plans should be developed with Department of Welfare to share this information as needed by professional personnel planning health services for the child.	E. Check the method the Welfare Department utilizes to share EPSDT screening information on students:	

Health Records

A. A health record should be started when the child enters school and should follow the student as he moves from grade to grade and from school to school. Confidentiality of all health and mental health records should be respected. All personnel should be very careful of sharing any information that might prove speculative or damaging to any student.	A. Does each pupil have a health record on file? Yes _____ No _____ Does your school use School Health Records, form 3613.13 Rev. 1974, from the Ohio Department of Health? Yes _____ No _____ If not, what form is used: Is the permanent health record transferred when a child changes schools? Yes _____ No _____	

428   Organization of School Health Programs

Standards and Recommended Practices	What are We Doing	Comments, Priorities, Proposed Plans, Time Schedule

Health Counseling

A. A definite plan of continuous follow-up should be established. The school nurse should be a liaison with school, parents and community resources.

A. Has your school established a plan of referral and follow-up?
Yes _____ No _____

B. Health counseling is one of the main functions of the school nurse, and important information should be shared with and utilized by school counselors, psychologists, teachers, etc.

B. Is the nurse given time for counseling?
Yes _____ No _____

C. The school nurse follows through to help the parent with remedial action. Upon discovering a health defect in a student, the school nurse should follow-up by assisting parents with a plan of remedial action. This could involve a team, such as: physician, psychologist, public health nurse, visiting teacher, speech therapist, school counselor, etc.

C. Does the nurse communicate with parents regarding child health defects and remedial action by:
Written note
          Yes _____ No _____
Telephone Yes _____ No _____
Home Visit Yes _____ No _____
Conference at school
Yes _____ No _____

D. The school nurse should have some training in mental health counseling. The school nurse and counseling psychologist should have agreed upon procedures for mutual referral and collaboration on students with significantly overlapping physical (somatic) and mental health problems.

D. Has the school nurse had any courses in mental health?
Yes _____ No _____
Are there mutually agreed procedures for referral by school nurse and by psychologist?
Yes _____ No _____

Teacher-Nurse Conferences

A. A teacher-nurse conference should be held at least once a year or as often as needed.

A. Is time provided for the nurse to schedule conferences with teachers?
1. Once a year
Yes _____ No _____
2. As often as necessary
Yes _____ No _____

Standards and Recommended Practices	What are We Doing	Comments, Priorities, Proposed Plans, Time Schedule

Children With Special Problems

A. Identification of and special provision for handicapped children; deaf and hard of hearing, crippled, visually impaired, neurologically and emotionally, educable mentally retarded, etc., is an important aspect of school health services.

The school should make special provisions for handicapped pupils in regular classes when this is the most appropriate placement.

Special facilities and/or programs should be made available to the children with any handicapping conditions.

A. Number of children with special problems in:
Elementary _____
Secondary _____
List types of handicaps:

What provision is made for children with special problems? Check:
1. Special Facilities:
Ramps _____
Special toilets _____
Rest areas _____
2. Special Services:
Occupational Therapy _____
Physical Therapy _____
Speech Therapy _____
Psychological _____
3. In-service education for teachers _____
4. In-service education for auxiliary personnel _____
Types:

5. Transportation provided _____
6. Other (list):

Dental Examinations

A. Examinations by a dentist for school purposes should be given to all pupils entering the system and at the beginning of the secondary school level.

A. Do pupils receive a dental examination upon entrance to school?
Yes _____ No _____
If yes, what percent? _____ %
1. Do pupils receive a dental examination at the secondary level?
Yes _____ No _____
If yes, what percent? _____ %

Organization of School Health Programs

Standards and Recommended Practices	What are We Doing	Comments, Priorities, Proposed Plans, Time Schedule
B. These examinations should be done by a dentist in his office or clinic with the parents of elementary children accompanying them.	B. Outline your plan for making a concentrated effort to have all students visit their dentist regularly	

1. Check reasons why students are not receiving dental care:
   Lack of dental manpower   _____
   Lack of funds   _____
   Lack of transportation   _____
   Other (list):   _____

C. The school or the community should provide for the dental examinations of indigent pupils. The local Dental Society working with the school and community should formulate a program to provide services for indigent students.

C. What dental services are provided for children whose parents cannot afford such services?

   1. What arrangements are made for the examination of indigent children?

D. All students involved in inter-scholastic contact athletics should be provided with mouth protectors. The local dental society should be contacted for assistance.

D. What arrangements are made for mouth protectors for students involved in interscholastic contact athletics?
   Provided by student
   Yes _____ No _____
   Provided by schools
   Yes _____ No _____
   Provided by local dental society
   Yes _____ No _____
   Provided by other (list):

E. The community water supply should be fluoridated.

E. Is your community water supply fluoridated?
   Yes _____ No _____
   1. If not, why?

F. In a good school health program, oral hygiene should be observed by the teacher, school nurse and other personnel involved in the health of the student. Pertinent information should be recorded on the cumulative health record. Evidence of dental neglect should be reported by the school nurse or teacher to parents. Follow-up of this referral should be done by the responsible person.

F. Pertinent dental health information is filed in the cumulative health folder?
Yes _____ No _____
Referrals from dentists
Yes _____ No _____
Recorded by nurse
Yes _____ No _____
Other (list):

G. Dentists, Dental Auxiliaries or affiliated groups are resources that can be utilized in a dental health education program.

G. Check the resources listed below which have been utilized in your dental program in the past.
Dentists
Yes _____ No _____
Dental Hygienists
Yes _____ No _____
Dental Auxiliaries
Yes _____ No _____
P.T.A. or P.T.O.
Yes _____ No _____
Others (list):

Future Plans:

Health of School Personnel

A. Pre-employment health examinations should be required of all school personnel.

A. Pre-employment examinations are required for all school personnel?
Yes _____ No _____

B. Periodic medical examinations of school personnel are recommended.

B. If periodic medical examinations are required, state the time intervals:

Standards and Recommended Practices	What are We Doing	Comments, Priorities, Proposed Plans, Time Schedule

Communicable Disease Control

A. There should be well defined school health policies developed in cooperation with local health departments and/or with School Health Services and approved by the Board of Education.

A. Does your school have written school health policies?
Yes _____ No _____

B. School personnel and parents should be informed regarding these policies.

B. Parents and teachers are informed regarding these policies by:
Meetings   Yes _____ No _____
Newsletters Yes _____ No _____
Other (list):

C. School nurses should report cases of communicable diseases, including pediculosis and scabies, to local health department.

C. Check the method the school nurses use in reporting communicable diseases to the local health department:
Phone   _____
Written form   _____

D. All students should comply with the law of Ohio regarding immunizations as stated in Section 3313.671 of the Ohio Revised Code. This law requires a pupil to be or in the process of being immunized against polio, rubeola, diphtheria, rubella, pertussis and tetanus. This is the responsibility of the administrator.

D. Does your school have a formal plan for enforcement of this law?
Yes _____ No _____

PART III
Healthful School Living

The health of the students and school personnel is affected by the environment in which they work and play. Environment influences the health, the habits, the attitudes, the comfort, the safety, and the working efficiency of school personnel. The environment is the responsibility of the school administration, helping to maintain it is the responsibility of all school personnel, and inspecting for environmental deficiencies is the statutory responsibility of the local department of health.

Standards and Recommended Practices	What are We Doing	Comments, Priorities, Proposed Plans, Time Schedule

Inspection

A. Semi-annual inspections of the school facilities are made by the local health department sanitarians and school health personnel (custodial staff—school administrators).

A copy of the School Environment Inspection Form is on page 441.

A. Date of School Inspection:

School Official
Name and Title: _____
_____

1. Progress of inspection recommendations:

*Copy of "Sanitation in The School Environment" No. 2116.32 is available from the Ohio Department of Health.

B. Semi-annual inspections of the school food service operation (if provided) are made by the local health department's sanitarian and school personnel (cafeteria supervisor-school administrators).

B. Date of Food Service Inspection:

School Official
Name and Title: _____
_____

1. Progress in correcting (remedying) inspection violations:

C. Procedure has been established to insure that inspection reports are properly interpreted to school authorities.

C. The inspection results are reviewed and explained with recommendations to the school officials at the time of the inspection.
School Officials consulted:
1. Superintendent or Principal _____
2. School Administrator _____
3. Custodial Supervisor _____
4. Cafeteria Supervisor _____
5. Others _____

Standards and Recommended Practices	What are We Doing	Comments, Priorities, Proposed Plans, Time Schedule
D. Copies of the inspection reports are sent to the appropriate persons.	D. Copies of the inspection reports are sent to: 1. Board of Education _____ 2. School Administrator _____ 3. Health Supervisor/Coordinator _____ 4. Custodial Supervisor _____ 5. Cafeteria Supervisor _____ 6. Others: _____	
E. Plans for any new physical structure, (including all major improvements) are submitted to the appropriate agencies prior to construction.	E. Plans are submitted to: 1. State Department of Industrial Relations _____ 2. State Plumbing Unit, Ohio Department of Health _____ 3. Local Health Department _____ 4. Others as required _____	
F. Periodic in-service education programs sponsored jointly by the health department and the school system for custodial and food service employees are recommended.	F. Check the in-service education programs for custodial and food service employees during the last 12 months. 1. A program conducted by the Health Department for custodial and food service employees. Yes _____ No _____ 2. Personnel attended workshop in Columbus conducted by the Department of Education. Yes _____ No _____ List future plans for in-service education programs for the next 12 months.	

Standards and Recommended Practices	What are We Doing	Comments, Priorities, Proposed Plans, Time Schedule
G. The school environment should stimulate learning and the development of good sanitation practices such as: 1. Food handling instructions for students assisting in the lunch room. 2. Students to learn and appreciate good food handling practices. 3. Maintaining a more attractive lunch room. 4. Proper storage of food.	G. Check any activities initiated by school officials which serve to motivate environmental sanitation practices. 1. Enlists the help of student patrols to make inspections of the environment to check for good sanitation and safety practices. Yes _____ No _____ 2. Food handling class conducted for students assisting in the lunch room. Yes _____ No _____ 3. Group of students works with lunch room personnel in improving attractiveness of lunch room. Yes _____ No _____ 4. Invites local sanitarian to discuss sanitation and safety practices to school personnel and/or health classes. Yes _____ No _____ 5. Others (list):	

Safe School Environment

Accident prevention is a vital part of semi-annual inspections conducted by local health sanitarians and school health personnel. These inspections place considerable emphasis on maintaining, planning and developing safety practices within the school environment and especially at specific locations.

A. The sanitarian's inspection of safety of the environment should include the following major areas: *School grounds *Parking area *Playground and equipment	A. 1. Parking kept away from playground equipment? Yes _____ No _____ 2. Playground equipment maintained in good repair? Yes _____ No _____	

*Athletic field and equipment
*Floor areas, stairs, ramps
*Classrooms
*Dressing/shower rooms
*Gymnasium
*Vocational areas/chem labs/ home economics rooms
*School cafeteria/kitchens
*Restrooms
*Fire fighting equipment/exits
*First aid emergency rooms

3. Has soft, absorbent surface been provided around playground equipment?
   Yes _____ No _____
4. Are floor surfaces kept clean, free of tripping, slipping hazards?
   Yes _____ No _____
5. Classrooms arranged for best traffic patterns, least amount of congestion?
   Yes _____ No _____
6. Classroom furniture kept in good repair, adequate lighting provided?
   Yes _____ No _____
7. Adequate supervision provided for organized/ unorganized activity on the school grounds and in the gymnasium?
   Yes _____ No _____
8. Necessary safety precautions taken in vocational shop, chem labs, home economics areas, i.e.:
   *protective eyeware provided
   Yes _____ No _____
   *faucet for eye lavage if chemically burned
   Yes _____ No _____
   *fire extinguisher close to heating elements
   Yes _____ No _____
9. In-service safety programs presented for food service personnel in school kitchen?
   Yes _____ No _____
   Date of last in-service workshop?
   Projected date for next food safety program?
10. Restroom floors kept dry, free of debris?
    Yes _____ No _____

Standards and Recommended Practices	What are We Doing	Comments, Priorities, Proposed Plans, Time Schedule
	11. Fire extinguishers checked monthly to determine operability? Yes _____ No _____ Date of last fire extinguisher check?	
	12. Proper class of extinguishers provided according to type of fire hazard, i.e., electrical, paper, chemical, etc.? Yes _____ No _____	
	13. Health department sanitarian meets with school personnel or safety committee to discuss findings of the school inspection and needed or recommended corrections? Yes _____ No _____ Comments:	

B. An effective school safety program encompasses many areas within the school system:
1. Constant awareness to potential hazards of new products being introduced into the school environment.
2. Special training, and drills of school bus drivers and children in school bus safety practices along with regular school vehicle inspections.
3. School safety concerns integrated into appropriate curriculum designs.
4. Fire drills
5. Safety education
	B. Check any special safety in-service education programs during the past school year for:
	Bus Drivers Yes _____ No _____
	Lunch room personnel
	        Yes _____ No _____
	Teachers Yes _____ No _____
	Custodians Yes _____ No _____
	Safety Patrol
	        Yes _____ No _____	

Standards and Recommended Practices	What are We Doing	Comments, Priorities, Proposed Plans, Time Schedule

C. Safety concerns should be integrated into the health education curriculum.	C. Check safety concerns that have been integrated into the curriculum this past year, such as:
	  1. Accident Etiology
	     Yes _____ No _____
	  2. Bicycle Yes _____ No _____
	  3. Home (urban/suburban)
	     Yes _____ No _____
	  4. Home (rural)
	     Yes _____ No _____
	  5. Toy Safety
	     Yes _____ No _____
	  6. Pedestrian Safety
	     Yes _____ No _____
	  7. Vacation Yes _____ No _____
	  8. Poisons Yes _____ No _____
	  9. Firearms and Hunting
	     Yes _____ No _____
	  10. Automobile and seat belt
	     Yes _____ No _____
	  11. Pets Yes _____ No _____
	  12. Fires Yes _____ No _____
	  13. Athletic and playground
	     Yes _____ No _____
	  14. Water and boating
	     Yes _____ No _____	

School Nutrition Program

A. There is a food service provided in the school and all pupils are encouraged to participate.	A. Is there a food service program in your school? Yes _____ No _____	
B. The lunch served meets the National "Type A" Standard.	B. Does it meet National "Type A" Standard? Yes _____ No _____	

C. Even though it is legal to sell candy and sweetened beverages in the school, it is recommended that this practice not be permitted during school or lunch hours. Sale of such items is in direct competition with a good lunch program.	C. Does your school sell:
	  1. Candy Yes _____ No _____
	  2. Soft drinks
	     Yes _____ No _____
	  3. Chocolate milk or drink
	     Yes _____ No _____
	  4. Other snack items
	     Yes _____ No _____	

Standards and Recommended Practices	What are We Doing	Comments, Priorities, Proposed Plans, Time Schedule

D. The school lunch program should be utilized as a learning laboratory for good nutrition in a child's life.	D. Check any of these activities related to lunch room and nutrition that are utilized in the health education program.
	1. Classroom units
	    Yes _____ No _____
	2. Pupils given an opportunity to evaluate menus to determine if they meet ''Type A'' School Lunch requirements.
	    Yes _____ No _____
	3. Pupils or art classes make posters for the lunch room.
	    Yes _____ No _____
	4. Classes plan menus and solicit the assistance of head cook in serving it to students.
	    Yes _____ No _____
	5. A class makes a survey of eating habits of students in lunch room to see foods rejected or wasted.
	    Yes _____ No _____
	6. Class tours the kitchen to observe dish washing, storage of food, etc. and to discuss why certain practices are necessary.
	    Yes _____ No _____	

E. School Food Service Personnel should be required (expenses to be paid by the Board of Education) to attend workshops and conferences sponsored by the State Department of Education for the lunch room workers.	E. In this school year, how many school lunch personnel attended the workshops and conferences sponsored by the State Department of Education? _____ 1. How many attended local workshops? _____	

School Environment Inspection Form

Health District

Name of School _____ Address _____
Clerk. Board of Education _____ Address _____
Superintendent or Principal _____ Address _____
Custodians _____

- ☐ Elementary
- ☐ Junior High
- ☐ Senior High

Enrollment _____

No. Classrooms _____
Food Service ☐ Yes ☐ No
Swimming Pool ☐ Yes ☐ No

- ☐ Municipal Sewage
- ☐ Public Sewage
- ☐ Municipal Water
- ☐ Public Water

Items marked by (x) are explained below with recommendations.

I Surroundings
  A. Location ☐
  B. Grounds, Walkways and
    Driveways ☐
  C. Playground Equipment ☐

II Building
  A. Structure ☐
  B. Floor Cleaning and Repair ☐
  C. Walls and Ceiling—Cleaning
    and Repair ☐
  D. Doors and Windows ☐

III Heating and Ventilation
  A. Thermostat and Thermometer
    Each Classroom ☐
  B. Temperature and Humidity ☐
  C. Ventilation and Dust Control ☐

IV Lighting
  A. Adequate Artificial Lighting ☐
  B. Maintenance of Fixtures ☐
  C. Quality and Proper Use
    of Lighting ☐

V Water Supply
  A. Source, Development and
    Treatment ☐
  B. Pressure and Chemical Quality ☐
  C. Plumbing, Maintenance and
    Design ☐
  D. Drinking Fountains ☐

VI Toilet and Locker Room Facilities
  A. Cleaning, Repair and Adequacy of
    1. Rooms ☐
    2. Showers and Toilet Fixtures ☐
    3. Lockers and Modesty
      Equipment ☐
    4. Handwashing Facilities ☐
  B. Ventilation ☐
  C. Rest Room Supplies ☐

VII Waste Disposal
  A. Sewage System Operation ☐
  B. Sewage System Maintenance ☐
  C. Refuse and Garbage Disposal ☐
  D. Refuse and Garbage Storage ☐

VIII School Room Facilities
  A. Adequate Equipment and
    Furnishings ☐
  B. Maintenance of Equipment and
    Furnishings ☐
  C. Room Population (Overcrowding) ☐

IX Accident Prevention
  A. Traffic Safety ☐
  B. Fire Exits Marked, Adequate ☐
  C. Fire Fighting Equipment ☐
  D. Rooms and Halls Free of Hazards ☐
  E. Stairways and Playgrounds Free of Hazards ☐
  F. Properly Equipped Emergency Room ☐

X Insect and Rodent Control
  A. No Evidence of Insect Infestation ☐
  B. No Evidence of Rodent Infestation ☐
  C. Proper Control Procedures Used ☐

Recommendations:

_____

_____

_____

_____

_____

_____

_____

_____

_____

_____

_____

_____

_____

_____

_____   _____
        Date   Sanitarian

PART IV

Health Education

Schools are the official community agencies for the education of children. They have the major responsibility for the health instruction of children, grades K through 12. Health education instruction should be organized to provide learning experiences which favorably influence understandings, attitudes, and behavior in respect to individual and community health. In addition, the program should be designed to teach the individual to assume an ever increasing responsibility for his or her own health status.

Careful and continuous planning on the part of the school is necessary for an effective health instruction program. Objectives must be established; a sequential curriculum K–12 must be developed or adopted; content should be appropriate to the needs, interests and intellectual ability of the pupils; adequate time and credit must be allotted; and, most important, well qualified, certificated and enthusiastic teachers must be assigned to teach the health classes.

Standards and Recommended Practices	What are We Doing	Comments, Priorities, Proposed Plans, Time Schedule

Administration

A. Authorities recommend that health be taught 15–30 minutes daily at the elementary level; a full year course taught daily at the 7th, 8th, or 9th grade; and a full year course on a daily basis at the 10th, 11th or 12th grade.

In the elementary schools, the Ohio State Department of Education requires a minimum of two 40 minute periods per week in grades 3 through 6, and two 45 minute periods per week in grades 7 and 8.

The Ohio State Department of Education requires a semester course or its equivalent be taught at the high school level (9–12).

A. 1. Time allotted/week

Grade
K _____
1 _____
2 _____
3 _____
4 _____
5 _____
6 _____

2. Health is taught as a separate course at the junior high level?
(Circle grade(s): 7, 8, 9)
Yes _____ No _____

3. Health is taught as a separate course at the high school level?
(Circle grade(s): 10, 11, 12)
Yes _____ No _____

Standards and Recommended Practices	What are We Doing	Comments, Priorities, Proposed Plans, Time Schedule

  4. How often do the classes meet?
     Junior High _____
     Senior High _____

  5. How much time is allotted per class period? _____

B. The number of pupils assigned to health classes should be no greater than those assigned to other classes.

B. 1. Average number of students per health class is _____ .
    2. Average number of students per all other classes is _____.

C. Most authorities recommend that health be taught in a natural setting and that the sexes should only be separated if they are separated for other courses.

C. 1. Which of the following is typical in your school?
       Separate classes, boys and girls
       Yes _____ No _____
       Coed classes
       Yes _____ No _____
       Usually coed, but separated for some classes
       Yes _____ No _____

       If yes, which topics:
       Human Sexuality
       Yes _____ No _____
       Feminine Hygiene
       Yes _____ No _____
       Other (list):

D. Scheduling for health instruction should be like all other disciplines.

D. Health receives the same status on scheduling as other disciplines? Yes _____ No _____

E. A staff member, specialized in health education (major in health education) should be designated health chairman or coordinator and assigned the responsibility for coordinating the entire health program.

E. A health chairman is designated?
   Yes _____ No _____

   1. If yes, is the health chairman a specialist in health education by professional preparation?
      Yes _____ No _____

Standards and Recommended Practices	What are We Doing	Comments, Priorities, Proposed Plans, Time Schedule
	2. If chairman is not a specialist in health education, check any of the following that apply: a. Has taken some health education courses and had experience in teaching health? Yes _____ No _____ b. Has attended a School Health Workshop at a college or university? Yes _____ No _____	
F. An interdisciplinary committee of persons should be appointed to plan and evaluate the health program cooperatively. The health coordinator should chair this group.	F. A health committee is appointed? Yes _____ No _____ 1. How often does the committee meet? 2. The health coordinator chairs this committee? Yes _____ No _____ 3. The local health committee is represented by the following (check appropriate ones): Teachers _____ Parents _____ Administrators _____ Physicians _____ Nurses _____ Guidance counselor _____ Psychologist _____ Students _____ Others (list):	
G. The school administration should provide a setting conducive to health instruction, including an equipped classroom, moveable furniture, supplies and materials and tables for demonstrations.	G. Our school utilizes: Regular sized classroom _____ Moveable furniture _____ Materials and supplies _____ Tables for experiments and demonstrations _____	

Standards and Recommended Practices	What are We Doing	Comments, Priorities, Proposed Plans, Time Schedule
H. The school should provide in-service education programs for teachers to assist them in conducting health instruction in an interesting and sequential manner.	H. How many in-service programs on health education were offered during the past year? _____ 1. How many faculty attended each program? _____ 2. List the grades represented by teachers attending: _____ 3. Were the in-service programs evaluated? Yes _____ No _____ 4. Topics covered (check appropriate ones): General health knowledge _____ New materials reviewed _____ Teaching ideas shared _____ Organization and curriculum development planning of program by grade level _____ Demonstration of use of audio-visual and other equipment _____ Other topics (please indicate): 5. Were resource persons from universities, state and/or local health agencies utilized? Yes _____ No _____ 6. If yes, name participating agencies.	
I. The school administration should provide textbooks, charts, filmstrips, resource books, models, pamphlets, transparencies, and other aids which are authoritative, up to date, interesting and appropriate for the grade level in which they are used.	I. List source of textbooks? 1. When were the health textbooks printed? 2. Have resources been reviewed by health committee? Yes _____ No _____	

Standards and Recommended Practices	What are We Doing	Comments, Priorities, Proposed Plans, Time Schedule

3. Which of the following are readily available?

Textbooks	_____
Charts	_____
Filmstrips	_____
Resource books	_____
Models	_____
Pamphlets	_____
Transparencies	_____

Others (list):

Curriculum Planning

A. The health instruction program should be based on the problem solving conceptual approach to studying and meeting the health needs, interests and problems of the students.

A. 1. Check ways students were surveyed to find their needs and interests:

Questionnaires	_____
Tests	_____
Checklists	_____
Personal Essays	_____

2. List ways the community has been utilized to find local needs and interests:

3. Are morbidity and mortality statistics for the community studied and utilized?

B. Curriculum planning should be carried out by the interdisciplinary committee responsible for the school health program.

B. Is the interdisciplinary committee assigned the task of writing the health education curriculum?
Yes _____ No _____
1. If not, who is responsible for the curriculum?

Standards and Recommended Practices	What are We Doing	Comments, Priorities, Proposed Plans, Time Schedule
C. The health instruction program should utilize the conceptual approach such as: School Health Education Study, "A Conceptual Approach to Curriculum Design," the ASHA Curriculum, the Ohio Department of Education Comprehensive Drug Education Curriculum.	C. Is the conceptual approach utilized? Yes _____ No _____ 1. Of the following, check those which have been reviewed by the health committee: School Health Education Study, "A Conceptual Approach to Curriculum Design" _____ American School Health Association's Curriculum _____ Ohio Department of Education _____ Comprehensive Drug Education Curriculum, K–12 _____ 2. If none of the above are utilized, name others that have been used as references: 3. Check the grade levels in which the conceptual approach is used: 1–3 _____ 4–6 _____ 7–9 _____ 10–12 _____	

Standards and Recommended Practices	What are We Doing	Comments, Priorities, Proposed Plans, Time Schedule

D. The school system provides for use in the school a teaching guide, which contains:
1. A statement of philosophy upon which the school health education program is based.
2. Health education instructional content guide which includes a developmental scope and sequence approach to curriculum design, including the following:

    a. Concept Emphasis

    b. Content

    c. Suggested teacher methods and techniques

    d. Student learning activities

    e. Evaluation

    f. Student/teacher resources and materials

D. A health instruction guide is available and used in the school? Yes _____ No _____
1. Is a statement of philosophy included in the guide? Yes _____ No _____
2. Of the areas recommended in Column 1, for inclusion in the guide, check those which are presently available:

	K 3	4 5 6	7 8 9	10 11 12
a.				
b.				
c.				
d.				
e.				
f.				

E. A long range plan should be developed for implementing the health instruction program outlined in the teaching guide. A definite time plan should be included.

E. Is a plan available?
Yes _____ No _____
Three years _____
Five years _____

Standards and Recommended Practices	What are We Doing	Comments, Priorities, Proposed Plans, Time Schedule

Curriculum Content

A. In general, the health instruction program for the school includes the following large areas with careful consideration being given to proper grade placement and sequence.

A. Indicate in which grades each subject is taught by placing a check in the appropriate square. Please write in the grade level.

	K 3	4 5 6	7 8 9	10 11 12
1. Nutrition				
2. Dental Health				
3. Physical activity, sleep, rest and relaxation, recreation				
4. Personal cleanliness and appearance				
5. Body structure and operation				
6. Prevention and control of disease				
7. Safety and First Aid				
8. Drugs, Alcohol and Tobacco				
9. Community Health				
10. Consumer Health				
11. Health Careers				
12. Mental, Emotional and Social Health, including Aggressive Behavior				
13. Sex and Family Life Education				
14. Environment Health				

1. Nutrition
2. Dental Health
3. Physical activity, sleep, rest and relaxation, recreation
4. Personal cleanliness and appearance
5. Body structure and operation
6. Prevention and control of disease
7. Safety and First Aid
8. Drugs, Alcohol and Tobacco
9. Community Health
10. Consumer Health
11. Health Careers
12. Mental, Emotional and Social Health, including Aggressive Behavior
13. Sex and Family Life Education
14. Environment Health

(Note: The above data should be analyzed and plans made for removing duplication and adding omitted topics to the curriculum.)

Methods and Instructional Aids

A. The students whenever possible should be actively involved in planning the health education program.

A. Of the following student-related activities, check those which are used:

Role-playing   _____
Group discussions   _____
Dyad (interaction between
2 students)   _____

Standards and Recommended Practices	What are We Doing	Comments, Priorities, Proposed Plans, Time Schedule

Debates _____
Panels _____
Case study _____
Independent studies and
  reports _____

B. The health instruction program should include a variety of teaching techniques. Instruction should be geared towards skill development in seeking information, analyzing it carefully, drawing conclusions, and making behavioral decisions.

B. Of the following methods, check those which are used:
Lecture _____
Field trips _____
Resource speakers _____
Demonstrations and
experiments _____
Surveys _____
Problem solving
  discussion _____

C. The school library should contain current periodicals and other reading matter as resource material for health classes.

C. Of the following, check the ones available to the students and staff:
"School Safety" _____
"Today's Health" _____
"Journal of School
Health" _____
Public Affairs Pamphlets _____
Science Research Associates
  booklets _____
Materials from American
  Medical Association _____
Ohio Department of Education
  Media Centers _____
"Ohio's Health" _____
Materials from Drug/Health
  Education Curriculum
  Center _____
Materials from AAHPER _____
Materials from the Ohio
  Department of Health _____
Materials from Voluntary Health
  Agencies (heart, lung, cancer,
  etc.) _____
Supplementary texts _____
Others (list):

Standards and Recommended Practices	What are We Doing	Comments, Priorities, Proposed Plans, Time Schedule

D. Projection equipment, tape recorders, and record players should be available for use in the classroom.

E. Educational media is utilized in the teaching of health education.

D. The following are available within the school for use in the classroom:

16mm projectors _____
Record players _____
Tape recorders _____
Slide projectors _____
Filmstrip projectors _____
Transparencies _____

E. Which of the following instructional television and/or film series are available:
"Inside Out" NIT-AIT _____
"Self-Incorporated"
NIT-AIT _____
"Knowing About
Growing" BGSU _____
"Feeling Good"
NIT-AIT PBS _____

Evaluation

A. The school makes periodic evaluation of the health instruction program to determine if behavioral objectives for pupils are being met. This includes an appraisal of knowledge gained, interests and values modified and behavior changed.

A. The health instruction program has been evaluated within the last three years?
Yes _____ No _____

B. Evaluation of the school physical and emotional climate is also included.

B. An effort has been made to appraise the school atmosphere?
Yes _____ No _____

C. The evaluation includes the interdisciplinary committee or program for health, the combined efforts of classroom teachers, health educators, administrators and, where appropriate, pupils.

C. The team approach has been used in the program evaluation?
Yes _____ No _____
1. A North Central or similar team has evaluated the health program in the last five years?
Yes _____ No _____

Standards and Recommended Practices	What are We Doing	Comments, Priorities, Proposed Plans, Time Schedule
D. The results of the evaluation are used as a basis for curriculum revision and program improvement.	D. The results of evaluations are being used? Yes _____ No _____	

SOME RESOURCES FOR MATERIALS IN SCHOOL HEALTH PROGRAMS

Ohio State Medical Association
600 South High Street
Columbus OH 43215
"Suggested Procedures for School Emergencies"

American Medical Association
535 North Dearborn Street
Chicago, Illinois 60610
"Health Appraisal of School Children"
"Suggested School Health Policies"
   Prepared by Joint Committee on Health Problems in Education of the NEA and the AMA

American Academy of Pediatrics
P.O. Box 1034
Evanston, Illinois 60204
"School Health: A Guide for Physicians"

American School Health Association
ASHA National Office Building
Kent OH 44240

American Alliance for Health, Physical Education and Recreation
1201 Sixteenth Street, N.W.
Washington D.C. 20036

Mental Health Materials Center
419 Park Avenue South
New York, New York 10016

Ohio Department of Education
Division of Elementary and Secondary Education
65 South Front Street
Columbus OH 43215
   and
Ohio Department of Education
Division of Special Education
933 High Street
Worthington OH 43085

Ohio Department of Mental Health and Mental Retardation
Office of Communications
2929 Kenny Road
Building A, Room 101
Columbus OH 43221

The following materials are available from the:

Ohio Department of Health
P.O. Box 118
Columbus OH 43216

1100 Hours—film
   15 minutes, 16mm, sound—showing aspects of sanitation in the school environment. Suited for school officials and interested adult groups.
   Health Education Section

"School Accident Report Form" 4966.32
"Summary Form for School Accident Report Form" 4965.32
  Accident Prevention and Product Safety Unit

"Sanitation in the School Environment" 2116.32
"Food Service Operation" 2231.32
  Bureau of Environmental Health

"Communicable Disease Information—A Guide for Schools" 0945.11
  Division of Communicable Diseases

"School Health Record Form" 3613.13 Rev. 1974
"Teacher Worksheet for Student Health Observation" 3611.13 Rev. 1967
  Division of Maternal and Child Health

*Recognized National, State and Local Voluntary Health Agencies Addresses and phone numbers are available in local telephone listings or Directories of Health Agencies.

Acknowledgements

Committee members who prepared this publication are:

Wesley P. Cushman	The Ohio State University
Doris Drees	University of Dayton
William Grimm	Ohio Department of Health
Robert Holland	Ohio Department of Education
Richard Mackey	Miami University
Helen Massengale (Chairman)	Ohio Department of Health
Kathy Scholl	Ohio Department of Health
Vincent Walker	Ohio Department of Health

The committee appreciates the assistance given it by other personnel of the State Departments of Education, Health, and Mental Health and Mental Retardation, the Committee on School Health Education of the Ohio State Medical Association, and the many individuals who read and made comments on the Pretest Copy.

Appendix

General Criteria for Evaluating Health Instructional Materials and Comparative Text Analysis

GENERAL CRITERIA FOR EVALUATING HEALTH INSTRUCTIONAL MATERIALS*

The following criteria are to help you evaluate health instructional materials. Indicate your judgment by circling the appropriate number. Each item must be rated. A separate evaluating sheet is necessary for each set of materials considered for recommendation.

NOTE: Comments that would add to this evaluation would be appreciated. Please use last page.

EVALUATED BY _____ DATE _____

COMMITTEE _____ SCHOOL _____

Data for materials evaluated:

Author _____

Title _____

Publisher or producer _____

Copyright date _____ Type of material _____

Grade level of material being evaluated _____

Is this material part of a series?   Yes ☐ Series grade level _____

                                      No ☐

Title of series _____

Cost per item _____

* Modified from: *Handbook I: Guidelines for the Development of Instructional Materials Selection Policies,* Olympia, Wash., State Office of Public Education.

Source: H. Cornacchia, L. Olsen, C. Nickerson: *Health in Elementary Schools,* St. Louis: C. V. Mosby Co., 1992, pp. 531–537.

Summary of Evaluation

	High				Low	M*	NA†
I. Text format	5	4	3	2	1	0	0
II. Audiovisual format considerations	5	4	3	2	1	0	0
III. Organization and overall content	5	4	3	2	1	0	0
IV. Bias content	5	4	3	2	1	0	0
V. Teacher's guide	5	4	3	2	1	0	0
VI. Additional support materials	5	4	3	2	1	0	0
VII. Purchase priority	5	4	3	2	1	0	0

I. Text Format	High				Low	M*	NA†
1. General appearance	5	4	3	2	1	0	0
2. Size and color practical for classroom use	5	4	3	2	1	0	0
3. Binding: durability and flexibility	5	4	3	2	1	0	0
4. Quality of paper	5	4	3	2	1	0	0
5. Readability of type	5	4	3	2	1	0	0
6. Appeal of page layouts	5	4	3	2	1	0	0
7. Usefulness of chapter headings	5	4	3	2	1	0	0
8. Appropriateness of illustrations	5	4	3	2	1	0	0
9. Usefulness of references, index, bibliography, appendix	5	4	3	2	1	0	0
10. Consistency of format	5	4	3	2	1	0	0

II. Audiovisual Format and Considerations	High				Low	M*	NA†
1. Sound quality	5	4	3	2	1	0	0
2. Picture quality	5	4	3	2	1	0	0
3. Emotional impact	5	4	3	2	1	0	0
4. Other qualities: vitality, style, imagination	5	4	3	2	1	0	0
5. Authoritative and well-researched, free of propaganda	5	4	3	2	1	0	0
6. Length suitable to audience and content	5	4	3	2	1	0	0

*Missing; material should have had item but does not.
†Not applicable.

Summary of Evaluation—*continued*

	High --------------- Low	M*	NA†
7. Durability	5 4 3 2 1	0	0
8. Usefulness in more than one subject area: write areas here	5 4 3 2 1	0	0

_____

_____

_____

_____

	High --------------- Low	M*	NA†
III. Organization and Overall Content: Coverage of Health Areas (How comprehensive is the coverage?)			
1. Anatomy and physiology	5 4 3 2 1	0	0
2. Community health (e.g., noise, chemical, water pollution control; community resources)	5 4 3 2 1	0	0
3. Consumer health (e.g., evaluating health products, use of medicines, components of health examinations, health care delivery system)	5 4 3 2 1	0	0
4. Disease prevention (e.g., life-style and disease, emotional illness, cancer, cardiovascular disorders, immunizations, diseases of interest to ethnic groups; oral health)	5 4 3 2 1	0	0
5. Adult life-style (e.g., changing roles; decisions about sex, marriage, and family; careers)	5 4 3 2 1	0	0
6. Fitness (e.g., benefits of fitness, fitness regimen, grooming and self-concept, fatigue, balanced diets, obesity, ethnic foods)	5 4 3 2 1	0	0

*Missing; material should have had item but does not.

†Not applicable.

	High --------------- Low					M*	NA†
7. Growth and development (e.g., reproduction process, prenatal concerns, tools of inheritance, birth defects, genetic counseling, effects of drugs and nutrition on developing embryo and fetus)	5	4	3	2	1	0	0
8. Mental health (e.g., coping skills, stress, human needs and emotions, self-concept, mental illness, psychologic growth and development, stereotyping)	5	4	3	2	1	0	0
9. Safety and first aid	5	4	3	2	1	0	0
10. Smoking, drugs, and alcohol (psychoactive drugs, medical use prescription and over-the-counter drugs)	5	4	3	2	1	0	0
11. Nutrition (e.g., basic necessities; balance; metabolism; changing needs; facts, fads, and fallacies; preparation)	5	4	3	2	1	0	0

IV. Bias Content

	High --------------- Low					M*	NA†
1. Presents more than one viewpoint of controversial issues	5	4	3	2	1	0	0
2. Presents accurate facts when generalizations are made	5	4	3	2	1	0	0
3. Includes all socioeconomic levels and settings and all ethnic groups	5	4	3	2	1	0	0
4. Gives balanced treatment of the past and present	5	4	3	2	1	0	0
5. Promotes the diverse character of our nation by:	5	4	3	2	1	0	0
(a) Presenting the positive nature of cultural differences	5	4	3	2	1	0	0

*Missing; material should have had item but does not.
†Not applicable.

Summary of Evaluation—*continued*

		High ---------------- Low					M*	NA†
(b)	Using languages and models that treat all human beings with respect, dignity, and seriousness	5	4	3	2	1	0	0
(c)	Including characters that help students identify positively with their heritage and culture	5	4	3	2	1	0	0
(d)	Portraying families realistically (one parent, two parents, several generations)	5	4	3	2	1	0	0
(e)	Portraying the handicapped realistically	5	4	3	2	1	0	0
6. Includes minorities and women by:		5	4	3	2	1	0	0
(a)	Presenting their roles positively but realistically	5	4	3	2	1	0	0
(b)	Having their contributions, inventions, or discoveries appear alongside those of white men	5	4	3	2	1	0	0
(c)	Depicting them in a variety of occupations and at all levels in a profession	5	4	3	2	1	0	0
(d)	Having their work included in materials	5	4	3	2	1	0	0
(e)	Presenting information from their perspective	5	4	3	2	1	0	0
(f)	Having appropriate illustrations	5	4	3	2	1	0	0

*Missing; material should have had item but does not.
†Not applicable.

Summary of Evaluation—*continued*

V. Teacher's Guide for Texts or Audiovisual Materials	*High* ---------------- *Low*					*M**	*NA†*
1. Easy to use	5	4	3	2	1	0	0
2. Answers provided	5	4	3	2	1	0	0
3. Background information	5	4	3	2	1	0	0
4. Teaching strategies	5	4	3	2	1	0	0
5. Ideas for motivation, follow-up, extension	5	4	3	2	1	0	0
6. Guidelines for evaluation	5	4	3	2	1	0	0
7. Inclusion of script	5	4	3	2	1	0	0
8. Bibliography	5	4	3	2	1	0	0

VI. Additional Support Materials
that Accompany Text
Please list the materials,
(e.g., workbooks, tests, and
use separate form for each
one listed)
USE THIS SPACE FOR COMMENTS:

*Missing; material should have had item but does not.
†Not applicable.

Organization of School Health Programs

COMPARATIVE TEXT ANALYSIS

The following form, entitled "Comparative Text Analysis," is included as an aid for those who may have the opportunity to review numerous texts in the process of selecting one for local adoption. It can also be used to build a case for replacing old health textbooks. Although the format is designed for facilitating comparison of texts, the items are appropriate for evaluating a single text.

Using the following rating scale, evaluate the material in each area identified.

High ----------- Low   Missing   Not Applicable
4   3   2   1   0   NA

Fill in *title, publisher,* and *copyright date* for each text.

A. *TECHNICAL QUALITY*
   1. General appearance
   2. Readability of type
   3. Quality of paper and binding
   4. Appropriateness of illustrations
   5. Format and general organization

B. *EFFECTIVENESS OF MATERIAL*
   1. Adapts to individual needs and/or interests
   2. Has appropriate sequential development
   3. Provides varied teaching and learning strategies
   4. Provides for measuring student achievement
   5. Provides management system for tracking student progress
   6. Provides clearly organized teacher edition

C. *CONTENT*
   1. Consistent with district, program, and course goals
   2. Reflects respect for personal worth
   3. Aids in building positive attitudes and understandings

Fill in *title,* *publisher,* and *copyright date* for each text.

4. Depicts cultural diversity

5. Deals effectively with issues and problems

6. Offers accurate and/or realistic treatment of subject

7. Incorporates balanced viewpoints

8. Makes provision for distinguishing between fact and opinion

9. Stimulates critical thinking

D. *CRITERIA FOR SEX BIAS*
1. Material divides qualities such as leadership, imagination, intelligence, and courage approximately evenly between male and female characters.

2. Females and males are equally represented as central characters in story and illustrative materials.

3. Both men and women are shown performing similar work in related fields.

4. Males and females are shown working together.

5. People are referred to by their own names and roles as often as they are referred to as someone's spouse, parent, or sibling.

6. Stereotyping language such as ''women chatting''/''men discussing'' is avoided.

7. Biographic or historic materials include a variety of male and female contributions to society.

Organization of School Health Programs

Fill in *title, publisher,* and *copyright date* for each text.

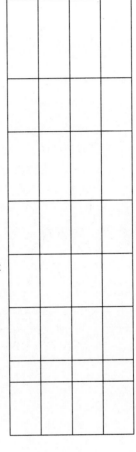

8. Both males and females are given credit for discoveries and contributions to social, artistic, and scientific fields.

9. Groups that may include both males and females are referred to in "neutral" language such as "people, mail carriers, fire fighters, or legislators."

E. *CRITERIA FOR RACIAL/ETHNIC BIAS*
   1. Materials contain racial/ethnic balance in main characters and in illustrations.

   2. Oversimplifications and generalizations about racial groups are avoided in illustrations and in text material.

   3. Minority characters are shown in a variety of life-styles in active, decision-making, and leadership roles.

   4. The vocabulary of racism is avoided.

   5. Minority characters are given credit for discoveries and contributions to social, artistic, and scientific fields.

Using the following rating scale, evaluate the material in each area identified.

High ----------- *Low*   *Missing*   *Not Applicable*
 4   3   2   1   0   NA

Fill in *title, publisher,* and *copyright date* for each text.

SUMMARY INFORMATION

List total points for each area by Publisher and Title.

A. *TECHNICAL QUALITY*

B. *EFFECTIVENESS OF MATERIAL*

C. *CONTENT*

D. *SEX BIAS*

E. *RACIAL/ETHNIC BIAS*

Grand total scores

Additional rationale for selection of these materials: _____

_____

_____

Appendix

Criteria for Evaluating Health Instruction Textbooks

CRITERIA FOR EVALUATING HEALTH TEXTS

Name of Textbook: _____

Author of Text: _____

Publisher and Copyright Date: _____

Name of Rater: _____

Identification of Rater (Educator/Lay): _____

Overall Rating of Text (Excellent, Good, Unsatisfactory): _____

Comments:

Criteria for Evaluating Health Texts
     E = Excellent
     G = Good
     U = Unsatisfactory

	E	G	U
I. AUTHOR AND PUBLISHER			
A. Does the author have credentials in areas covered in the field of health education?			
B. Is the publisher established at publishing educational materials in the field of health education?			
C. Does the copyright indicate a current publication?			

E = Excellent
G = Good
U = Unsatisfactory

	E	G	U

II. INCLUSIVENESS OF PROGRAM
  A. Does the series provide thorough information in the following areas:
      1. Mental Health—Dealing with the learning process.
      2. Emotional Health—Learning to use one's instinctive drives for expressing one's self in a constructive manner. (Behavior)
      3. Social Health—An understanding of those instinctive drives affecting social relationships.
      4. Physical Health—The physical aspects of health presented in such a way as to show the interdependence of the various systems and its relation to total health.
  B. Does the series overemphasize any one phase of health? (i.e., too much physical health)
  C. Does the series have needless repetition?
  D. Can the learning activities be carried over to promote good health habits in adult life?
  E. Does the series teach health as opposed to a technical medical approach?
  F. Is the series free of undesirable stereotypes? (i.e., sex roles, racial, occupational, etc.)

III. CONTENT
  A. Is the information current?
  B. Does the series present the following phases of health in a comprehensive manner? (The grade levels indicate introduction according to the State Health Guide. An * indicates it is not in the State Health Guide.)
      1. Accident Prevention K–3
      2. Alcohol, Smoking, Drugs, and Narcotics 4–6
      3. Personal Hygiene K–3
      4. Community Health Programs and Disease Prevention K–6
      5. Community Helpers (Health Delivery Systems) K–8

E = Excellent
G = Good
U = Unsatisfactory

	E	G	U
6. Dental Health K–3			
7. Environmental Health 4–6			
8. Physical Fitness and Relaxation K–6			
9. First Aid and Safety K–3			
10. Food and Nutrition K–8			
11. Mental Health and Personal Adjustment K–8			
12. Noncommunicable Diseases and Medical Problems 4–6			
13. Physical Changes During Growth and Development *			
14. Boy–Girl Relationships *			
15. Sex Education *			
16. Venereal Disease 6			
17. Anatomy and Physiology K–6			
18. Vision and Hearing K–3			
19. Consumerism *			

IV. APPROACH

	E	G	U
A. Does the series take a positive approach to health?			
B. Does the series avoid all-inclusive statements? (i.e., We are always good sports.)			
C. Does the series take examples from all walks of life rather than just the ideal situation?			
D. Are questions and situations, as well as experiments, provided at frequent intervals throughout each chapter to motivate class discussion and help students relate what they know to what they just read?			
E. Do useful activities appear at the end of each chapter?			
F. Are there numerous subheadings to help the pupil understand what he/she is reading?			
G. Are opportunities for student decision-making provided?			

$$\begin{aligned}&\textbf{E} \ = \ \text{Excellent}\\&\textbf{G} \ = \ \text{Good}\\&\textbf{U} \ = \ \text{Unsatisfactory}\end{aligned}$$

	E	G	U

V. TEACHING AIDS

   A. Are the complete pupil texts included in the Teacher's Editions?

   B. Are the suggested teacher presentation activities broken down into lesson topics?

   C. Are the health terms introduced at the beginning of each unit to eliminate reading problems?

   D. Is the teacher given the following?
      1. Material that helps preview the unit.

      2. Points to emphasize.

      3. Preparation for such lesson.

      4. Extra projects for extension of activities.

   E. Are reference books, visual aids, and resource materials presented at the end of each chapter in the Teacher's Edition?

VI. GENERAL

   A. Illustrations—do they stimulate interest in the study of health and do they have color and eye appeal?

   B. Diagrams—are they large enough to ensure clear and concise interpretation?

   C. Print—is it easily read?

   D. Is the textbook durable?

   E. Is there a table of contents, an index, a glossary?

   F. Is the reading level appropriate for grade level?

   G. Is the comprehension level appropriate for the grade level?

OVERALL RATING:

Excellent	
Good	
Unsatisfactory	

Index

Angel Dust, 205
Animal Intelligence, 289
Anorexia nervosa, 192–95
Anorexia Nervosa and Associated
  Disorders (ANAD), 195
Anvil, 111
Apache Junction Unified School
  District, 348
Appearance, 102
  evaluation of, 410
  and medical problems, 93
Appraisal
  of existing health education
    curriculum, 296
  health, 91–128
  of health attitudes, 379–80
  of health practices, 380
  and self-appraisal, 371, 413–54
Approving, 158, 159
Aqueous humor, 97
ARC. *See* AIDS-related complex
  (ARC)
Arizona, and health education,
  264–70, 310–11, 345, 346
Arizona Comprehensive Health,
  essential skills, 346
Artery disease, 120
Arthritis, 180
Arthropod infections, 138–39
Artificial immunity, 142
Ascariasis, 137
Assessment, of health instruction
  material aids, 382–83
Assigning tasks, 158, 159
Association for the Advancement
  of Health Education, 250, 285,
  400
Association of State and Territorial
  Directors of Public Health
  Education, 250, 285
Asthma, 183–84
Astigmatism, 100–101
Ataxia cerebral palsy, 187
Atherosclerotic coronary artery
  disease, 120
Athetoid cerebral palsy, 187
Athlete's foot, 131, 136
Attending, 158
Attitudes, appraisal of, 379–80
Auburn University, 260

Audiometer, 112, 113, 115
Audiometry, 113
Audiovisual aids evaluation form,
  405–6
Audiovisual materials, 409–10
Auditory nerve, 111
Auricle, 111
Autobiographies, and informal
  autobiographies, 371–72

Bacillus, 130
Back-to-basics movement, 245,
  263, 295
Bacteria, 129–34
Baffi, C. R., 380
Baker, D., 195
Barbiturates, 202
Barbs, 202
Basic, 245, 263, 295
Bayer, A., 195
Beatings, and child abuse, 226
Behavior, 102
  and anorexia nervosa and bulimia
    nervosa, 194
  and child neglect, 235–36
  and medical problems, 93
Behavioral objectives
  and unit development, 328
  writing, 313–16
Bender, S. J., 309
Benzedrine, 203
Berkeley Project, 340–43
Bicycle routes, 53
Big C, 203
Big H, 201
Binary fission, 130
Binocular coordination, 96
Biphetamine, 203
Black, J. L., 218
Black Beauties, 203
Blackham, G. J., 151, 158–59, 160
Black Tar, 201
Blepharitis, 102
Blind spot, 97
Blood pressure, 118–20
Bloom, B., 252, 316
Blow, 203
Blue Devils, 202
Blue Heaven, 205
Body louse, 138–39
Body odors, 62

Boehringer Mannheim Reflotron,
  121
Boils, 130
Bonvechio, L. R., 28
Botulism, 132
Bowditch, H. P., 19
Bower, G., 289
Brain, 20
Brainstorming, 317–18
Breathing, and asthma, 183–84
Broad fields health instruction, 247
Brookbeck, M., 309
Brown Sugar, 201
Brucellosis, 132
Building, and physical plant,
  50–51
Bulimia nervosa, 192–95
Bumblebees, 203
Bureau of Health Education, 392
Bureau of Health Professions, 400
Bush, George, 245
Buttons, 205
Buzz groups, 324
Byler, R., 307

CA. *See* Chronological age (CA)
Cactus, 205
Cafeterias, and food sanitation,
  71–75
CAI. *See* Computer-aided
  instructions (CAI)
California Framework, 346
California State University, Long
  Beach, 260
Canal of Schlemm, 97
Cancer, 351
Cannabis. *See* Marijuana
Capute, A., 189
Cardiac defects, 132
Cardiopulmonary resuscitation
  (CPR), 171
Care, 366
Carnegie Council on Adolescent
  Development, 311
Carnegie Foundation, 291
Carroll, C. B., 246
Center for Health Promotion and
  Health Education, 392
Centers for Chronic Disease
  Prevention and Health
  Promotion, 392, 393

Facilitative conditions for
counseling, 157–58
Family
  and child neglect, 236, 237
  and curriculum responsibility,
    291–92
  and development, 22–24
  and family life, 251
  and family socioeconomic status,
    20
Farsightedness, 98, 99
Fat, and cholesterol screening,
  120–21
Faye symbol chart, 106
FDA. *See* United States Food and
  Drug Administration (FDA)
Federal government, 392–94
Feet, 124–25
Feldhusen, J. F., 315
Fentanyl, 202, 208
Fernandopulle, G., 154
Fever, 130, 133, 138
Field trips, and excursions, 325
First aid, 170
Fission, 130
Flake, 203
Florio, A. E., 165
Flukes, 137, 138
Fodor, J. T., 252, 306, 307, 313,
  381, 395, 399
Follow-up
  procedures, 367
  and referral, 125–27
Food
  poisoning, 132
  sanitation and cafeterias, 71–75
  service personnel, responsibilities
    of, 32
Food Service Sanitation Manual,
  73
Food: Your Choice, 352
Foot. *See* Feet
Footballs, 203
*Forms and Indicators of Child
  Abuse,* 227
Foundations, 14–44
Fountains, and water supply, 67–68
Fovea, 97
*Framework for Health Education,
  A,* 346

*Framework for Health Instruction
  in California Public Schools,*
  346
Free association, 317
Freebase rocks, 203
From the Inside Out, 344
Fully functioning persons, 153
Fungi, 129, 131, 136
Fungicides, 136
Fused health instruction, 247

Gaines, J. M., 34
Games, educational, 325
Garbage, 64–65
Gateway drug, 207
General condition, and medical
  problems, 93
General criteria for evaluating
  health instructional materials
  and comparative health
  analysis, 455–64
German measles, 132, 143
Germs, 129
Gestalt theory, 290
Gilman, S., 184
Glands, and medical problems, 93
Glare, 58
Glasses, use of, 106
Goals
  long-range, 312–13
  and objectives, 29
Gonorrhea, 132
Good Samaritan law, 173
Government, federal, 392–94
Grade placement, 86
Grades, in health instruction, 384
Grading, 85–86
Grafton School District, 348, 349
Grand mal, 177–78, 179
Grass, 206
Green Dragon, 205
Greulich-Pyle, 118
Gronlund, N. E., 314, 315
Grossman, H., 188
Grounds, and physical plant, 49
Group reports, 326–37
Groups, and buzz groups, 324
Growing Healthy, 293, 340–43,
  393
Growth
  and medical problems, 93

TGE. *See* Theoretical growth
  evaluation (TGE)
Guest speakers, 327
Guided discovery, 326
Guidelines for Sex-Fair Vocational
  Education Materials, 407–10
Gymnasiums, 70

Hair
  diseases of, 131
  and medical problems, 92
Hallucinogens, 198, 199, 200–204,
  205, 208
Hamburg, M., 389
Hammer, 111
Hand/eye coordination, 96
Handicapped students
  and mainstreaming, 191–92
  and physical plant, 52
Hand-washing, 68, 69
Hanlon, John, 27
HAP. *See* Health Activities Project
  (HAP)
Harmon, M., 319
Harrelson, O. A., 361
Hash, 206
Hashish, 198, 206
Hashish Oil, 206
Hash Oil, 206
Haslam, R., 180
Have a Healthy Heart, 343–44
Hazards, 164
HBV, 143
Head louse, 138–39
Health, defined, 9
Health Activities Project (HAP),
  353
Health advising, defined, 10
Health agencies
  official and voluntary, 293
  responsibilities of, 33
  See also Health-related agencies
Health analysis, 43
Health appraisal, 91–128
Health attitudes, appraisal of,
  379–80
"Health Concepts: Guides for
  Health Instruction," 284
Health coordinators,
  responsibilities of, 31–32

Hospitalization, 144–45
HOTV screening, 107, 110
Hubbard Scientific Company, 353
Human immunodeficiency virus
    (HIV), 216–19, 220, 298, 391,
    393
Humors, 97
Humphrey, J. H., 34
Hurt, T., 170, 173–74
Hygiene, 283
Hyperopia, 98, 99

IDDM. *See* Insulin-dependent
    diabetes mellitus (IDDM)
Illinois, legislation in, 345
Illness, 20, 169–71
Illumination, 57–59
Illustrated presentations, 326
Imhoff tanks, 64
Immunity, 141–44
Immunization, schedule for
    children, 143
Implementation, of curriculum, 299
Inadequate shelter, and child
    neglect, 233
Incest, 231
Incubation, 140, 145
Incus, 111
Indirect transmission, 140
Individual reports, 326–37
Individuals, identifying needs, 297
Industry, private, 293–94
Infections
    and arthropod infections, 138–39
    body defenses against, 141–44
    of eye, 102
    and hearing, 112, 113
    and infectious disease process,
        139–41
Infectious mononucleosis, 135
Infectious parotitis, 132
Inflammation, 130, 141–44
Influences, and development,
    22–24
Influenza, 130, 135
Informal autobiographies, and
    evaluation, 371–72
Informing, 158, 159
Inhelder, B., 328

Injuries
    and child abuse, 226
    and injury prevention, 251
Inkblot test, 150
In loco parentis
Inner ear, 111
Instructing, 158, 159
Instruction, 242–404
    criteria for evaluating textbooks,
        465–68
    evaluation of, 367–73
    grades in, 384
    and health instruction, 243–73
    textbook sources, 411–12
    traditional and direct, 245–46
Instruction material aids,
    assessment of, 382–83
Instruction methods, evaluation of,
    383
Instruction programs, selected,
    339–54
Insulin-dependent diabetes mellitus
    (IDDM), 184–85
Integrated health instruction, 247
Intelligence quotient (IQ), 148,
    149, 188, 189
Intelligence testing, 148–50
Intensity, defined, 63
Interdisciplinary teamwork, 191
Interests, and needs, 34–35
Interferon, 135
Interpretation, and counseling,
    147–62
Interpreting, 158, 159
Intervention, medical, 144
Interviews, and evaluation, 371
Ionamin, 204
IQ. *See* Intelligence quotient (IQ)
Iris, 96
Isolation, 144–45

JDRP. *See* Joint Dissemination
    Review Panel (JDRP)
Jean, Sally Lucas, 283
John Barleycorn, 277
Johns, Edward B., 2, 3, 4, 260, 296
Johnson, R., 148, 149, 150
Joint Committee on Evaluation of
    School Health Programs, 359

Joint Committee on Health
    Education Terminology, 8, 243,
    250, 285, 311
Joint Dissemination Review Panel
    (JDRP), 337–39, 393
Journal of School Health, 4
JRA. *See* Juvenile rheumatoid
    arthritis (JRA)
Junk, 201
Juvenile rheumatoid arthritis
    (JRA), 180

Kansas Sunflower Project, 348,
    349–50
Kass, C., 189
Kempe, R. S., 236
Kidneys, 20
Kilander, H. F., 37
Killer Weed, 205
Kime, R., 375
Kiwanis International, 293
Knowledge
    health, 375–79
    of learner, society, and discipline
        content, 305, 306
Kohlberg, Lawrence, 17–18
Kolbe, L., 4, 6
Krathwohl, David, 253
Kryspin, W. J., 315
Kwell, 139
Kyphosis, 121

Lady, 203
Language, 407–8
Lantagne, J., 307
Larimore, Granville, 259
Lavatory facilities, 68, 69
Lazy eye, 100
Lead, and poisoning, 66–67
Leading, 158, 159
Lean, 185
Learner, knowledge of, 305, 306
Learning, PAL, 340
Learning activities, selection of,
    316–28
Learning centers, 320
Learning disabilities, 189–91
Learning for Life, 344
Learning opportunity, 316, 328,
    329
Learning theory, 289–90

Lectures, 323
Legal responsibilities, 33–34, 171–74
Legal trend, and child neglect, 236–38
Legislation, 345, 389
Lens, 97
Leprosy, 132
Lesson plans, 329–30
Lewis, G., 307
Liability, 33
Librium, 202
Lice, 138–39
Life Education, 348
Ligaments, and eye, 97
Lighting, 57–59
Lions Club, 293
Litwack, L., 152, 157
Liver, 20
Locally based programs, 347–50
Location, of physical plant, 48
Locke, John, 276
Locker rooms, 69
Lomotil, 202
Long-range goals, and curriculum, 312–13
Longree, Karla, 72
Lookalike drugs, 207
Looking at Children, 366
Lordosis, 121
Los Angeles Area School Health Education Evaluative Study, 27
Louis Harris and Associates, 390
Louse. See Lice
Lovato, D., 278, 298
Loveboat, 205
Lovely, 205
LSD. See Lysergic acid diethylamide (LSD)
Ludes, 202
Lungs, 20, 131
Luther, Martin, 276
Lyme disease, 133–34
Lysergic acid diethylamide (LSD), 205

MA. See Mental age (MA)
McGarry, R., 377
Macula lutea, 97
Mager, R. F., 289, 315
Magic mushrooms, 205

Magrab, P., 148, 149, 150
Mainstreaming, and handicapped students, 191–92
Maintenance, 57–76
Malaria, 131
Malfeasance, 33, 173
Malleus, 111
Management, of epileptic, 179–80
Mandate, 389
Mann, Horace, 277
Marijuana, 198, 199, 204–7
Mary Jane, 206
Maslow, Abraham, 153, 290
Massachusetts, and history of health instruction, 276–77
Mastoid cells, 111
Matching items, 378
Matching symbol test, 107, 110
Material aids, assessment of, 382–83
Material child neglect, 233
Materials
  general criteria for evaluating, 455–64
  resources for, 453–54
Materials center, 321–22
Mayshark, C., 8, 31, 247
MDM, 208
MDMA, 208
Means, Richard K., 260, 275
Measles, 132, 134, 143
Measles virus, 132
Measurement
  and evaluation, 359
  of health knowledge, 375–79
Medical indicators, of child neglect, 235
Medical intervention and prevention, 144
Medical practice, private, 292–93
Medical problems
  indicators of potential, 92–93
  of school-age students, 177–96
Membership
  of community health council, 41–42
  of school health council, 38–39
Me-Me Drug Prevention Education Program, 340
Meningitis, 130, 131, 143

Mental age (MA), 149
Mental habits, 150
Mental health, 251
  criteria for, 152–54
  teachers and administrators and, 156–61
Mental retardation, 187, 188–89
Mepergan, 201
Meperidine, 201, 208
Mesc, 205
Mescaline, 205
Mesomorph, 19
Metazoans, 129, 131, 137–38
Methadone, 201
Methadose, 201
Methamphetamines, 204, 208
Methaqualone, 202
Methedrine, 204
Methods
  evaluation of, 383
  selection of, 316–28
  and unit development, 328, 329
Metropolitan Life Foundation, 347, 348, 390
Metropolitan Life Insurance, 366
Michigan model, 347
Microdot, 205
Microorganisms, 129
Middle ear, 111
Mild emotional problems, 154–55
Milton, John, 276
Miltown, 202
Minnesota Multiphasic Personality Inventory (MMPI), 151
Misfeasance, 33, 173
Mixed symptoms cerebral palsy, 187
MMPI. See Minnesota Multiphasic Personality Inventory (MMPI)
Modes of transmission, 140
Mononucleosis, 135
Moral development, 17, 18
Morphine, 201
Motivation, 206, 317
Mouth, and medical problems, 93
MPPP, 208
MPTP, 208
Mroz, J. H., 163
Mud, 201
Mulcaster, Richard, 276

Organizational patterns for curriculums of health instruction, 245–50
Organization plan, selecting, 305–8
Organ of Corti, 111
Ossicles, 111
Otitis media, 112, 113
Outer ear, 111
Oval window, 111
Overweight, 185–87

Packaged Activities for Learning (PAL), 340
PAL (Packaged Activities for Learning), 340
Palsy, 187–88
Pancreas, 20
Panels, 324
Paragoric, 201
Paramyxovirus, 132
Paraphrasing, 158
Parasites, 129, 131, 138–39
Parasitic worms, 129, 131, 137–39
Parcel, G., 184
Parent-nurse conference, 126–27
Parents
  and emotional climate, 86
  responsibilities of, 32
Parent-Teacher Association (PTA), 294
Parent-Teacher-Student Association (PTSA), 294
Parepectolin, 201
Pathogens, 129–38
Patterns of health instruction, 243–73
Pavlov, Ivan, 289
PCE, 208
PCP. See Pencyclidine (PCP)
PCPy, 208
Pectoral syrup, 201
Peers, and development, 23–24
Pencyclidine (PCP), 205
Pennsylvania Association of Health, Physical Education, Recreation, and Dance, 345–46
Pennsylvania Health Curriculum Progression Chart (PHCPC), 345–46
PEPAP, 208
Pep Pills, 203

Perception checking, 158, 159
Percocet, 202
Percodan, 202
Performance tests, 376, 379
Peripheral awareness, 96
Personal health, 251
Personality testing, 150–51
Personnel, training points, 2
Pertussis, 132, 143
Pethidine, 201
Petit mal, 178, 179
Peyote, 205
PGHCP. See Primary Grades Health Curriculum Project (PGHCP)
PHCPC. See Pennsylvania Health Curriculum Progression Chart (PHCPC)
Phencyclidine (PCP), 208
Phenix, P. H., 309
Philosophy
  development of, 297
  and safety and emergency care, 165–69
  of school health program, 27–28
  and selecting content, 310–11
Physical abuse, 225–30
Physical appearance, evaluation of, 410
Physical child neglect, 232
Physical considerations, of school rooms, 80–81
Physical development, 17–22
Physical examination, 123
Physical plant, planning of, 47–55
Physicians, responsibilities of, 31
Physiology
  of hearing, 111–12
  of vision, 96–97
Piaget, Jean, 22, 290, 328
Pigg, R. M., 31, 254, 270, 294, 307
Pinworms, 131, 137, 138
Pitch, defined, 63
Planning
  curriculum, 305–33
  and horizontal planning, 253–54
  of physical plant, 47–55
  and vertical planning, 252–53
  who plans the curriculum, 290–94

Plans, lesson. See Lesson plans
Plaque, 132
Play, and social stage, 21
Plegine, 204
PMA, 208
Pneumonia, 130, 132, 133
Poisons, 66–67, 131, 132
Policy
  and AIDS, 219, 220
  and drug-related school policy, 212–15
  and safety and emergency care, 165–69
Poliomyelitis, 130, 132, 143
Polio Plus, 293
Poliovirus, 132
Pollock, Marion B., 260, 361, 389
Pollutants, and environment, 65–67
Pondimin, 204
Popham, W. J., 372
Positive mental health, teacher and administrators and, 156–61
Post-secondary health education program, defined, 11
Posture, 93, 121–23
Pot, 206
Practicality, 373–75
Practices, appraisal of, 380
Predispositions, 150
Pregnancy, 132, 197, 219–22
Preludin, 204
Prescription drugs, 198
Presentations, and illustrated presentations, 326
President's Committee on Health Education, 392, 393
Pre-State, 204
Prevention, 1–2
  and control of disease, 251
  counseling as, 152
  of drug abuse, 209–11
  education as, 218–19
  and injury prevention, 251
  medical, 144
Primary disseminated fungal infections, 136
Primary Grades Health Curriculum Project (PGHCP), 341
Primary health education definitions, 9–10

Primary prevention, 144, 152
Principles for development of curriculum, 294–99
Principles of Public Health Administration, 27
Private health agency, defined, 9
Private industry, 293–94
Private medical and dental practice, 292–93
Prizing, and valuing, 318
Probart, C. K., 66
Problems, medical. *See* Medical problems
Problem solving, 160, 316, 317–19
Prodromal stage, 141, 145
Professional preparation, 394–99
Professional societies, 292–93
Programming Learning Disabilities, 190
Programs
  commercially prepared, 352–54
  criteria for evaluating (Ohio), 413–54
  educational, 367
  evaluation of, 357–88
  and health-related agencies, 350–52
  locally based, 347–50
  and Role Delineation Project, 400–401
  selected, 339–54
  state-based, 344–47
Projective techniques, 150
Projects, of students, 321–22
Project SCAT (Skills for Consumers Applied Today), 340
Proliferation, 130
Protozoans, 129, 131, 137
Psilocybin, 205
Psychiatric disorders, 151
Psychodynamic indicators, and child neglect, 237
Psychological dependence, 199
Psychologists, responsibilities of, 31
Psychomotor seizures, 178, 179
PTA. *See* Parent-Teacher Association (PTA)

PTSA. *See* Parent-Teacher-Student Association (PTSA)
Pubic louse, 138–39
Public Health Education, 400
Public health officials, responsibilities of, 33
Pupil, of eye, 97
Pupil-to-pupil relationships, 82
Puretone audiometer, 112, 113, 115
Purposes of Education in American Democracy, The, 279

Q-fever, 130
Quaaludes, 202
Questionnaires and evaluation, 370
Questions and answers, 323–24

Rabelais, Francois, 276
Rabies, 130
Radon, 65–66
Rash, J. K., 31, 254, 294
Raths, L. E., 319
Reaction, 143
Reasonable man, 172
Recognition, 143
Records
  and evaluation, 370
  of experience, 324
  and health records, 125
Red Cross, 170, 344
Red Devils, 202
Red Dragon, 205
Reefer, 206
Reexposure, 143
References, and unit development, 328, 329
Referrals, 91, 95, 125–27
Reflectances, 60
Reflecting, 158
Reflotron, 121
Refractive errors, 98–99
Refuse waste disposal, 64–65
Rehabilitation Act, 192
Relationships
  administrative, 84–85
  and emotional climate, 81–85
  pupil-to-pupil, 82
  school-community, 43
  teacher-to-pupil, 83–84
  teacher-to-teacher, 84

Reliability, 147, 373–75
Renaissance, 276
Report of the Sanitary Commmission of the State of Massachusetts, A, 277
Report on the Seven Cardinal Principles of Education for Secondary Schools, 279
Reports
  individual and group, 326–37
  and written reports, 378–79
Resource people, 327
Resources for materials, 453–54
Responsibility, 6–8, 29–33
  and child abuse and neglect, 238–39
  and curriculum, 291–94
  and safety and emergency care, 165–69
  of school health council, 38
Resuscitation, CPR. *See* Cardiopulmonary resuscitation (CPR)
Retardation, 132, 187, 188–89
Retina, 97
Rheumatic fever, 133, 180
Rheumatoid arthritis, 180
Rhinitis, 181
Ribonucleic acid (RNA), 134
Rickettsia, 129, 130, 138
Rigidity cerebral palsy, 187
Ringworm, 136
Ritalin, 204
RNA. *See* Ribonucleic acid (RNA)
Rock, 203
Rocky Mountain spotted fever, 130, 138
Rodriguez, A., 154
Rods, 97
Rogers, Carl, 153, 160, 161, 290
Role Delineation Project, 400–401
Roles, occupational and social, 408
Roman Empire, 276
Roosevelt, Theodore, 278
Rorschach test, 150
Rotary International, 293
Round window, 111
Roundworms, 137
Rubbish, 64–65

Rubella, 132, 143
Rubella virus, 132
Russell, Robert D., 260, 262

Safety, 251
  and emergency care, 163–75
  and physical plant, 49–50
St. Pierre, R., 319
Samuel Bronfman Foundation, 259
Sandrex, 204
Sanitation, food and cafeterias,
  71–75
Saturated fat, 120–21
Scabies, 138–39
Scarlet fever, 130, 133
SCAT (Skills for Consumers
  Applied Today), 340
Schaller, W. E., 365
Schlaadt, R., 375
School
  and curriculum responsibility,
  292
  and development, 23
School-age child, 15–25
School-age students, special
  medical problems of, 177–96
*School-Based HIV Prevention: A
  Multidisciplinary Approach*,
  393
School-community relationships,
  43
School day, organization of, 77–80
School environment, 47, 367
School health council (SHC),
  37–44
School Health Curriculum Project
  (SHCP), 340–43, 393
School health education, 400
  current status of, 389–404
  defined, 11, 286
School Health Education
  Evaluation (SHEE), 307, 343
School Health Education Study
  (SHES), 257, 259–63, 282, 310,
  345
School health educator, defined, 11
School Health in America, 345,
  389
School health instruction programs,
  selected, 339–54

School health program
  criteria for evaluating (Ohio),
  413–54
  development bases of, 27–36
  evaluation of, 357–88
  of Johns, 2, 3
  of Kolbe, 4, 6
  of Nader, 4, 5
  organization of total, 28–35
  philosophy of, 27–28
  and responsibility, 29–33
School health services
  defined, 11
  evaluation of, 365–67
School health team,
  responsibilities, 6–8
School rooms, physical
  considerations of, 80–81
Schools for the Sixties, 281
School teachers, professional
  preparation of, 394–99
Sclera, 96, 97
Scoliosis, 121–22
Screenings, 91–95
  and blood pressure screening,
  118–20
  and cholesterol screening, 120–21
  and dental health screenings,
  123–24
  and hearing screening, 112–14
  and height and weight, 114–18
  and ocular muscle balance test,
  108
  and tympanometry screening,
  113–14
  and visual screening, 104–10
Seattle Project, 341
Seconal, 202
Secondary prevention, 152
Secondary school teachers,
  preparation of, 395–99, 396–97
Sedatives, 198
Seizures, 177–80, 187
Self-appraisals, 371, 413–54
Sensitization, 143
Septic tanks, 64
Serax, 202
Serono Laboratories, Inc., 115
Service clubs, 293

Services, 90–240, 365–67
Set, 199–200
Setting, 199–200
Severe emotional problems,
  154–55
Sewage disposal, 64
Sex-Fair Vocational Education
  Materials, guidelines for,
  407–10
Sexual abuse, 231–36
Sexually transmitted disease
  (STD), 392
Shattuck, Lemuel, 277
Shaw, D., 8, 247
SHC. *See* School Health Council
  (SHC)
SHCP. *See* School Health
  Curriculum Project (SHCP)
SHEE. *See* School Health
  Education Evaluation (SHEE)
SHES. *See* School Health
  Education Study (SHES)
Show-and-tell time, 327
Shower facilities, 68–69
Sidewalks, and physical plant, 52
Simon, S., 319
Simulations, educations, 325
Sinsemilla, 206
Site, and physical plant, 49
Skill-based health instruction,
  248–49, 263–71
Skilled building components, 209
Skills, essential, 346
Skills for Consumers Applied
  Today (SCAT), 340
Skin
  diseases of, 131
  and medical problems, 92
Sliepcevich, Elena M., 246, 260,
  335
Smack, 201
Smoking, 215–16
Smolensky, J., 28, 42
Snellen chart, 103, 104–7, 108
Snow, 203
Snowbirds, 203
Social development, 17–22
Social roles, 408
Social stage, and play, 21

Social workers, responsibilities of, 31
Societies, professional, 292–93
Society, knowledge of, 305, 306
Society for Public Health Education, 250, 285, 400
Society of State Directors of Health, Physical Education, and Recreation, 250, 285, 400
Sociodramas, and evaluation, 371
Socioeconomic status, 20
Solid waste disposal, 64–65
Sopors, 202
Sorochan, W. D., 309
Sound, 62–63
Sound mental health, criteria for, 152–54
Sources of textbooks for health instruction, 411–12
Southern Illinois University, 260
Spastic cerebral palsy, 187
Speakers, and guest speakers, 327
Special group requirements, and physical plant, 52–54
Specialists, and content specialists, 311–12
Special medical problems, of school-age students, 177–96
Special People, 351
Speech, problems of, 188
Speed, 203, 204
Spinal meningitis, 143
Spine, and posture, 121–23
Spleen, 20
Sponges, students as, 308
Stafford, G. T., 165
Stages of Development of Man, Erikson's, 15–17
Standardized, 147
Standardized tests, 380–82
Stanford-Binet intelligence scales, 148, 149
Stanford University, 209, 210, 212, 213, 214
Stapes, 111
Staphylococci, 102, 131, 132–33
Starga's World, 351
Starvation, 194
State-based programs, 344–47

Status
  family socioeconomic, 20
  of school health education, 389–404
Status epilepticus, 178
STD. *See* Sexually transmitted disease (STD)
Stimulants, 198, 199, 200, 203–4
Stirrup, 111
Stomach, 20
Stories, open-ended, 320
STP, 208
Strabismus, 100
Streptococcal pneumonia, 133
Student-nurse conference, 127
Student projects, 321
Students, responsibilities of, 33
Sty, 102
Subjective evaluation, 368–69
Subjective tests, 378–79
Substance use and abuse, 251
Suffield Public Schools, 348
Sugar Cubes, 205
Summarizing, 158, 159
Sunflower Projects, 348, 349–50
Supporting, 158, 159
Surface brightness, 59
Surgeon General's Report on Health Promotion and Disease Prevention, 286
Surveys, 325–26, 370
Suspensory ligaments, 97
Swayback, 121–22
Sweep test, 112
Symbiosis, 129
Symbol chart, 106
Symbol text, 107, 110
Symposia, 324
Synthetic Heroin, 208
Syphilis, 130, 132

Taba, Hilda, 296, 308
Talwin, 202
Tanner, 118
Tapeworms, 131, 137, 138
Task assignment, 158, 159
TAT. *See* Thematic Apperception Text (TAT)
TCP, 208
Teachable moment, 246

Teacher
  and emotional problem awareness, 154–56
  and positive mental health, 156–61
  professional preparation of, 394–99
  responsibilities of, 30
Teacher effectiveness training (TET), 156–57
Teacher-nurse conference, 126
Teacher-nurse referral form, 95
Teacher observation, 91, 366
Teacher-to-pupil relationships, 83–84
Teacher-to-teacher relationships, 84
Teaching aids, and unit development, 328, 329
Teamwork, interdisciplinary, 191
Teeth, and medical problems, 93
Tenuate, 204
Tepanil, 204
Terminology, 8–12, 243, 250, 285, 311
Tertiary prevention, 152
Testing, 147–51
Tests
  essay, 376
  objective, 376–78
  performance, 376, 379
  standardized, 380–82
  subjective, 378–79
TET. *See* Teacher effectiveness training (TET)
Tetanus, 132, 143
Tetrahydrocannabinol (THC), 205, 206
Textbooks
  and content, 321
  criteria for evaluating, 465–68
  sources of, 411–12
TGE. *See* Theoretical growth evaluation (TGE)
Thai Sticks, 206
THC. *See* Tetrahydrocannabinol (THC)
Thematic Apperception Text (TAT), 150